A DEVELOPMENTAL ANALYSIS OF CUBA'S HEALTH CARE SYSTEM SINCE 1959

A DEVELOPMENTAL ANALYSIS OF CUBA'S HEALTH CARE SYSTEM SINCE 1959

Theodore H. MacDonald

Studies in Health and Human Services
Volume 32

The Edwin Mellen Press
Lewiston•Queenston•Lampeter

Library of Congress Cataloging-in-Publication Data

MacDonald, Theodore H. (Theodore Harney), 1933-
   A developmental analysis of Cuba's health care system since 1959 /
Theodore H. MacDonald.
       p. cm. -- (Studies in health and human services ; v. 32)
   Includes bibliographical references and index.
   ISBN 0-7734-8049-8
   1. Medicine, State--Cuba. 2. Public health--Cuba. 3. Medical
care--Cuba. 4. Social medicine--Cuba.   I. Title.   II. Series.
RA413.5.C9M33   1999
362.1' 097291--dc21   99-22943
                                                                                          CIP

This is volume 32 in the continuing series
Studies in Health & Human Services
Volume 32 ISBN 0-7734-8049-8
SHHS Series ISBN 0-88946-126-0

A CIP catalog record for this book is available from the British Library.

        The Edwin Mellen Press   The Edwin Mellen Press
              Box 450   Box 67
        Lewiston, New York   Queenston, Ontario
        USA 14092-0450   CANADA L0S 1L0

                    The Edwin Mellen Press, Ltd.
                    Lampeter, Ceredigion, Wales
                    UNITED KINGDOM SA48 8LT

                Printed in the United States of America

To all health care workers in the Third World this book is
humbly dedicated

Table of Contents

PREFACE

"Health is politics, politics is health"

Rudolph Virchow (1821-1890)

Professor Théodore MacDonald is that rare being, a true polymath. Having held Chairs in Education, Medicine and Mathematics he has published in excess of 30 books and over 170 research papers. He has worked in a range of developed and underdeveloped countries, including: Korea, Vietnam, the Caribbean, Central and South America, Australia, Canada, the USA, Britain and both eastern and western Europe. He is a committed socialist. This book can be used as a companion to one of his other Cuban studies : *Schooling the Revolution: An analysis of developments in Cuban Education since 1959* : London, Praxis Press (1996); although it stands perfectly well on its own.

The book deals with Cuba's health care system, including its caring and preventative aspects, since the overthrow of the dictator Fulgencia Bastista on January 1, 1959. But there are strong underlying themes which assume importance in the world today. These go a long way in explaining why Cuba has survived as a socialist state, despite the loss of economic support from the former Soviet Union and the simultaneous tightening of the US embargo. One of the most significant indicators of socialist intent was the announcement by Fidel Castro, on assuming power, that the first three revolutionary priorities were to be: agrarian reform, universally available schooling and a comprehensive health care system free of charge at point of access. The Cuban revolutionaries were resolute in their goal of eradicating the prevailing levels of deprivation, still a feature of many other third world countries. They also explicitly acknowledge that gaining power was only the beginning of the revolution and that the real challenge would be to be able to maintain and further it. One of Cuba's unique strengths, very early in its revolution, was the degree to which it was able to look outwards and establish itself as an international presence.

The main thrust of this book focuses on the extraordinary improvement in Cuban public health over the past four decades. Most of the statistics are those used by the WHO in assessing the efficacy of national health programmes, and they are impressive. They show that in such important aspects as Infant Mortality and Life Expectancy, Cuba has achieved first world standards and ranks better that the USA in some key measures. For instance, in Washington, DC, Infant Mortality is twice that of Cuba. In Harlem, New York, infant mortality rates among black Americans are much higher than Cuba's figures and equal to those of Bangladesh – one of the poorest nations on earth.

The results cited for preventive measures of public health, such as immunisations, vaccination and health examinations in Cuba are also remarkable. Cuba has had no cases of poliomyelitis since 1963, malaria has been eradicated since 1968, diphtheria disappeared from the scene in 1971. Gastroenteritis, a common enough killer of third world infants, caused the deaths of 4,157 Cuban children in 1962, but by 1975 this figure had dropped to 761.

Despite all of this, MacDonald does make some trenchant criticisms. He picks up on two important points – the fact that the Cuban health care system leaves itself open to serious destabilisation by its heavy reliance on high tech medicine and that there has been a possible over-production of doctors leading to a tendency for health promotional initiatives to be too heavily medicalised. He also takes exception to Cuba's slowness in recognising and effectively responding to the hazard that smoking poses to health. Cuba, of course, is a major tobacco producer.

On the home front Cuba has an outstanding record in the training of doctors and is justifiably renowned for its success in setting up primary health care systems in other third world countries. The first of Cuba's international health and education brigades was sent to Algeria in 1963 to help organise rural health centres and to establish a literacy programme. By 1984 there were 2,000 Cuban health workers and 3,500 Cuban educationalists involved in projects in 25 countries. More recently medical help has been accorded to Ukraine as a result of the Chernobyl disaster. Angola and Mozambique were also recent recipients of massive Cuban medical aid. Often, indeed, children in need of specialist medical attention are welcomed to Cuba itself, where they live for as long as their treatment requires. In this regard, 12,000 Ukrainian children from Chernobyl spent nearly a year in Cuban care centres as did 60 victims of last year's volcanic eruptions on Monserrat.

All of this good work is increasingly threatened by the US embargo of Cuba, which now directly interferes with other countries trying to trade with the island. This even poses barriers to attempts to gain access to needed food and pharmaceutical supplies. From 1992 onward, beginning with the infamous Cuba Democracy Act (the Torricelli Law), the embargo has been tightened until now – with the 1997 Helms Burton Act – Cuba's health care system is being seriously undermined. In October 1996, a group of US doctors, representing the American Medical Association visited Cuba to give a first hand report of the magnitude of this assault on the integrity of Cuba. Among other things, they concluded that the US embargo has "drastically harmed the health and nutrition of large numbers of ordinary Cuban citizens ..... a humanitarian catastrophe has only been averted because the Cuban government is so highly organised and effective in responding to its people's needs."

MacDonald is a most energetic writer - teacher, doctor, musician and socialist. I often wonder what gives him his formidable drive. Perhaps it is outrage at injustice around the world. Harold Pinter's article on the Cuban embargo "Caribbean Cold War", in the May 1996 issue of Red Pepper provides an appropriate closing comment to this Preface. He says:

"There exists today widespread propaganda which asserts that socialism is dead. But if to be a socialist is to be a person convinced that the words 'the common good' and 'social justice' actually mean something; if to be a socialist is to be outraged at the contempt in which millions and millions of people are held by those in power, by market forces, by international financial institutions; if to be a socialist is to be a person determined to do everything in his or her power to alleviate these unforgivably degraded lives, then socialism can never be dead because these aspirations will never die."

Professor David A. Player;
FRCP (Edin), FRC Psych, FRCM.
Edinburgh
November 1998

ACKNOWLEDGEMENTS

Much more difficult than trying to decide who to acknowledge in the authorship of a book is deciding who not to acknowledge! There are simply too many people to list whose help, encouragement, wisdom and patience made this book possible.

Certainly the Cuban people themselves, with their vivacious good humour, have had totally undeserved sufferings gratuitously visited upon them by the United States, yet they have persisted. That ability to stand up for social principles and not give in has acted as an immense incentive to me to do what I can to let people know the truth of the situation.

I thank all of the various media outlets (the World Wide Web was enormously helpful) and contributors - each acknowledged in the text - whose permission has made possible the inclusion of their comments.

Individually Cubans have given me freely of their time and hospitality while I conducted long and detailed interviews with them concerning the Cuban health care system. This is also true of the numerous local branches of mass organisations such as the FMC (Cuban Federation of Women) and the CDR (Committees in each block for the Defence of the Revolution), whose directors (all voluntary posts) were unfailingly generous with information and helpful, sometimes strenuously so, in making sure that I was able to contact individuals and institutions appropriate to my needs.

With respect to the professional medical aspect, personnel at all levels in the Cuban Ministry of Public Health in Havana went to great lengths to let me gain access to medical establishments, authorities, research workers, teaching hospitals, specialist units, etc., up and down the length of Cuba. In particular I wish to record heartfelt thanks to Dr Nelson Patallo Hererro, first vice Director of the National Research Hospital Hermanos Ameijeiras in Havana; Dr Jeremias Hernandez Ojito, Director of the Advisory Panel on Health and Biomedical information, and Dr Jose Mendez Rodriguez, National consultant in Epidemiology at the National Centre for Medical Information. Not only did these busy people frequently make themselves available to me at short notice, but were energetic in scaring up obscure statistical details, facts and publications, as and when my research for this book made such necessary. They also generously read and commented on various chapters of the manuscript itself.

iv

Perhaps it is routine for authors to allude to the forbearance of their families in the authorship of a book, but in this case the sentiments are all too genuine. Who but saints could put up with a paterfamilias coming home every night after work to a small flat and saying "Please don't talk to me to even to each other. I have to finish this chapter!"? Therefore, to my wife, Chris, and son, Matthew, I accord the most heartfelt thanks. Both share with me - and exemplify it with more purity than I - a commitment to social justice worldwide and a profound respect for the people of Cuba.

It goes without saying that all errors in the text are the responsibility of the author alone.

Professor Théodore H. MacDonald

Brunel University
London, England.

September 1998

WHY THIS BOOK HAD TO BE WRITTEN?

In May 1998, the G8 Nations (that is, the G7 nations, with Russia added as both a courtesy and in the hope of stimulating a rational solution to its own economic problems) met in Birmingham, England, to deal with various issues. Outstanding among these was the devastating problem of Third World debt and popular were the great expectations that the G8 would make some radical move to reduce that progress-stifling debt. In fact, no such thing happened, but the whole scenario did bring the issue to the public mind and widespread concern was engendered in the issue of what options really are open to third world societies in pursuits of human dignity. Cuba is an outstanding example of such a society.

It is a small, third world country, under a classical communist administration. It bears all of the stereotypical marks of what we in the West have come to associate with that sort of scenario - totalitarianism, massive disregard for the "rights" of free speech and press, freedom to worship or to form non-government secular organisations and freedom from the fear of arbitrary arrest. Life there is further encumbered by such petty irritations of communism as lack of variety of consumer goods, a stodgy bureaucracy which intrudes in a thousand and one ways into daily living, restrictions on the possibility of travel to other countries, etc.

Most such administrations have ignominiously collapsed in the last few years. Why then should Cuba be of interest?

For a variety of reasons that will become apparent in this book Cuba has, since its revolution in 1959, actually delivered the goods as far as social policy is concerned. In this regard they have been spectacularly successful and astonishingly innovative in the two critically important public policy areas of education and health. No other Latin American country, indeed very few other countries altogether, routinely has all of its children in full time schooling from age six through age fifteen. Cuba's entire pre-school system (formerly referred to as "circulos infantiles") provides almost every parent in the country with high quality, day-long childcare facilities, something that if it were widely known about in the US and UK - would be the envy even of parents in those countries. On top of that, I am hard pressed to think of any other small nation that offers such comprehensive and socially responsive health care. As the reader will see on reading this book, this not only embraces fully the principle of "medical care free at point of access to any citizen" but includes a range of highly innovatory health promotion initiatives generated at the grass roots level, along with astonishing research and development enterprises in high technology medicine.

In the areas of health and education, success has already served as a model to other developing nations; more so in health care possibly because education is by its very nature more "language bound." Revolutionary Cuba, until 1993, has aggressively followed a policy or extravagance in its readiness to provide corps of teachers and health workers for other third world countries unable to afford to pay for them. It has, since the early 60's been an educational Mecca for these same countries, who have sent armies of their own nationals to study in Cuba in order to return to their own countries as teachers and health workers. This latter would not have happened had Cuba not had something of value to offer. For instance, it cannot be attributed to some devious trick of communist propaganda because many of the countries which have so taken advantage of Cuba's largesse are not aligned with Cuba politically. In this regard, one can list many of the Latin American nations, India, Pakistan, and a number of non communist African states, etc.

I have already written a booklength account of Cuba's versatile educational system.[1] I felt well qualified to pen such a volume as I had worked in Cuban education at all levels from pre-school to university and was thoroughly acquainted both with the development of its elaborately comprehensive system of schooling and with many of the psycho - social phenomena encountered in Cuba's singularly effective campaign against adult illiteracy.

In the pages of an earlier book[2], I referred to Cuba's extraordinary achievements in health care only in passing and only as they impinged on health education delivery and methodology. But I did comment that Cuba's health care system is, if anything, even more remarkable than its educational enterprise. At the time, I wrote as a professor of education, and I observed that Cuba's innovatory approach to medical care also called for reportage, but that it would require a medically trained narrator to do it justice. I had had some medical training, but had - years before - abandoned it part way through in favour of mathematics

---

[1] MacDonald, T. (1996) Schooling The Revolution: An analysis of development in Cuban education since 1959. London, Praxis Press.

[2] MacDonald, T. (1986) Making A New People. Vancouver, New Star Books.

and then of research into the psychology of how mathematics logic is understood. This in turn, led me into education and ultimately to a university chair in that discipline.

However, not long after completing "Making a New People", I gave up my professorship in education and completed my medical training. As a general physician I worked in Haiti and later taught at medical schools in the Dominican Republic and again in Cuba - this time in the medical arena. I am at present in charge of postgraduate studies in health at Brunel University in West London.

In this way, I find myself again uniquely qualified to narrate the present account. Whatever political fate befalls Cuba as a nation as a result of American machinations, attitudes in much of the third world have already been massively influenced by Cuba's example and in this, Cuba's health care system has played an even more dominant influence than have its successes in general schooling.

A FOREWORD

FOR WHOM THE BELL TOLLS

One would be hard-pressed indeed to think of a more apposite quote than the title of this foreword to sum up a widely accepted attitude to Cuba's fearful struggle against the US economic blockade. If the blockade is successful in its stated aim - the destruction of Cuba's social system - it will constitute an attack not only on Cuba but on the aspirations of poor people everywhere and of every nationality.

The extra-legal implications of this are extremely important. Embargoes, as far as international law is concerned, may be brought by one country (or several) against another in the event that the parties to be embargoed represent a military threat to the others. Use of the embargo never has been accepted as having as its main purpose the destabilisation of a domestic government. But on April 24, 1992, President Bush actually admitted, in a speech given in Maine, that the purpose of the US embargo was to isolate Cuba until it alters the domestic government in such a way as to render it acceptable to US regional interests.[3]

The President's remarks, on that occasion, were made in support of the "Cuban Democracy Act of 1992, introduced in February 1992 by Robert Torricelli (Democrat - New Jersey). This Act, rendered subsidiary trading with Cuba illegal. At the time, 70% of such trading was in medical supplies and foods! Various amendments already collected by the Bill in its passage through US legislation, also made it illegal for any third world country which has trade with Cuba, to also trade with the US.

During the 1980s and half-way through the 90's, we witnessed the ascendance of right-wing administrations in many of the metropolitan countries and, following on from it, the ineluctable erosion of the public sector, especially health, education, housing and transport. We became accustomed, in those years, to the visibility of the poor and homeless on our streets and even elaborated - with astonishing facility - all of those classical social responses which, for example set the atmosphere for many Victorian novels about life in England. These responses included a range of dismissive

---

[3] Murray, Mary (1992), Cruel and Unusual Punishment - The US Blockage Against Cuba. Ocean Press, Melbourne.

attitudes from "They are too lazy to look for work!" to "It's not really the concern of the government". A common enough, and more socially generous response, holds that the phenomenon does not represent any deep defect in the administration of the economy, but simply castigates the government for closing down too many residential mental illness facilities! Either way, whether the victims are regarded as the non-deserving poor or as crazy, such categorisation made it all too possible to dismiss them and to continue supporting political philosophies based on the exaltation of selfishness and on the denial of the dictates of a broader social morality. In the UK, in fact, even a change in political party in power (from Conservative to Labour) made little difference to these social attitudes.

The undignified collapse of the former communist empire may well have introduced yet a few million more losers into the equation world wide. To both of these repositories of misery can be added the great mass of poverty-stricken humanity found in what we refer to as "the third world." It is now estimated by several aid agencies that the percentage worldwide of the "profoundly poor"[4] has passed 20% of the world population.

Since 1959 Cuba has emerged as a beacon to these people - and as a powerful symbol to all poor people, even those living in the comparative luxury of unemployment in the UK and in the US! An affirming flame attesting to the possibility of confronting third world status and triumphing over it, the Cuban revolution, like none other before it, threw up a whole gallery of personalities who reflected an unswerving idealism manifested in a commitment to social justice and dignity. Che Guevara was doubtless the most famous of these but there were so many others that Cuba was able to sustain a policy of internationalism and support for the rest of the third world which involved it in exporting whole armies of teachers and medical workers to these countries in numbers far in excess of those sent by any other nation, including those which are leading economic powers. This highly visible altruistic activity of Cuba has made it almost impossible for the US to even think about trying to get rid of it by using direct military means.

---

[4] People who are without any means at all of protecting themselves from starvation and disease. New Internationalist, March 1993.

At this point, it might be worth quoting Che Guevara directly, since he was medically trained, from a comment he made in a speech "On Revolutionary Medicine". The entire speech is found in a book edited by John Gerassi.[5]

> "Except for Haiti and Santo Domingo, I have visited, to some extent, all the other Latin American countries. Because of the circumstances in which I traveled, first as a student and later as a doctor, I came into close contact with poverty, hunger and disease; with the inability to treat a child because of lack of money; with the stupefication provoked by continual hunger and punishment, to the point that a father can accept the loss of a son as an unimportant accident, as occurs often in the downtrodden classes of our American homeland. And I began to realize that there were things that were almost as important to me as becoming a famous scientist or making a significant contribution to medical science: I wanted to help those people.

> "How does one actually carry out a work of social welfare? How does one unite individual endeavour with the needs of society?

> "For this task of organisation, as for all revolutionary tasks, fundamentally it is the individual who is needed. The revolution does not, as some claim, stanardize the collective will and the collective initiative. On the contrary, it liberates one's individual talent. What the revolution does is orient that talent. And our task is to orient the creative abilities of all medical professionals toward the tasks of social medicine.

> **"The life of a single human being is worth a million times more than all the property of the richest man on earth... Far more important that a good remuneration is the pride of serving one's neighbor. Much more definitive and much more lasting than all the gold that one can accumulate is the gratitude of a people.**

> "We must begin to erase our old concepts. We should not go to the people and say, 'Here we are. We come to give you the charity of our presence, to teach you our science, to show you your errors, your lack of culture, your ignorance of elementary things.' We should go instead with an inquiring mind and a humble spirit to learn at that great source of wisdom that is the people.

> "Later we will realize many times how mistaken we were in concepts that were so familiar they become part of us and were an automatic part of our thinking. Often we need to   change our concepts, not only the general concepts, the social or philosophical ones, but also sometimes our medical concepts.

---

[5] Gerassi, J. (1961), Venceremos - The Speeches and Writings of Che Guevara. New York. Simon Schustes. Pp 112-119.

"We shall see that diseases need not always be treated as they are in big-city hospitals. We shall see that the doctor has to be a farmer also and plant new foods and sow, by example, the desire to consume new foods, to diversify the nutritional structure which is so limited, so poor.

"If we plan to redistribute the wealth of those who have too much in order to give it to those who have nothing; if we intend to make creative work daily, dynamic source of all our happiness, then we have goals towards which to work."

Virtually the only way of confronting such idealism is with a blockade. It is not sudden or spectacular. Destabilisation is hard to trace and is not newsworthy. It is widely understood that Chile was economically destabilised by the US government, leading to the domestic unrest and finally to the activation of the country's right wing military forces. This led ultimately to the destruction of Allende's government and to years of brutal suppression following it. Altogether the US has had plenty of practice in thus overthrowing Latin American regimes not to its liking, all of them with some claim to being, at least mildly socialist in their intentions! But Cuba - for all of the reasons already discussed - is powerfully symbolic. It is not too much to say, I believe, that if the economic blockade does succeed, the shock waves will be felt far beyond Cuba's shores. People in large numbers will just give up the struggle. If even Cuba can be destroyed, what chance does any other social revolution have?

The imperative, then, is to make the story of Cuba's achievements as widely known as possible, even as the jackals gather in preparation for its death throes. Some can hardly wait. Consider the following item from the April 1, 1993 edition of the widely read British broadsheet, **The Independent.**

"Cuba facing 'stone-age' economy

A report reputedly prepared by Cuban government officials predicts the island's economy will collapse by July and warns the army may be needed to keep order, AP reports from Miami.

The Cuban American National Foundation, a Miami- based exile group which released the 10 page summary, said it was obtained from Fidel

**Castro's inner circle. The report shows Cuba's economy has withered
to only 37 percent of 1986-1989 levels, total foreign reserves have fallen
to only $12.3m (£8.25m), the sugar harvest has tumbled and
transportation will grind to a halt by mid-1993.
The report concludes Cuba must be ready to implement "Emergency
Phase 1". Jorge Mas Canosa, chairman of the group, said. This
envisages a "stone- age economy" and military repression."**

Large numbers of people reading such an account in their daily paper would hardly be in a
position to realise that the AP, from which agency the story is derived, had a long track
record of unmitigated hostility to the Cuban regime and was renowned throughout the years
of the Vietnam War for the regularity of its releases predicting the imminent victory of the
American forces and the momentous collapse of the North Vietnamese administration!
Knowing all of that certainly puts the above quote in a useful perspective. Even more useful
to me is the fact that I read it while flying from London to Havana on April 1, 1993, to
spend two weeks in Cuba leading a group of 24 British health workers on a study tour of the
island's health care facilities.

But while the imminence of Cuba's economic destruction may be nowhere near as
precipitate as the quoted news item might have led us to believe, the danger of it becoming a
fulfilled prophesy must increase with each person who uncritically accepts that sort of thing
as true and who, in consequence, writes off the hope that is Cuba.

Considering the wretchedness and poverty from which Cuba has pulled its
population in only 40 years of revolution, it would be easy indeed to write a paean of
unstinted praise in describing the impressive development of its health system. In large
measure, this volume does praise it and does stress how remarkable it is that a poor third
world country should, in so many ways, be able to show more advanced nations how to run
a socially responsible health system. Obviously there are worries and there are criticisms
which can be levelled, and these will also be found in this volume.
Perhaps one criticism might productively be raised at this point. Cuba has every reason to
be singularly proud of its reputation, especially throughout the third world, in the medical
field. But it has severely distorted its own medical orientation - perhaps with an eye to

international acclaim - by embarking on intensive developments in medical technology and high tech diagnostic/treatment modalities. Initially much of the funding for this came from the former USSR, in its close relationship with Cuba but now that source has dried up. Moreover, such elaborate machinery as CAT-scanners are subject to the frequent need for parts and, of course, the more complex the replacement part required, especially if it involves computer features, the more likely it is to fall foul of the US embargo. Thus, although Cuba has - through considerable sacrifice - attained a high level of sophistication in medical technology, much of it is at present unusable. This includes, for instance, an inability to use fairly routine electrocardiograph equipment because of an inability to obtain ECG paper.

But there is a more serious philosophical issue to all of this -namely the matter of priorities. In Cuba we have a country which, again as a consequence of the blockade, is having trouble feeding itself. This constitutes a much more pressing health problem than does the ability to do heart transplant operations! Where are Cuba's priorities? Commentators antagonistic to Cuba have been quick to broadcast Cuba's own official accounts of an eye affliction which has recently caused widespread distress among Cubans. The Cubans have always blamed the US blockade for this and,
to a large extent, and given Cuba's present inflexible policies regarding land use, this must be seen as accurate. But Cuba could reject political ideology to a level sufficient to allow it to feed its own people. It does have the land, the know-how and the indigenous crops to do it. Thus the criticisms levelled at Cuba's communism by its enemies are by no means wholly invalid.

A more dispassionate account by WHO of this whole incident was reported in **The Guardian** of Thursday, September, 1993 as follows:

"The eye disease which swept Cuba earlier this year has been eliminated by the government's swift response, the world health organisation said yesterday, heaping praise on the country's medical system.

The disease - optic neuritis - which at its height between March and May claimed more than 4,000 victims a week, has been wiped out by

18,000 Cuban physicians dispensing advice and vitamin B complex pills to Cuba's 11 million people, Dr Bjorn Thylefors, a WHO blindness specialist, said in Geneva. "Cuba has invested more in health services than almost any other country," said Dr Thylefors, " and it has a higher health profile than the US." Doctors had been able to react remarkably quickly to the disease.

WHO also commended Cuban health care for preventing the disease's spread to vulnerable age-groups. "Cuba treats its children very well. The same goes for the old," said Dr Thylefors. The provision of free milk and other essential nutrients to these two age groups meant that the disease had been confined to the 25-65 age bracket.

But specialists from all over the world, including Britain, are still unclear about what exactly caused the illness, which, in the worst cases, resulted in a 70% loss of eyesight.

"After careful research we have come to the conclusion that the disease was probably caused by the effects of some sort of household toxin combined with poor nutrition levels," said Dr Thylefors. It was clear, however, that no virus or other microbe had been responsible.

The poor economic climate - worsened by the US embargo - had meant a deterioration in the Cuban diet, increasing most people's vulnerability to the harmful side-effects of household toxins, Dr Thylefors said.

Since the break-up of the Eastern bloc in 1989, average Cuban food consumption had fallen from 2,940 calories per person per day to 2,100 - the average in the West being 3,000. Many Cubans had been forced to switch from a protein-based diet to a sugar-dominated one. Under such conditions, the disease, which first surfaced in Cuba last December, had been able to claim more than 50,000 victims causing symptoms such as

blurred eyesight, loss of weight and, in some cases, partial paralysis. Luckily, only 1,300 cases have shown signs of retaining any permanent disabilities, the report said. However, similar epidemics have begun to surface in Africa."

To some extent, Cuban authorities have manifested a healthy non- ideological eclecticism. On my second to last visit to that country, in April 1993, I noticed that in their desperate search for hard currency, the authorities had pushed tourism to the limit and had instituted steps, such as minting token coins which tourists receive as change when they use - as they are expected to - US dollars. The idea behind this was to make sure that the tourists did not use Cuban currency. This effectively shut most ordinary retail outlets to them, confining them to shops and hotels specifically for tourists. In provincial areas, of course, it was sometimes necessary for tourists to patronise ordinary Cuban hotels. But in that event, the tourists were fed much better food and in greater quantity in segregated fashion in the same dining rooms as were used by local hotel customers - whose ration cards were scrutinised before they could eat. But in the fullness of time legislation was passed in 1996 enabling Cuban citizens to posses and use US currency.

The freak weather condition called 'El Nino' has brought drought to Cuba during the 1996-97 and 1997-98 growing seasons, causing food shortages exacerbated by the Blockade. The rationing now in Cuba is so severe that children on the street are starting to ask tourists for food. Surely the energies directed presently toward showcase medical technology might better be re-channelled into aggressive programmes for self-sufficiency in agriculture. The real and lasting dignity of the Cuban people as far as health is concerned, lies not so much in heart transplants as in a primary health care that operates on the basis that the Ministry of Agriculture can adequately feed the people and in Cuba having sufficient autonomy to be able to do this without imports - and therefore without fear of the blockade.

It is in terms of primary health care - the priorities targeted by WHO in its health for all 2000 objectives - that Cuba's achievements really stand out. These achievements are summed up in the epidemiological data found in appendix A of this book. Obviously such material will be of immediate and pressing interest to medically trained readers - the sort of information that such people would critically peruse before reading the book itself, perhaps. However, the lay reader also would benefit immensely from consulting that data from time to time as the main body of the book is read. It is primarily for the lay reader that it has been included.

Kidney transplants and genetic engineering make for good TV viewing and engrossing reading, but the long term real commitment of a society to human dignity is reflected in the slow and patient improvement of figures on infant mortality, maternal health and on the eradication of respiratory and cardiovascular diseases. Indeed, Cuba's ministry of public health (MINSAP) is aware of this for, not only did it freely make the material included in appendix A available (it is much more difficult to extract equivalent statistics from the appropriate authorities in the UK and the US!), it eagerly gave permission for it to be included in this book.

Let the reader then share my wonder and admiration at Cuba's remarkable health care system, remembering surely that such a system is a product not only of applied science and of high tech systems, but is also a product of a social policy. We might not like the ideology, but it is difficult indeed to see how Cuba would have accomplished what it has without it. If all of this achievement should be destroyed by socially reactionary forces over which Cuba has no control, ask not for whom the bell tolls. It tolls for all of us.

A Brief Chronology of the US Embargo and Especially its Impact on Cuban Health

1960

March 1960: President Dwight D. Eisenhower approves a plan of convert action and economic sabotage against Cuba. In the first months of 1960, the U.S. government waged a campaign to prevent Cuba from receiving loans and credit from Western European and Canadian institutions. A consortium of European banks, under pressure from the U.S., cancelled plans to negotiate a $100 million loan to Cuba.

July 1960: President Eisenhower cancelled the unfulfilled balance of the Cuban sugar quota to the U.S. for 1960.

August 1960: Cuba issued Resolution Number 1 under Law 851 which ordered the expropriation of twenty-six of the largest United States companies operating in Cuba.

October 1960: In what the media describes as a "quarantine" of Cuba, the Eisenhower Administration bans U.S. exports to that country - except for foodstuffs, medicines, and medical and hospital supplies. Companies wishing to sell such goods to Cuba can do so under a "general" licence (i.e. no specific license application is required). Imports from Cuba continue to be allowed.

1961

January 1961: The U.S. severs diplomatic relations with Cuba.

April 1961: The Bay of Pigs invasion is launched.

September 1961: The Foreign Assistance Act of 1961 authorizes the President to establish and maintain "a total embargo upon all trade between Cuba and the U.S."

1962

February 1962: The Kennedy Administration extends the embargo to prohibit Cuban imports into the U.S.

March 1962: The embargo is further tightened to prohibit imports into the U.S. from third countries of goods made from or containing Cuban materials.

August 1962: In order to dissuade third countries, Congress amends the Foreign Assistance Act of 1961 to prohibit U.S. assistance "to any country which furnishes assistance to the present government of Cuba."

1963   **February 1963:** President John F. Kennedy prohibits U.S. government-purchase cargoes from being transported on foreign flag vessels which after January 1, 1963, had called at a Cuban port.

July 1963: The U.S. Treasury Department produces the Cuban Assets ControlRegulations. These regulations embody the essential features of the U.S. economic embargo against Cuba that has been in effect ever since, including a freeze on all Cuban-owned assets in the United States and a prohibition on all non-licensed financial and commercial transactions between Cuba and the United States and between Cuban and U.S. nationals (including the spending of money U.S. citizens in the course of travel to Cuba).

1964   **May 1964:** The Commerce Department revokes its prior general license policy for export to Cuba of foods, medicines and medical supplies. The Commerce Department adopts a broad policy of denying requests for commercial sales of food and medicine to Cuba and permits only limited humanitarian donations.

July 1964: The Organization of American States (OAS) passes a resolution obliging its members to enforce a collective trade embargo on Cuba. The resolution excludes sales of foodstuffs, medicines and medical equipment. The United States, however, persists in its policy of denying licenses for such sales.

1974   **July 1974:** The Treasury Department liberalizes its Cuban regulations, among other things, to allow the importation of Cuban books and records and to liberalize restrictions on travel to Cuba by scholars and journalists.

1975   **July 1975:** The OAS repeals its regional trade embargo against Cuba, prompting the Ford Administration to end the ban on third-country subsidiary trade with Cuba and instead requiring only that U.S. companies obtain individual licenses for transactions involving their overseas subsidiaries.

1977   **March 1977:** The Carter Administration removes restrictions on travel to Cuba by U.S. citizens.

1982   **April 1982:** The Reagan Administration severely restricts the travel of U.S. citizens to Cuba.

1992   **October 1992:** President George Bush signs the Cuban Democracy Act (CDA) which outlaws subsidiary trade with Cuba and imposes severe restrictions on foreign ships that visit Cuba before attempting to enter U.S. ports. The CDA gives the Treasury Department for the first time the authority to levy civil fines to $50,000 for violations of the embargo.

996   **March 1996:** The Cuba Liberty and Democratic Solidarity Act (the "Helms-Burton Act") becomes law. The Act seeks to impede economic recovery under the present Cuban government by deterring foreign investment. Among other measures, the Helms-Burton Act allows foreign companies to be taken to court in the United States if they are "trafficking" in former U.S. citizen-owned properties in Cuba nationalized by the government of President Fidel Castro. ("Trafficking" is expansively defined to include not just direct investment in such properties but also any activities involving such properties that "benefit" that so-called "trafficker.") In addition, the Act "codifies" the existing Cuban Asset Control Regulations. Any modification of those regulations is intended, henceforth, to require an act of Congress.

CHAPTER ONE

CUBA - A MEDICAL PARADOX

Some Vignettes

At the graduation ceremony for medical personnel at Cuba's Santa Clara University in
the summer of 1992, Fidel Castro commented:

> **"Even if we stop building hospitals and health care centres until 1997,
> Cuba will retain its privileged position as having by far the most
> successful public health system of any other third world country".**

Again, at a Conference convened in Copenhagen, Denmark, in June 1995, Fidel
stated[1]:-

> "Despite the grievous loss of economic support from the former Soviet
> Union and other socialist economies and despite the agonising severity
> of the US Blockade, Cuba has not yet closed a single school or shut
> down even one hospital."

Both of these comments are proud boasts indeed, but how true are they?

Any survey of the Cuban "health system" (more accurately a "condominial
enterprise", as it is so thoroughly linked with both the public education system and the
social welfare as to be indistinguishable at its peripheries from either) confronts one
with a matrix of contradictions:

Item - Cuba has pioneered in the management and restoration to health of
schizophrenics, yet spends a lower proportion of the total medical budget on mental
health than does Tanzania!

---

[1] UNESCO (1995): World Summit for Social Development - Cuba National Report.
Pg. 103 . Copenhagen.

Item - Cuba now leads Latin America in research in the field of HIV+ infection, yet as late as 1986 was officially stating that AIDS was a homosexual phenomenon and that homosexuality had no place in a healthy socialist society!

Item - Cuban schools push the "anti-smoking" message and yet this author watched with amazement as two doctors, both smoking into the face of their prostrate patient, worked at trying to revive someone who had collapsed in a corridor of Havana's leading hospital.

Not only is the practice of Cuban medicine beset with anomalies such as illustrated by the foregoing vignettes, but the interaction of ideology on the one hand, and of realpolitik on the other have invested the whole health care enterprise with policy contradictions. Probably the best way of appreciating this is to present a brief overview of some of Cuba's medical achievements since the revolution under three headings: Medicine as a commercial enterprise, High Tech medicine and Community Health care. These three categories are not mutually exclusive, of course, nor are they exhaustive of Cuba's rich panoply of initiatives in the field of health, but they reflect the complexity of the topic.

Medicine as a Commercial Enterprise

Cuba has been singled out uniquely for " economic quarantine" by the US since the Bay of Pigs invasion. Whatever the rights and wrongs of this in terms of international law and diplomacy, it is a fact and it is a fact which constitutes the bottom line in almost any discussion of Cuban domestic policy. The long and the short of it is that Cuba is desperate for dollars, like any other Latin American country, as it was before the revolution as well. However, there were then no ideological barriers to obtaining dollars through the running of gambling casinos, various rackets involving the American underworld, prostitution, etc. There was also no ideological barrier to trade with the US, whose tourists kept those dollar generating activities running.

Now ideology has rendered such enterprises unacceptable and, at the same

2

time, has excluded much of the access to American tourism.

However, as mentioned elsewhere in this book, Cuba does have a long tradition - certainly antedating the revolution - of creativity and ingenuity in the medical business! From the end of the Second World War up until 1959, private 'clinics' abounded in Cuba. These generally did not treat Cubans - unless they were very wealthy indeed - but catered for American clients. They offered services, sometimes highly technical services, at much lower prices than prevailed in the US and thus attracted relatively large numbers. Moreover, they were unrestricted by the American Medical Association (AMA) regulations governing ethics and safety and could therefore be much more daringly innovative than could their private sector American counterparts.

Along with routine surgical and medical practices, such clinics could - and did - carry out radical cosmetic surgical procedures that could not be obtained at any price in the US because they were proscribed on safety grounds by the AMA. In those years from 1954-1959, a lot of Americans must have wanted bits cut off, reshaped or put on, sufficiently desperately to forsake the conservative clinical safety offered by the AMA and to take their chances with Cuban scapel wielders, for cosmetic surgery in Cuba generated an average of 5 million dollars a year from 1948 through 1958[2]. This is discussed in greater detail elsewhere in this book.

The reader must not imagine that this sort of thing is common, either among Latin American countries generally or third world countries generally. Some countries run small enterprises of this type, a steady supply of clients being guaranteed by the high costs of private medical care in the US. But the Cubans have always been especially adept at it. It has to be seen as one of those fortuitous "national characteristics". They also boast a proud tradition of eminence in surgery. One only has to look at the US register of surgeons to appreciate how high a proportion of them

---

[2]Life Magazine: 28 August 1964. No source for the figure given in that article, but the author has heard similarly unreferenced figures ranging from 4-8 million dollars per year, so the Life one is probably not too far out.

trained at the University of Havana Medical School before the revolution.

With that in mind, the reader will not be surprised to find that revolutionary Cuba was not slow in organising this sort of thing as a dollar generator when the blockade began to bite deep in the early 60's. Of course, it creates logistic problems for Americans wishing to use the services because to do so violates US laws under the rubric of "trading with the enemy". However, as one Florida businessman I met in Havana in 1993 said - he was there for two weeks to undergo kidney surgery - "Rules are challenges and ways are meant to be found around them!" One such way is for an American client to go to Canada for a few weeks. While there he can visit the Cuban Economic Mission in Ottawa and obtain the necessary travel documents to Cuba without his passport being marked. Mexico is similarly involved in ferrying Americans to and from Cuba.

I was amazed, when staying in Cuba in 1993, at the range and extent of the medical services thus offered to foreigners and also by the fact that Americans are by no means the only customers. Germans also occupied a high profile as did Greeks. Canada itself provides a steady, if small, stream of clients. The only Cubans I met in any of these clinics were on the staff. I saw dollars being handed over in cash and in travellers cheques. The latter represent a problem as the Trading with the Enemy Act renders it impossible for Cuba to cash travellers cheques drawn on American banks. My Florida acquaintance mentioned above, paid in Thos. Cooke Sterling Travellers Cheques. It is all so open that it must be government-run, although when questioned about it by me no-one in the Ministry of Public Health actually admitted it.

There are a great many implications to this aspect of Cuba's medical activities. One obvious point is that, were it not for the blockade, there is no doubt that Cuba would flourish in a normalised relationship with the US. The ideological disadvantages seem to bite both ways, for it is difficult to see how any number of American enterprises would not find the lifting of the blockade mutually advantageous.

But at an ideological level, this process of making money out of medicine creates philosophical and moral problems. One meets many articulate medical professionals in Cuba who castigate it roundly, claiming that it uses up resources that could otherwise be applied to community health care. Counter arguments put to me by the director of a private medicine clinic in Havana include that it allows Cuban doctors to purchase expensive, high tech clinical and diagnostic apparatus which can then also be used by the public sector. I did, in fact, see direct evidence of this in Havana's Almeijiras Hospital, a show-piece of Cuba's medical system and the largest hospital in Latin America. This hospital is primarily part of the public health matrix. But each of its specialist departments also runs "international clinics" and, with the money thus generated, have purchased state-of-the-art diagnostic machinery which is also available for use on public patients. This in turn raises other serious difficulties which will be dealt with later.

Other arguments used to justify this flourishing branch of private enterprise in a socialist context are that it generates much needed hard currency and that it provides an avenue for Cuban medical personnel to gain a diversity of medical experience not often encountered by third world doctors.

High Tech Medicine in Low Tech Cuba

In Mantanzas, I was recently being shown over a maternity hospital. Off on one side I saw a rather unprepossessing little single storey building with the words (in Spanish) "Research and Investigation Unit" painted on the door. Uncertain as to whether it was someone's idea of a joke, I tentatively asked about it. I was ushered in, to find myself confronted by a row of 8 cubicles, in each of which were foetal monitors, sonographs and 1992 Japanese computerised utero scanners. In each cubicle was a patient undergoing what was referred to as a "routine ante-natal check"!

As the Director of the unit made clear, obviously not every pregnant Cuban is accorded that level of antenatal investigation, but that particular unit had been doing research on a wide variety of epidemiological issues related to foetal development since 1989 and was one of 9 in Cuba that had been earmarked by MINSAP for research in the area. Their team had already published in various international journals and had been visited by other investigators from the UK, Sweden and various other industrially advanced nations.

One of their staff was at that moment on a year's leave in Stockholm refining his skills and furthering his research.

When one has lived and worked in Cuba, this sort of thing no longer comes as a surprise, but a general view of Cuban health care often held by medical people in such places as the US and the UK, is that they operate a universal socialised health care system, but almost at the "barefoot doctor" level. This is not so. Although a third world country itself, Cuba has made a number of internationally acclaimed breakthroughs in high tech medicine, to say nothing of its widely acknowledged achievements in low tech community medicine and primary health care. As pointed out by American medical observers of Cuba (Chapter Sixteen) the continued US Blockade is beginning to undo many of Cuba's achievements in public health.

However, let us consider some positive examples, most of which will be discussed in greater detail in Chapter Twelve. In 1991 two Cuban endocrinologists at Santiago Medical School, Drs. Hector Lazarus and Guillelm Ortez Franks, working with a computer technician, Luisa Evangelina Cortes, came up with a non-invasive device for detecting minute changes in thyroid activity. It arose out of attempts to ascertain whether people applying for entry to a local agricultural college were likely to develop disabling allergies - apparently a worrying cause of attrition of student numbers. But their preliminary investigations went far beyond this to the development of what is now referred to internationally as the Ultra Micro Analytical System (UMAS). Its range of applications at the prognostic and diagnostic levels has proven to be immense.

In several other instances recently Cuba has distinguished itself in the area of computerisation and laser technology, principally as a spin-off from the care of track and field athletes suffering muscular injuries. Cuba has a long tradition of excellence in competitive athletics and in such team sports as baseball. The communist regime was not slow in building on this and in giving athletes representing Cuba abroad the very best of medical and physiotherapeutic care. It is therefore natural that any medical

6

intervention associated with the biomechanics of sport and muscle tone should be of interest at the highest medical levels in Cuba.

One could go on at much greater length, but the issue is discussed in detail in Chapter Eleven. For present purposes it is enough to observe that Cuba is now at the forefront of high tech medical research in encephalogram interpretation, computerised diagnosis of neurological pathologies and the monitoring of laser neurosurgery. This is easy to state but almost unbelievably remarkable for a third world country beleaguered by the most stringent economic quarantine ever imposed on any country and for a greater length of time.

While I find much to criticise, as a priority strategy, with Cuba's almost obsessive preoccupation with carving an international reputation for herself in high tech research and development in medicine, it has unquestionably helped to establish Cuba's moral leadership in the third world through her policy of sharing the fruits of such initiatives with other developing nations. Cuba cannot be said to have let many propaganda opportunities slip by here!

In time for the July 26 celebrations[3] in 1990, Cuba announced to the world the opening of the Iberian and Latin American Centre for Nervous System Transplant and Regeneration. Since then its clientele have included some leading people from a range of other countries as well as a steady supply of more humble citizens from the same countries who are never charged for the service and whose travelling costs to and from Cuba are even usually paid for often by Palestinian sources as a means of according their Middle Eastern struggles a favourably humanitarian image.

---

[3] July 26 is Cuba's national day, for on that date in 1953 Fidel Castro led his small band of rebels on the now famous Moncada Barrado in Santiago, a large and - as it unfortunately turned out - well defended outpost of the Batista Dictatorship.

Community Health Care

No matter how spectacular Cuba's successes in commercial medicine and/or high tech research, her unimpeachable fame will always lie in the more prosaic - but certainly of wider applicability - field of general practice and its contextual matrix of community health care. Cuba's deeds in this arena are now so widely acknowledged that a mere litany of them would be superfluous. The intersectoral mix of social and governmental forces required to sustain it all, though, is exhaustively analysed in Chapter Ten. As an introductory comment, though, we are talking about a third world country, with a population of 12 million, whose standardised Mortality Ratios, Infant Mortality Figures, Maternal Morbidity Figures and Life Expectancy (routine epidemiological data used for comparing health indices) all rank it with the most fortunate of the industrialised nations. What this boils down to is the fact that Cubans are people who are born in a third world economy and who sicken and die of first world pathologies!

Although this phenomenon will be analysed in detail, a few comments about it at this stage are in order. Firstly, Cuba now has a doctor-patients ratio of 1:300. This is a much better ratio than prevails even in the UK and the US. It is all the more remarkable in that almost all of their doctors are GP's (about 83% by my Byzantine calculations from MINSAP data!) and (as of 1998) about 60% of those either are now, or are becoming, further qualified as Family Physicians.

The first impact of such statistics is on both the character of medical work that these doctors routinely carry out and on the role they occupy in the community. Unavoidably, one finds the greatest concentration of this medical expertise in urban areas, but not to the extent that this occurs in a free market economy or even in other 'socialist' societies.

No citizen of Cuba is without access to a doctor, either geographically or for financial reasons. At the operational level, every GP lives in the community he serves and, in a city, such a community would be no more than 2 or 3 city blocks! This means that people are always in contact with their doctor. He/she, in fact, often spends a part of each day making unsolicited calls on his/her patients - rather like the old-style parish priest doing his rounds. More than once I have been sitting socialising with a Cuban family in their apartment when someone suddenly says: "Aqui tiene medico" (Here comes the doctor) as a figure parks a bike at the curb and walks in without so much as a by-your-leave. On such occasions the doctor characteristically is welcomed in the standard laid-back Cuban style, with a drink and a bit of social banter. The doctor will always look at any baby in the family, if one is there, and may pass a comment or two (which would be classified as "Health Promotion" in the context of the UK GP contract!) about eating, smoking, etc., and then saunters off. People still attend their doctor's surgery, but only for specific problems. Many Cuban GP's have told me that they rarely confront real illness because the level of routine preventive medicine is so high!

As the reader will also be doubtless aware, Cuban medical schools produce a super-abundance of medical graduates. While communities within Cuba may be over-saturated with medical care at the ratio referred to, excess doctors serve all over the world in countries much less fortunate in terms of medical provision, than Cuba. In the context of Cuba's third world status, the question might well be asked as to how such a state of affairs came about. We in the industrialised first world struggling as we are with what appears to be an impossible equation of rising medical costs and the need to impose a ceiling on the percentage of the GNP we can accord health care, the Cuban scenario seems to break all of the rules. Within our own social political contexts, we tend to respond to such problems by such aphorisms as: "You don't solve social problems by throwing money at them." The Cuban experience suggests that that is exactly how you solve them, with the caveat emptor that, if you don't have much money, you prioritise what you do have. Such a view, of course, obviates the operation of a free-market economy. This is virtually akin to suggesting that a socially responsible programme of community health care cannot be run outside of a socialist context. Whether this is true or not as a general rule remains to be seen, but there is no doubt that Cuba's success in this sphere is inimitably interlinked with the ideological vade mecam of socialism. Analysis of this fact forms a significant part of this book, but a brief overview of the nexus between the two is appropriate in this chapter as a scene-setter, so to speak.

Let us begin by quoting Article 49 of the Socialist Constitution of the Republic of Cuba.

> **"Everyone has the right to the care and protection of their health. The State guarantees this right: By offering free hospital and medical services... By offering free dental treatment; By developing plans for sanitary efforts, health education, periodic medical exams, general vaccination, and other preventive medical means. In these plans and activities the entire population participates through the social and mass organizations."**

Many personal accounts were published in the early days of the Cuban revolution, reflecting the sense of relief felt by ordinary people who, for the first time in Cuban history, had been accorded these rights. Representative of that reportage is a quote from Terence Cannon's[4] book on Cuba, in which the words of a peasant Enrique Otero Fernandez are given prominence:

> **"He who was seriously ill was just stuck. To be treated one had to go to Cienfuegos, which in the spring, took 15 hours. One travelled by horse or on foot along a terrible path toward Gavilanes, the boat to the Guanaroca lagoon, and from there to the Bay of Cienfuegos. We saw many people die on the road. Today one makes the trip by highway, direct, in less than an hour.**
>
> **We guajiros of the Escambray didn't have the right to be born and not even the right to die decently. The women gave birth naturally, without any help, just like the cows in the pasture. Today the rural women have all their treatment guaranteed from the first moment to the birth, and even our cows now have veterinary doctors. If our women in those days had even the attention that our cattle do now, it would have saved the lives of many children and pregnant women."**

Those remarks were made in 1974 and reflect the astonishing fact that in its first 15

---

[4]Cannon, Terence: "Revolutionary Cuba". José Marté Publishing House, Havana (Foreign Language Section), 1983.

years, the revolutionary regime had gone a long way to overcoming two huge problems which had together conspired to keep rural Cuba in a state of medievalism, as far as medical facilities were concerned. The two problems were;

     a)   Distribution of doctors and of primary health care facilities.

     b)   Actual numbers of doctors and paramedical staff.

Since the elaboration of Cuba's now renowned system of public health necessitated the hurdling of these two major obstacles, and since the details of how this has been done and the stages of its development constitute a major theme in the book, a few preliminary remarks are called for.

Cuba is a delight for those who are given to such punitive pursuits as rock-climbing and hill walking in that a large proportion of it was until recently inaccessible to ordinary transport. Peasants living in the mountain fastness of the Sierra Maestra, or even in the swampy lowlands of Giron, existed for past generations without significant contact with mainstream life in Cuba. Whole settlements had remained untouched by the social forces of education and orthodox health care - until the revolution took power in 1959. In its first two years in power, the great bulk of these "forgotten people" had been given access to both schooling and modern health care. This was accomplished partly by an aggressive road-building programme, along with the establishment of a comprehensive network of rural boarding schools, holding in excess of 1000 students each and which were also equipped with medical and paramedical staff. The Great Literacy Campaign for which Cuba is so justly famous [5] also had penetrated into all of these hitherto neglected pockets of Cuban society and had in many ways, prepared the people psychologically to forsake their superstitious practices and to embrace orthodox medical care when it became available.

What doctors there were in pre-Revolutionary Cuba were heavily concentrated in the two cities of Havana and Santiago. These two centres of population accounted

---

[5]This took place in 1960-61 and was the first nationwide adult literacy programme initiated since 1945 and classified by UNESCO as a success. See MacDonald, T. (1984) "The Two Illiteracies". University of Newcastle Press Monograph in Education.

11

for 65% of the general practitioners. It goes without saying that no specialist would be practising in an area bereft of advanced technical facilities and a reasonably well-integrated GP matrix. Likewise, nurses and the paramedical personnel did not, in pre-Revolutionary Cuba, work independently in small rural clinics as they often do now, but invariably worked either as part of some specialists "team" or as staff at a medical institution. Thus many areas of rural Cuba - even accessible areas - were routinely not serviced by health workers. The geographical barriers to which reference has already been made, certainly accounted for part of this, but it was no means the only reason. Medical care in pre-Revolutionary Cuba was almost exclusively private. Doctors did not practice in rural areas because a decent living could not be made there. There was no government health care to speak of, and what existed was principally confined to Havana. The Catholic Church also ran various medical facilities on a charitable basis, but again largely ignored the rural poor. In this respect it is interesting to note how different Cuba was from many other Spanish-speaking nations with regard to religious influence. Pre-Revolutionary Cuba was only 10% Catholic! Moreover, Protestant denominations were barely represented at all, and then mainly in Havana. The implication is that most of Cuba's population were non-Christian. Various Voodoo cults of African origin constituted the main focus of religious expression.

Thus, until the revolution came to power, medical care was very much an urban business enterprise. Even in the cities, pre-Revolutionary medical care was inaccessible to all but the wealthy. There was a Ministry responsible for health care (The Ministry of Health and Social Assistance) but it was typically a corrupt outfit. Accounts abound[6] of the way in which it was used by politicians and others as a means of enrichment through embezzlement, padded accounts and rake-offs. In fact, a common enough practice was the garnering of votes in exchange for hospital beds. In return for a physician's recommendation that a person be admitted to hospital, the patient handed over his/her voting card. Doctors collecting enough of these could then use them for

---

[6]See, for instance, Hugh Thomas' balanced account "The Cuban Revolution" Wiedenfield and Nicolson, London, 1986 (pp. 120,121)

personal gain from venal politicians!

The total roll of physicians and surgeons in Cuba in 1959 was 6,000[7]. About 1500 fled to Miami within a week of Batista taking the same route. It is said that two enterprising Ministry officials stayed behind long enough to transfer 1-2 million dollars (US) from the Cuban Hospital Fund into personal bank accounts in Miami[8]. Doctors kept leaving Cuba throughout the first 6 months of the revolution, especially when it became plain that medicine as a business occupation was finished, that they would have to work as public servants for low salaries and that they might be sent anywhere in Cuba! Thus, and here paradox rears its quizzical head yet again, at the very time when Cuba's new legislation made medical care available to anyone, the number of doctors became half of what it had been when they had only been serving, say, 10% of the population. This did call for strenuous and highly innovatory action on the part of the new government, and the detailed account of how they did it is examined thoroughly in subsequent chapters.

Suffice to say, they met the challenge by a series of temporary measures, including the use of doctors volunteering from other countries (including the USA - Fidel Castro was regarded as a folk hero in the US for almost a year after he came to power in Cuba!), using medical students in their last two years of training etc. A serious blow to the entire enterprise was the fact that Cuba had only one medical school (that at the University of Havana) and most of its leading staff fled with Batista. Fortunately a number of medical professors from other countries - some of them Spanish! - lent their services. I have been regaled by a number of accounts of Russian, German, Canadian and French medical professors trying, with a dictionary in one hand and a frightful level of dependence on hand-waving, to teach Cuban medical students in those early days. Cuban medical personnel who were students then still talk about it

---

[7]This figure is approximate, but all sources agree that it was about that. See Thomas, Ibid. 2.

[8]Personal conversation with Dr. Augusto Hernandez Batista, Director of Health Administration For Havana province. 1993.

with ribald good humour. I have heard the story so many times of a foreign professor (his nationality changes with whoever is telling the story!) who confused the neck with the cervix in Spanish that I suspect that the story must be apocryphal!

A new generation of doctors was gradually trained, dedicated to spreading medical care to the entire country. Beginning in 1960, the Ministry of Public Health (MINSAP) sent teams of doctors to towns and villages where no doctor had ever been seen.

Though they believed in preventive medicine, these early teams could do little more than attack the worst ills of a peasantry suffering from parasites, malnutrition, anaemia, polio, gastroenteritis, respiratory diseases, malaria, typhoid, and whooping cough. The doctor usually set up shop in a corner of the home of a campesino, travelling to the surrounding area by horse or mule or on foot. He treated a daily stream of people, sometimes able to do little more than sympathise, knowing that poor sanitary conditions, overwork, too little food, and poor nutrition were the real causes of their ills. He dispensed pills, delivered babies, gave advice on sanitary habits, and argued against those who believed that magic or potions or God were the means to health. 58 year old Dr. Garcia Lorca, now Registrar General of Benitez Hospital in Oriente (1998) recalls:

> **"In the countryside it had been the custom, and in this area even more, for doctors to charge for a birth in proportion to the number of miles he had to travel, in addition to the medical care. One morning at six a campesino arrived on muleback asking me to go to his house to care for his wife. She was having contractions and he couldn't take her to a hospital.**
>
> **We made the journey on foot in three hours. The woman gave birth, happily, at three in the afternoon. When it was over, she asked for the campesino to take me back to the dispensary, since I didn't know the road. The man appeared at five in the afternoon, very worried.**
>
> **"Doctor," he said to me, "I'll bring you the money early tomorrow. I left to sell a cow, but they aren't going to pay me until tomorrow morning."**
> **I felt so embarrassed. I put my arm around him and told him,**

**"My friend, you're mistaken. I'm a doctor that the Revolution
sent to take care of you, not to rip you off."**

The true enemy of public health, a 1969 MINSAP report noted, had been "economic underdevelopment, feudal exploitation, the latifundia and its consequences: illiteracy, the hundreds of thousands of unemployed, the terrible tiempo muerto with its inescapable companions: misery, hunger, and death." To deal with the problem at its root meant agrarian reform, public education, roads, communications, hygiene, full employment.

In that sense it was the Revolution itself that contributed most to health in the early years. Slowly things improved. Sanitary practices took root. The Revolution spread a network of roads, schools, medical posts. Agrarian reform gave land to the peasants and unemployment shrank.

The rural doctor began to be freed from his daily consultations, to plan with the villagers for the long-range needs of the community - to co-ordinate vaccination campaigns, to improve sanitary conditions, to hold classes on preventive medicine.

Mass campaigns were begun in 1962 against polio, malaria, and tetanus. The CDR (Committees for the Defence of the Revolution), the Federation of Cuban Women, and other organizations held vaccination drives in every section of the country: 2,216,022 children were immunised against polio that year, using the Sabine vaccine; 4,000,000 inoculations against diphtheria, tetanus, and typhoid were carried out in a four-month period. As a result, there have been no cases of polio in Cuba since 1963. Malaria, which before had struck some 3,000 persons a year, was eliminated in 1968. Diphtheria was eradicated in 1971. Gastroenteritis, a major killer of children in underdeveloped countries, killing 4,157 Cuban children in 1962, 80% of them under the age of one, was curbed, causing only 761 deaths in 1975.

Behind these efforts lay a profound philosophical assumption: under socialism - "the protection of people's health is the obligation of the socialist state," in the words of a 1969 MINSAP statement. The quality and availability of health care should in no way be affected by one's ability to pay or one's geographical location.

15

This constituted an enormous achievement in the North American/South American context. Nothing like it had ever been accomplished in the western hemisphere before, although Canada finally developed a comprehensive health service not many years later.

To carry out this obligation, the Cuban Revolution had within 15 years, created a remarkable network of medical services that now reaches every Cuban man, woman, and child with comprehensive, preventive, and curative medical care, equal in quality and free of charge. The rural hospital or polyclinic is the basic unit of the health system. Here is where most of the people of Cuba receive medical care. The polyclinic offers general medicine, paediatrics, gynaecology, obstetrics, dental care, control of communicable diseases, hygiene, and health education.

This is an important facet of Cuba's public health care system and reflects a number of unique features. The whole issue is dealt with in detail in Chapter Eleven and elsewhere in this book. Obviously it did not fall into place overnight or entirely as a consequence of revolutionary fiat. Rather it was the product of thought, experimentation and thoroughly grass-roots consultation. What is staggering is that, in form, the polyclinic system was fully operational within 15 or 16 years of Fidel Castro's accession to power. To quote Cannon[9] again:

> "In 1975 I visited such a rural hospital, the Mario Munoz
> Hospital, named for the doctor killed in the attack on the
> Moncada garrison. The hospital lies near a sugar mill deep in the
> countryside north of Holguin, almost at the sea. The country is
> rolling, with sudden precipitous hills and stretches of pasture and
> cane. I had expected a small building, like a community clinic in a
> city, and was surprised to find a large modern hospital.
>
> The social workers from the hospital, I was told, fan out over the
> rural area, visiting sick people in their homes, arranging for
> transportation to the hospital. When a mother needs to be
> treated, they arrange for the children to be housed by other
> families or at a day-care centre while she's gone. When any
> prolonged treatment is called for, the social worker helps settle the
> home problems that may arise: providing a guaranteed salary

---

[9]Cannon, Terence Ibid. 9.

16

> **from the Ministry of Work, school arrangements, child care, a j**
> **for another member of the family, special care for older depend**
> **members of the family."**

The energy and commitment with which these changes were brought into being can be appreciated if one compares the WHO figures on Cuba from 1958 (just prior to the revolution) with those which the same agency recorded for 1974 - a mere 16 years later. See Table 1.1.

Table 1-1: Health Data From Cuba 1958 and 1974[10]

	1958	1975
National Health Budget	**$22,000,000**	**$400,000,000**
Hospital Beds	28,536	46,402
Blood Banks	1	22
Medical Schools	1	4
Physicians	6,000	10,000
	(3,000 left Cuba	
	after the Revolution)	
Nursing Schools	1	34
Polio	300 cases/year	0
Malaria	3,000 cases/year	0
Diphtheria	600 cases/year	0
Gastroenteritis	4,000 deaths/year	761
Infant Mortality	60 per 1000 live	28.9
	births	
Life Expectancy	55 years	70

A question must arise about the reliability of these figures, as indeed with all other statistical detail presented in this volume. Communist regimes have never been

---

[10]Health Provision in the Caribbean, WHO, Geneva. 1975.

renowned for the integrity attendant upon their statistical presentations. However, these are WHO figures, rather than, say, UNESCO figures. Cuba is of profound interest to WHO, as it is to the worldwide health community generally. It is at any one time host to hundreds, if not thousands, of health care workers from Europe, Africa and Asia who study it closely. WHO has representatives in Cuba several times a year and these people have direct and friendly access to senior officials in MINSAP. UNESCO, on the contrary, sends a team for a short visit every few years. Figures quoted by UNESCO are, in most cases, data given to them by Cuban government officials and they are rarely queried.

The International Connection

Any account of the medical paradox that is Cuba must include its role as a health care benefactor to so may other countries while unable to provide its own citizens with enough to eat!

As will be discussed in subsequent chapters, one reason for this anomaly is that Cuba's startling development as a "medical nation" came about because of the revolution, but largely outside of its control. To a lesser degree the same sort of maverick anarchy attended some of its more novel educational initiatives. Could this be because the revolution gained ground in those two areas faster than the party bureaucrats - also new to the job in the western hemisphere - could evolve controls over it all. One certainly gained the impression that that was happening during the Literacy Campaign.[11]

Cuba's international reputation today is certainly rendered evident by the fact that her network of health services now routinely extends beyond her frontiers. This began within three years of the revolutionary forces coming to power. Cuba's first medical mission was sent in response to a request to newly independent Algeria in June

---

[11]MacDonald, Theodore. Ibid. 1.

1962. This has now evolved into a permanent programme of medical training and technical training.

During the bombing of North Vietnam, twenty-one Cuban doctors and medical workers treated both victims of war and the general population. After the war, Cuba maintained a director and several physicians at the Vietnam-Cuba Friendship Hospital, in Hanoi, training Vietnamese medical personnel.

Cuba has sent other medical teams to Peru, Guatemala, Nicaragua, and Chile to help during earthquakes and disasters. At present, Cuba maintains medical missions in Vietnam, Ethiopia, Yemen, Somalia, Laos, Tanzania, Algeria, Guinea, Angola, Equatorial Guinea, Guinea-Bissau and the Congo. An American doctor, Dr. Percival Rimmer, who travelled to Cuba in 1982 with a group from the American Public Health Association had high praise for the spirit of the doctors he met there:[12]

> **"Everyone I met seemed to be making their life decisions around what the community needs and wants. Doctors would frequently say, "I will work where the Revolution needs me." After completing their obligatory three years of rural medical service following medical school, they would, I think, be perfectly happy to stay on another five years if it was necessary. They receive satisfaction out of the group success and the group experience. That's a really exciting feeling, and to see it embraced by just about everybody I met made me think that socialism was a success in Cuba."**

The internationalism of Cuban medicine, though, has not relied solely on her capacity to overproduce doctors at home and thus be in a position to make foreign service after graduation a pre-condition for full registration.

People from medical missions and enterprises crowd into Cuba to be instructed in everything from arcane micro-surgery techniques, basic medical education and epidemiology. Cuba has been the venue of numerous international gatherings, the most recent being the International Association of Medical Endocrinologists, which met in

---

[12]Rimmer, Percival. "Can Caring Be Taught As A Medical Skill?" Journal of the World Educational Fellowship, Oregon. Aug. 1982.

Havana in the summer of 1998.

In the arena of public health medicine, then, unlike the situation in Commercial Medicine and high Tech Medicine, perhaps Cuba has demonstrated what can happen when the "healing art" is unfettered from the market forces which traditionally bind it. While one quickly becomes inured to the transparent cant of many propaganda statements put out by communist governments for public discussion, there does remain something eloquently forceful, and forceful because so many Cuban doctors seem to believe it, about a summary statement made by the Cuban Institute of Family Doctors in 1968. It contained the following:

> "Our medical service must be made more humane and scientific;
> each sick person should be cared for as if they were our own
> father, mother, spouse, or child. In this way, we will enrich
> ourselves, being more human to others."

CHAPTER TWO

THE POLITICAL / PHILOSOPHICAL CONTEXT

The Cuban Revolution - A Brief Resume

Back in 1944 I recall sitting in a physics lesson on the electric motor. In trying to make a point, the teacher said: "Now, where do we have one revolution per minute?" His question was greeted by that languid silence so dreaded by pedagogues until the class wag answered: "In South America, sir!" If nothing else, this bon mot (which is not apocryphal, by the way) illustrates something about both Third World history and about First World perception of it. Desperately wretched economic and social conditions do, when combined with a wide-felt sense of despair that things will never improve, lead to periodic episodes of violence directed against the power structure. Lay people in the democratic and technologically advanced nations, however, often interpret this phenomenon as stemming from the national or racial characteristics of the people concerned. Thus, the popular stereotype of the Latin American revolutionary, with his (it is always a man!) extravagant gestures and romantic oratory, is very deeply rooted in the lay mind.

Most of the Latin American nations have a history of revolutions, repression and autocratic tyrannies going back to the early days of Spanish, Portuguese, English and French colonisation of the region. Cuba is no exception. It resisted Spanish colonial domination periodically throughout the 17th and 18th centuries, its principal literary hero in this regard being the prolific author and philosopher José Martí, who died defending his country from Spanish domination in 1865. But whether these uprisings failed outright (the usual scenario) or succeeded in bringing about the downfall of whatever tyranny was in force at the time, they cannot properly be called "revolutions".

21

Revolutions Vs Palace Coups

A 'revolution', as political scientists now understand the term, has to involve a drastic realignment of all of the social structures in society, and not merely be a violent substitution of one leader by another! Looked at in that light, there really have not been many revolutions. For instance, it can be argued that Mexico never had one. As for Cuba - it suffered a number of hideously violent episodes of civil unrest, resulting in changes of caudillo, interspersed with weak but more or less democratic governments. But it has only had one revolution.

That one achieved military power on January 1, 1959 led by Fidel Castro. The tyranny it replaced had been headed by Fulgencia Batista. His regime had certainly not been the most diabolically repressive in Cuban history (probably Machado is owed that honour!), nor was it the most enlightened. As Latin American dictatorships go, it started off as relatively benign (but hideously corrupt and implacably oppressed to even elementary social reforms) but became progressively more repressive and indiscriminately violent. It has to be said that this was largely in response to the undercurrents of revolutionary thought and action. Indeed it changed from a self-seeking, corrupt and inefficient dictatorship into an ideologically revanchist, more efficient dictatorship whose 'public policy' increasingly became `public terror', as it desperately tried to contain the revolutionary ferment.

Another attribute that political scientists use to differentiate between a palace coup and a revolution is that the latter is broadly supported by various sectors in the society. The person generally regarded as the prime initiator and leader of the Cuban revolution is Fidel Castro. As has often been the case in these things, Castro himself came from the comparatively wealthy classes (so did Lenin, Trotsky, Mao Tse Tung and Ho Chi Minh - to name but a few other revolutionary leaders) and at first saw Cuba's needs in the idealistic terms encouraged by his acquaintance with the Christian gospel and with 18th century anarchist thought. The writings of José Martí influenced him profoundly.

Fidel Castro's Role

His own experiences with various levels of the power structure -beginning with the over-formalised and bureaucratic administrations he ran up against in school and university all the way up to the naked oppression he encountered in his dealings with the police - moved him from idealism to communism. In the confined compass available to this author in writing about it, Castro's development as a philosophical revolutionary cannot be accorded justice. The interested reader can find more detailed accounts in various sources right across the political spectrum, almost all of which give Batista an exceedingly poor press.[13] Suffice to say, Fidel Castro came to realise that several important criteria would have to be addressed before any substantial reform could be brought to fruition in Cuba, most of which eventually would have implications for health care.

These are:

1.   A revolution would have to be total. That is, it could not be brought about by a benevolent dictatorship at the top doing the "right thing" by the people - the enlightened despot model. Thus, a people empowerment model in government might be expected to reflect itself (with respect to health issues) in the relationship between community, doctor and patient.

2.   It could not be exclusively political or administrative, leaving other areas of national life unaffected. Instead it would have to involve a widespread change of attitude about the meaning of human dignity - nothing less - and this would of necessity involve the arts, moral considerations, health care, religion,

---

[13]Miller, W : The Last Plantation, Secker & Warburg, London, 1961 gives a rather rightwing view, but at that time was still essentially "pro-Castro". By 1962 or 1963, most accounts of events in Cuba were "pro" if written from the left, and "anti" if written from the Right e.g. Huberman, L & Sweeney, P. "Socialism in Cuba", Monthly Review Press, New York, 1969 gives a leftwing account, while Thomas, H. "The Cuba Revolution", Wiedenfeld & Nicolson, London, 1986 is much more even-handed.

- every aspect of national life and feeling.

3.   It could not be achieved by normal "democratic" due processes because this would clearly have to involve powerful and privileged interests conniving in their own downfall! The clear implication of this, of course, is that force would be necessary and hence idealism would constitute an inadequate basis for it. One of Castro's strongest allies on promoting this view was Che Guevara, who was also a fully qualified medical doctor. The ideas, then of "revolutionary purity" and "commitment to peoples' health" early became established in the Cuban popular mind.

4.   It could not be accomplished by people taking orders, but would have to provide its own intrinsic motivation for each person's involvement and commitment. This implies the necessity of educating people ahead of time which, in turn, constantly would expose the developing revolution to the possibility of infiltration, sabotage and betrayal. If people were going to commit themselves to it, they had to know what they were doing and why.

5.   Such an undertaking could not confine itself to one social class (i.e. students and intellectuals) but would have to embrace workers, peasants, bureaucrats, soldiers, etc. This would have to involve a relatively long period of subversive activity and education of various types. It also inexorably cast the guerrillas in the role of caring teachers and health care workers, among whom they carried on their precarious and illegal activities.

6.   Finally, any enterprise encapsulating all of the fore-going attributes would have to be extremely well organised, with coherent structures for command and response. It was not the sort of thing that a "brilliant charismatic leader" could do on the basis of issuing inspired slogans, but would require the sort of party-structure and party-discipline, a careful articulation of planning and responsibility, for which the Soviet Union had already had a working model. This is reflected with astonishing fidelity in the administrative structure of health care in Cuba today.

As previously stated, this did not all come to Fidel in a flash of inspiration or out of a book, but as a result of direct, practical experience in trying to confront power structures at different levels in the name of such ethical goals as "justice". His years at first as an arts student and then as a postgraduate law student at the University of Havana gave him ample time to read the social and political classics and to educate himself in the theory. It also gave him an opportunity to practice public speaking. He won a number of oratory prizes and was leader of the University Debating Union. His political evolution toward 'orthodox' communism continued even after he first assumed power.

On September 5, 1957, a direct attempt was made by students to oust Batista from the presidential palace, but it was neither well organised in execution nor did a subsequent plan of action as to what to do should they succeed seem to have been worked out. Fidel Castro's group was involved in that attack. But at that point Fidel was still thought of very much as a utopian idealist because he had been known throughout his university years as a brilliant orator with respectably middle-class liberal ideas about constitutional democracy, etc! What is indisputable is that there is no question that many people in Cuba came to the conclusion from the brutality of Batista's reprisals that a revolution was called for. Even foreign observers were rapidly coming to that conclusion.[14]

Philosophical Aspects of Revolution

One obvious lesson from such fiascos is that a revolution has to establish its credentials initially at the peripheries of power and then relentlessly move in, gradually isolating the power centre from the rest of the society. Once people perceive a leadership to be, at best, irrelevant to their daily lives, the actual take-over comes fairly easily - or so history would suggest. The problem with a direct, focused attack on the leadership at

---

[14]Wyden, P., Bay of Pigs, Jonathan Cape, London, 1979.

the beginning is that, if it succeeds, the surrounding matrix of social institutions which had, either tacitly or otherwise, been part of that leadership's power structure, would not know what was expected of it when a new leadership required its support. This would force the new leadership also to rule arbitrarily. Thus the history of Latin America can, to a large degree, be expressed in terms of one palace coup replacing another in a succession of cut and thrust arrangements between army officers and wealthy landowners - with American business interests usually prominent in the background, with or without CIA involvement.

Fidel Castro's politics developed increasingly on the basis of what he read and what he observed and reflected less and less his previous preoccupation with Christian social justice. He and his closest collaborators gradually built up a clandestine, but broadly-based infrastructure throughout the country. In retrospect it can be seen that it was disproportionately student-run, had only tenuous links with trade union leaders (but few actual workers) and had no peasant representation at all. There is insufficient scope in these pages to describe how Fidel Castro's first attempt at a major revolutionary action went so badly wrong.

Moncada!

Suffice to say, on July 26, 1953, Fidel's group tried to attack the military barracks at Moncada near Santiago (at the other end of Cuba from Havana). The general idea was to hold the barracks long enough to demonstrate to the people of Cuba that a revolutionary group did exist and was able to attack and hold isolated outposts of the dictatorship and, also, to arm the revolutionary forces with supplies from the Moncada barracks itself. But, as indicated, the whole thing went drastically wrong.

Through a breakdown in communications, various bands of the attackers - who were supposed to converge at strategic points in and around Santiago - lost their way or arrived at incorrect times. As well, the intelligence gathered by the revolutionaries to the effect that only a few soldiers would be on duty at Moncada on July 26, turned

26

out to be grossly incorrect. There were over 1,000 soldiers there, just returned from a special 3 month training course in the U.S. on counter-insurgency techniques![15] One could go on.

In any case, the attack was quickly repelled - and then came the repression. Batista personally ordered the eradication of the young revolutionary movement which had thus flexed its muscles too soon. As the police and army closed in, blood literally flowed in the streets of Santiago. Many accounts exist giving details of subsequent events - mass torture to extract names of other evolutionary supporters, gratuitous butchery, rape and denial of any form of normal human rights. Somehow Fidel Castro and 24 others escaped capture and retreated into the hills. Subsequently they were all captured, but only after widespread condemnation of Batista's police had made those instruments of repression a bit more hesitant to openly violate human rights. As well, the army, under the Batista regime, tended to have a much better reputation than the police for respecting due legal processes and constitutional rights. When he was ready, Fidel made sure that he was arrested by the army, not by the police!

Creating Fidel the Hero

This ensured that he was charged, convicted and duly sentenced to 15 years of prison. The trial at which Fidel was convicted attracted international media attention and he was able to use the witness stand as a podium for his now famous speech "La Historia me Absolverá" (History will absolve me). This impassioned document laid out the moral authority behind the idea of a Cuban revolution. It has been widely read and continues to inspire the fight for justice all over the third world. Even the manner of its written form (because, of course, in court it was only spoken) was sufficiently dramatic to help ensure its immortality. It was written on tiny scraps of paper and smuggled out in bits in the cuffs of visitor's trousers, etc. Once outside of prison, people painstakingly reconstructed it - itself a highly perilous activity in the teeth of the Batista

---

[15] Cannon, James: Revolutionary Cuba, Casa de las Americas Publishing, Havana, 1984

tyranny and one for which more than one life was paid.

In 1955, Batista badly needed to clean up his act. The Cuban government was trying to extract development finance from the World Bank and the International Monetary Fund - both largely controlled by the U.S. American public opinion had been rudely shocked by the tyranny's excesses - which had included such features as gruesome tortures and hangings from street light posts! - and, in the U.S. there would not be much support for American government financial assistance to Batista.[16] Advised accordingly, Batista gave the appearance of having turned over a new leaf. He brought an end to the gratuitous abuses of power perpetrated by the police and declared an amnesty for political prisoners. Fidel Castro, and a number of his revolutionary colleagues, were released. He correctly divined that residence in Cuba might not be particularly good for his health and fled to Mexico. There he set about systematically planning the revolutionary overthrow of the Batista regime.

The Revolution - Politics and Spectacle

The Cuban archetypal revolutionary not only embodied the appropriate social and political elements, but in so many respects he/she reflected all of the romantic and heroic features that we ordinarily associate with folk heroes like Bonnie Prince Charlie. One such figure, who played a decisive role in the Cuban revolution and who after his death entered deeply into popular consciousness of social justice, was Ernesto 'Che' Guevara. He was an Argentinean doctor and revolutionary idealist, wandering about Latin America observing and looking for a cause to which he could commit himself body and soul. Then he met Fidel Castro, and his little group, in Mexico in 1955! As Che was to write later: [17] "It would have taken very little to persuade me to join any

---

[16] As much is candidly admitted by Urrutia, M "Fidel Castro & Co. Inc - Communist Tyranny in Cuba". Frederick Praeger, New York, 1964. pg.36-37.

[17] Franqui, Carlos 1959 " Cuba: Le Livre des Douge" Gallimaid, Paris

28

revolution against a tyranny". The price he paid was his first marriage. His first wife, Hilda Gadea, was quoted as saying "I lost my husband to the Cuban revolution".[18]

Fidel Castro and his revolutionaries may have learned much as a result of the ill-fated attack on Moncada, but events soon showed them that they had not learned enough! Having gathered and trained a highly committed group of 82 guerrilla fighters, Castro set off from Florida for Cuba with his entire force in a motor launch called, rather picturesquely, "Grandma" (by its former American owner) in November 1956. The boat, now on display at the Museum of the Revolution in Havana, turned out to be a poor purchase. It kept breaking down and was swamped by storms. During one such storm, the only person in the group who knew how to navigate was lost overboard. As a result, instead of the boat landing in a pre-arranged safe spot, where it would have been met by resident revolutionaries, it landed in the wrong place and was immediately attacked by government troops, as it had been spotted some miles offshore. The force of 82, surrounded by ground troops and attacked by ten aircraft, as it tried to take cover in the hills, was reduced to 12 men. Even at that reduced level, they continued to make amazingly elementary mistakes and, when one speaks today to any of those original fighters, none can explain how they weren't completely wiped out. They had three things going for them:

a.   They had a patriotic mission to fulfil and hence felt a higher sense of commitment than did the tyranny's forces.

b.   By heading for cover in the hills, they entered country quintessentially hostile and unfamiliar to any previous Cuban government. Batista's groups had only ever entered those remote and inaccessible areas in violent pursuit and they had never made common cause with the peasants. Fidel's group did do so.

c.   The revolutionaries gradually won not merely acquiescence from the peasants but immense popular support. The rural peasantry acted as Fidel Castro's eyes and ears as far as movements of Batista's troops is concerned . In return, the rebels dispensed rudimentary health care and taught some peasants to read.

---

[18]Sinclair, Andrew, 1970 "Guevara" p.16, Fontana/Collins, London

29

In time peasants actually joined Castro's group, causing its numbers to grow. An urban guerrilla movement had also been organised. Early in 1957 they made another attempt on a barracks, but this time nothing as large as Moncada. They took the rural Plata Barracks, occupying it for long enough to remove guns and ammunition and to get back to safety. As Fidel later said: "When we re-assembled after the decimating attack on us as we landed, we had only 12 people and 7 rifles. After the attack on Plata, we had 12 rifles and 28 people!"[19]

Without going into all the details of the revolutionary war prior to 1959,[20] it is clear that one of the lessons learned in the Sierra Maestra campaign of guerrilla activity, was that a prerequisite to a successful revolution is involvement and support of the peasantry. By, on the one hand, becoming utterly dependent on peasant support during those early days in the hills, and, on the other demonstrating to the peasants by their actions that the guerrillas themselves were people of integrity who had no interest in stealing land or crops for themselves, the trust of large sections of the peasant community was finally won over.

Peasant Support

As well as peasant passive support, there were some incidents in which peasants actually joined the rebels. Those who did so were vital to the success of the entire enterprise. They could organise reliable food supplies, keep Fidel and the other leaders advised as to the movements of Batista's forces, etc. As well, they taught urban

---

[19]Ibid. 3

[20]To devote space in this account to this vitally germinal topic would be to swamp its primary purpose - namely to describe and interpret the Cuban health care system. But the interested reader is strongly urged to consult books such as Che Guevara "Notes on the Revolutionary War in Cuba", Pelican Books, 1968, for a real insight into any of Cuba's achievements is probably impossible without knowledge of the revolutionary background to it.

recruits techniques of survival in the bush. In fact, there was a two-way exchange of teaching going on, with the rudimentary lessons in rural hygiene and first aid being provided by Che. Undoubtedly, it is these experiences which lie at the base of the continuing revolutionary commitment to health and education provision in the countryside. As reference to Che's diaries and his account of the revolution make clear, the impact of peasant influence on subsequent development of the revolution had even deeper ideological roots:

> **We began to grow more conscious of the necessity for a definitive change in the life of the people. The idea of agrarian reform became clear and unity with the people ceased to be theory and was converted into a basic element of our being... We became part of the peasants and they became part of us. As for me as a doctor, my attempts to treat peasant illnesses in the Sierra converted my spontaneous feelings into a force that was sounder based than idealism. Those suffering and loyal inhabitants of the Sierra Maestra have never suspected the role they played in forging our revolutionary ideology.[21]**

In yet other ways, experience turned out to be the best of teachers. In fighting against the soldiers and police of a cruel and corrupt regime, it is easy enough to forget the importance placed, by people who have been denied it, on human dignity. Fidel quickly perceived that the peasants responded positively to cases in which captured Batista soldiers were treated humanely. Along the peasant grape-vine the reputation of the guerrillas for compassion grew in contrast to the general brutalities gratuitously inflicted by Batista's forces.

Once widespread peasant support had been gained, the rebels began to win one

---

[21]Ibid. 3, It is in comments such as this that one comes to appreciate the essential inseparability of Cuban attitudes towards health care policy and ideological purity. Indeed, the bond in this respect is even stronger than it is in Cuban educational policy.

skirmish after another, taking over an increasing number of rural barracks and outposts. Government soldiers became rationally fearful of venturing off the trails or even into the countryside altogether. Many defected to the rebel side. This deteriorating state of affairs, from Batista's point of view, caused him to exercise even greater brutality in an attempt to counter it. Peasants suspected of "fidelista" sympathies were routinely tortured, leading previously neutral peasants to throw in their lot with the rebels. Likewise, in the towns, especially in colleges and universities, a direct attempt was made to eradicate fidelista support. Of course, young people being what they are, such a short-sighted policy had the opposite effect.

By the time the Batista regime had been defeated in the rural areas, it had also lost all credibility in the urban areas. In other words, it had lost authority and was psychologically defeated. Psychological defeat became actual defeat when Batista and his henchmen (along with two jumbo jets full of currency and valuables) fled to Florida in the final hours of 1958, leaving the army and police to try to stop the rebels. Inevitably, Fidel Castro's forces triumphed, first in Santiago and then in Havana. Records of those heady days all speak of the spontaneous ecstasy with which their victory was greeted within Cuba - and throughout the world. It is doubtful whether any revolutionary leader anywhere else has ever been accorded the international goodwill and adulation accorded Fidel .

As has often enough been observed, winning a revolutionary victory over reactionary and unpopular government forces is nowhere near as difficult as winning the revolutionary peace afterwards! Revolutions are fuelled by the existence of unacceptably high levels of social injustice, problems with access to education, health care and even food and shelter, and by the objective reality of a visible enemy. Getting the enemy to flee does not solve these problems. Any attempt to solve problems of such a magnitude that people had been willing to risk their reputations and/or personal safety to overcome them, must forfeit some of the general goodwill generated by the purely military defeat of the ancient regime.

The triumph of the Cuban revolution held on to a larger proportion of that initial goodwill, and still does even now, than is customary for several reasons. But one of the principal ones was Fidel's choice of priorities in making his first statement of revolutionary intent at 8 minutes into New Years Day, January 1, 1959. The first three revolutionary priorities he mentioned were: agrarian reform, universal access to education and comprehensive health care. It is almost universally agreed, even by his enemies, that the revolution has made remarkable achievements in these areas. When this author was in Cuba in 1988 the worst anti-government comment that he heard (whispered into his ear as he stood at a urinal in Cuba's Ministry of Education!) was:

"Look, maybe you don't understand, but there's more to life than health and education!". Such a proposition, if made in most other Latin American countries (where these things cannot be taken for granted) might well occasion the response: "Is there?"

Before detailing the achievements in health care, though, we should perhaps consider how Cuba fared in these respects in 1958 and get some insight into the magnitude of the task that Fidel's exuberant comments in that first victory speech had set the revolution.

References Used in Chapter Two

1. Huberman, Leo & Sweeney, Paul. " **Socialism in Cuba**" Monthly Review Press, New York, 1969.

    This is a straight out "apologia" and ideologically simplistic, although compellingly written. It is aimed at a politically naive American audience. It is very much a "period piece" in that it would be difficult today for such an unsophisticated and ideologically pure account to find a publisher. The Monthly Review Press was at one time the publishing company for the American Communist party.

2. Miller, Warren. **"The Last Plantation - The Face of Cuba Today"**

    This is a light weight contribution to the now growing Cubaniana literature, written in 1961 and published in London by Secker & Warburg. Although presented as embodying the views of ordinary Cubans about the revolution, it is really a rather self - indulgent travelogue by a British writer who had never before lived in a Spanish speaking country. It is, however, useful in conveying the popular (non-Cuban) attitude of near veneration with which cult - heroes like Che and Castro were held by ordinary non - Cubans in the immediate aftermath of the overthrow of Batista. Castro and his administration have long since been moved by the popular media in Britain and the US into the category of "baddies" with the result that it is difficult for non - Cubans to realise how singularly his administration is associated with altogether "positive" issues, such as universal health care. Many Cubans likewise find the diabolical image that the Cuban revolution presents in the mind of the British or American man in the street difficult to understand. Warren Miller's book helps to put things in perspective in that way.

3.   Thomas, Hugh: **The Cuban Revolution**. Wadenfeld & Nicolson. London 1986.

This is a good, non - partisan account, largely free of ideological bias either way.

Other useful references

4.   Chadwick, Lee. **"Cuba Today"** Lawrence Hill & Co, 1975.

Although written from a left wing, totally " pro - Cuba" stand point, the book gives an excellent overview of what life in Cuba really was like at the time. The book has a vigorous yet informal style and features good photographs and lots of interviews in schools, hospitals, prisons, etc

5.   Harnecker, Marta: **Cuba, Dictatorship or Democracy,** Lawrence Hill & Co 1975.

Marta Harnecker was (is?) a communist party member from East Germany, as it was in 1975. Her writing is entirely predictable and monotonously orthodox. Cuba is right because the party governing it is right. All opposition to it is linked to atavistic impulse and conscious anti - socialist conspiracy. This is a dull read, unless you are a party hack. However, it contains the most complete description up until that time of the structure of the Cuban government bureaucracy. Reading Harnecker will equip the reader with a good understanding of how and where the original idealistic attitudes toward health issues still survive and are given policy expression.

6.   Santamaría, Heydée: **Moncada - Memories of the Attack that launched the Cuban Revolution.** Lyle Stuart, Inc, New Jersey 1980.

A remarkable little book if you want an "inside" account. Heydée was one of the Fidelistas involved in the attack on Moncada. The story of her survival of

35

the prolonged and brutal suppression following it would be of particular interest to health - focus readers, as her main commitment was to the socialist philosophy of health care management.

7.   Urrutia, Manuel: **Fidel Castro & Co Inc. - Communist Tyranny in Cuba.** Frederick Praeger, New York 1964. Urrutia was a judge in the Cuban supreme court during the Batista tyranny. He avidly supported the overthrow of Batista and was made Minister of Justice in Fidel Castro's first revolutionary government. In 1961, he defected to the US claiming that Castro had betrayed the revolution and that Cuba had simply moved from a right wing to a left wing totalitarianism. Compellingly written.

CHAPTER THREE

FROM SOCIAL CHAOS TO HEALTH FOR ALL

The Social and Educational Context

When the Revolution triumphed, Cuba represented a mixture of social conditions. Although its illiteracy rate was high, almost total in the rural areas, it had the highest average literacy rate in Latin and Central America (74%) because the literacy rates in the two main cities, Havana and Santiago, were much higher than that in other Latin American cities. Likewise, although it had the best medical school in all of Latin America, so good in fact that the American Medical Association recognised it as being on a par with those in the US, Cuba's rural infant and maternal death rates were the second highest in Latin America. In cultural terms, Cuba was nominally Catholic, yet only 10% of the population were even listed as Catholic. Again, the discrepancy was due to the vast difference between rural and urban life.

In the urban areas, Catholicism was virtually universal, with a small scattering of other Christian denominations represented but catering mainly to expatriates. However, in the more remote rural areas, one ran across anomalous mixtures of Catholicism and Voodoo with people having very limited access to systematic confessional information. For instance, in 1956 the present author, while camping in the Sierra Maestra, found himself invited into a peasant hut. On the wall was a picture postcard showing Mary, Joseph and Jesus with the title printed above it 'La Sagrada Familia' (The Holy Family). Under it was a rather rusty soup tin from which an objectionable smell seemed to arise. When I asked about it, I was told that the three figures in the picture were powerful gods who had to be placated if one's children were not to die. The printed title meant nothing as none of the people living there could read it.

It was necessary to do two things if your previous children had died in babyhood and you produced another son (daughters did not matter as much!) whose survival you wanted to guarantee. Firstly you had to get it baptised. Only a priest could perform this magic rite, but it cost 5 pesos out of a total disposable income of maybe 100 pesos per annum. Once the priest had done his bit, you had to honour the 'three gods' in the picture by keeping a certain quantity of goat's blood under the picture for a year after the baptism had been done. The people there had never attended Mass, as no church was available, and only saw a priest if one happened to come that way to do some baptisms.

In the case of this particular family, the child for whose protection these elaborate and costly precautions had already been taken did not seem to have benefited much from them. Although ten months of age, he appeared deathly pale, although much of his body was covered in a brilliant pink rash, and he made no noise and not much movement the whole time I was there. He was fed out of a tin, similar to the one with the goat's blood in it, which contained a greyish - yellow semi-liquid. I was told that it was "soup". This was not heated up or otherwise prepared, but was simply uncovered and several spoonfuls fed to him, before it was covered over and replaced on the floor at the back of the hut. Both parents expressed great pride in Christofo, the baby, and told me they had previously lost 3 children, two just after birth (a boy and a girl) and a little girl who had lived "until she could talk". Then, when their fourth baby came along, the Obeah man (a local medicine man) had told them about the necessity of baptism.

A similar mix of Catholic and Voodoo religious practices was common throughout rural Cuba. For instance, it was frequent practice for people employed on the cane harvest to touch their upper right arm and machete blade to a crucifix before work, to protect against accidents and/or to insure productive labour.

The Rural/Urban Contrast

Not surprisingly, schooling was accorded sharply different status in the Cuba of 1959, depending on whether it was rural or urban. For instance, a survey carried out in 1957 showed that 65% of rural children never even started primary schooling, while in the cities, only 27% did not complete primary schooling. There would thus appear to be an inconsistency with the figure quoted previously of a literacy rate of 74%. However, there is no inconsistency. Even in industrially advanced nations, schooling regrettably does not guarantee literacy nor does lack of schooling necessarily preclude it. This is discussed at great length in my book "Perspectives on Illiteracy".[22] In that same book, I also analyse the criteria used by UNESCO in determining levels of `functional literacy'. Suffice it to say that schooling is neither a necessary nor sufficient condition for `literacy' as so measured. Obviously, education and health care go hand-in-hand. The focus of this book, of course, is on the latter, but an account of the education side of the equation can be found in a previous book by the same author.[23]

One could go on at some length, but a random selection of just a few more statistics will serve to make the point clear. When Fidel Castro came to power, the following was true of Cuba.

75% of the rural huts were one room dwellings, with earthen floors, one door and one window and no power or running water. They were made of mud and sticks and were called `bohíos'. During four months of the year, rural work was available on the sugar cane latifundia. It was poorly paid work, but at least it was work. The rest of the year was referred to as `tiempo muerte' (dead season) when , once the money had run out, life in the bohíos became even more wretched, as peasants foraged about trying to find edible plants, etc. Typically, there was little light in the bohíos during the

---

[22]MacDonald, T. (1968) "Perspectives On Illiteracy". Newcastle University Press, Newcastle, Australia.

[23]MacDonald, T.H. (1996) "Schooling the Revolution." Praxis Press, London

tiempo muerte, once the money had gone and people could no longer buy oil for their lamps.

Most of the land on which the sugar cane was grown was divided up into large latifundia owned by a small minority - less than 3% of rural Cubans owned the land on which they worked. These owners often allowed bohíos to be built on their land, guaranteeing them access to a pool of cheap labour for the four months of intensive work required of sugar cane agriculture. The diet of peasants living under such conditions was both monotonous and inadequate, consisting principally of beans and lard during the working season and beans (if they were lucky enough to have any left) without lard during the tiempo muerte.

Family life in the Countryside

Accounts of family life under such circumstances are unrelievedly depressing. A pregnancy was a disaster, but contraception was not available for financial as much as religious reasons, so that births were frequent. A huge infant mortality served as an effective population control and indeed, the fact that the high rate remained as high as it did is a testimony to the durability of the human race! Boys stood a much better chance of survival than girls, because parents knew that once a boy was 6 or 7 there was at least the possibility that he could earn money on the sugar cane fields. Girls, on the other hand, represented a serious economic burden and had little going for them. Huberman[24] gives an account of how a few very fortunate families might be approached by men from Havana who brought up young girls to train as `hostesses' for night clubs, gambling casinos and whore-houses catering to the wealthy American tourist trade. Such a transaction brought some real cash to the family and for the girl it usually meant a much better life socially and materially, although many were atrociously exploited and never saw their families again.

Isolation of the peasantry was an accepted fact of life in pre-Revolutionary

---

[24]Huberman, L. (1962) `Cuba: Anatomy of A Revolution', Monthly Review Press, New York.

Cuba. Not only were they largely illiterate and hence cut off from newspapers, etc., and wretchedly poor and so not in a position to travel around, but the general lack of roads and of transport would have made such travel next to impossible. Figures for 1985 show that in Cuba as a whole there was only one doctor for every 1,950 people and that most doctors lived in Havana or Santiago. This left health care virtually by default in the hands of untrained herbalists and/or voodoo medicine -men. A common proverb in Batista's Cuba was "In Cuba more cows than people get vaccinated". A cow, after all, represented a valuable financial investment!

Health - Some Valuable Statistics

Only 4% of Cubans in the rural areas regularly ate meat, only 1% ate fish, 3% ate bread(!), 11% had milk after weaning, less than 2% ate eggs, and green vegetables were, curiously, not part of the natural diet. Appalling as such figures are, at least two of them cannot be fairly ascribed altogether to economic privation - the figures for fish and for greens. Cuba is surrounded by some of the richest fishing waters in the world. In fact fishing is so good in Cuban waters that it has always represented a major tourist attraction. However, it was not until Czech nutritional advisors strongly urged the revolutionary government to consider developing a fishing industry, both for trade and for domestic consumption, that the bulk of Cubans incorporated fish into their diets. Even then it took some doing. Although some Cubans certainly eked out a living as fishermen (e.g. see Ernest Hemmingway's "The Old Man and The Sea"), fish was simply not a very popular food with Cubans. Persuasion on health and nutritional grounds to eat more of it was not easy. In 1965, for instance, Cuban residential schools - just about all rural children attend boarding schools in revolutionary Cuba - offered only fish for the main meal several times a week until the children had conditioned themselves to eat it! In a similar drive in the urban areas, meat was heavily rationed while fish was not, in a successful effort to force Cubans to incorporate more fish into their diets. Green vegetables likewise have never featured strongly in Cuban

41

culinary culture. Even now, one does not often see spinach, Brussels sprouts, etc. offered with Cuban meals, and the lettuce on which various bean salads are served in restaurants, is frequently left uneaten.

UNESCO data for 1958 showed that 35% of Cubans in the countryside were victims of parasitic diseases. The same figures list an average annual rural income of $91. Although Cuban geography has blessed it with something in excess of 82% of its land being arable, in 1958 only 22% of it was being used for agriculture. The lion's share of this was devoted to sugar, mainly for export as Cuba's major source of income. This, of course, put pre-Revolutionary Cuba in the unenviable position of all such monoproduce economies of being entirely at the mercy of fluctuations in the international market for the price of that one product. For the first six years of the revolutionary government (up until 1964) Cuba bent its efforts to escape the tyranny of the `one crop economy' by diversifying widely, and using agricultural resources inefficiently for alternative crops which could have been used more efficiently for sugar.

Then, with a vengeance, it swung back almost exclusively to sugar production in 1965, but with the former Soviet Union, rather than the USA, as its trading partner. In fact, the production of sugar cane for 1965 almost reached 10 million tonnes, a higher figure than had ever been reached under pre revolutionary conditions. In those old pre-Revolutionary conditions, American sugar companies directly controlled 93% of Cuba's sugar land and 75% of Cuba's unused arable land.

Foreign Control To Autonomy

In fact, American `economic participation' in Cuba generally, on January 1st, 1959 when Fidel Castro came to power, was as close to total as it is anywhere in Latin America. US interests owned 95% of the telephone services, 92% of the electrical services, 60% of the railways and half of the sugar processing mills.

All of this was the debit side of what the rebels inherited when the Batista regime was driven from Cuba. On that New Year's day victory, it is said that Fidel

42

Castro's entire guerrilla army amounted to no more than 803 men. A French journalist, Régis Debray, observed at the time: "Fidel's victory was not a real military victory in the classical sense. It was primarily a moral victory of the people."[25]. And the new regime has, by and large, honoured its promises. Especially in the early years of the revolution, the emphasis was very much on the `moral victory of the people' theme mentioned by Debray. It was in this context that Cuba's spectacular and internationally respected achievements in both health and education were initiated.

Glancing only briefly at education, we note that, from the end of World War II until 1960, approximately 42 national literacy programmes had been mounted by UNESCO (or under its auspices) in a number of third world nations. None of them managed to raise the national literacy rate for more than a short time - they made no long-term impact- none of them, that is, except the Cuban one. For details about the magnitude of the Cuban success story with literacy see MacDonald.[26] - [27]

Developments in Public Health

A similar story can be told about Cuba's achievements in public health and health promotion. The reader will recall that the author mentioned the University of Havana Medical School. It was the only medical school in Cuba before the revolution and its credentials were impeccable. Not only was it recognised as being equivalent to the best American schools by the American Medical Association as far as basic medical education was concerned, but it was active in postgraduate medical research and the elaboration of medical specialities. However, the basic medical training, relying almost exclusively on textbooks used in American medical schools, prepared doctors better for

---

[25]Williams, E. (1970), From Columbus to Castro : The History of the Caribbean 1492-1969', Andre Deutsch, London.

[26]MacDonald, T. Ibid. 1

[27]MacDonald, T. Ibid. 2

American medical realities than for those which prevailed in Cuba. As most graduates of the medical school aimed to establish lucrative practices in the urban areas, where they could gain a clientele wealthy enough to pay, this was not too serious an obstacle. The modern urban environment anywhere in the world is congenial to the best of American medical practice, with its emphasis on good pathology lab services and attention to conditions associated with an urban life-style.

It should also be noted that the educational standard required to gain admission to the University of Havana Medical School was as high as that required for entry to most US medical schools - namely possession of a first degree, preferably in science (with a strong major in biochemistry or some other pre-clinical discipline). The average state-run secondary school in Cuba could not hope to prepare students adequately even for entry to such an undergraduate degree programme. For one thing, there were comparatively few state-run secondary schools in Cuba before the revolution and those which did exist would not have had the sophisticated laboratory and teaching apparatus required for a first rate pre-college science course. From where, then, did the medical students come? They came largely from expensive privately run schools and colleges, accessible only to the ultra wealthy.

Medicine Under Foreign Control

Indeed it is worth examining this question of the relative irrelevance of the medical education provided there to Cuba's needs. Up until 1959, the major causes of childhood death in rural Cuba were three:[28] parasitic infestation, usually intestinal; gross malnutrition (starvation mainly) and enteric infections in the first two years of life which lead to uncontrolled diarrhoea and hence to death by dehydration. These conditions certainly would have been enough to keep any department of paediatrics at any medical

---

[28]Lomax, P.(1960): Child Health in the Caribbean 1948-1958. Forum -J of the American Paediatric Council.Vol 3 No 1. January 1960 University of Chicago Press

school busy with research projects. Did the University of Havana Medical School have a Paediatrics department? It did indeed, and a postgraduate faculty as well, which could qualify doctors as specialists in paediatrics.

Enquiries carried out by the new government in 1960 - and all that was required was consultation of old prospectuses and lecture programmes - showed that the department of Paediatrics had never addressed any of the three main causes of childhood death mentioned. It had an ongoing, and successful, research programme in two areas, hyperactivity and leukaemia. Use of Ritalin in the control of hyperactivity in children aged 9 to 12 was not a major worry in the Cuban system when such a reduced proportion of children that age were in school anyway. Leukaemia research may have been of some relevance, but it was not even in the top twenty causes of death in Cuba in 1959.[29]

As for parasitilogy, it was not even a required element of the basic medical degree course, but was an elective. It is difficult to believe that in a tropical country with a good medical school, no postgraduate provision had existed for research or study in the area of parasitology. The large number of Cuban children who died of starvation might have benefited from the nutrition course which was a required part of every fourth year medical student's curriculum. Let us look at that unit of study in some detail. It consisted of 16 lectures and prepared students to answer the sort of nutritional questions that regularly featured on the US Medical Board Registration Examinations. Starvation itself was never addressed. The three lectures that dealt specifically with childhood malnutrition were derived from standard American nutrition textbooks and dealt with vitamin and mineral deficiencies attendant upon excess intake of `junk foods' - hardly a major problem for Cuba's destitute!

Again, enteric diseases in children also somehow missed the boat. The material was covered in a required third year course in the basic programme, Internal Medicine.

---

[29]This material is still widely available for impartial scrutiny. For instance, prospectuses for the of Havana Medical School (in English) for the years 1951-1959 are available at the British Library as well as in the libraries of many medical schools.

Curiously, the emphasis was on enteric diseases in the US. The only two diseases covered that were a problem in Cuba dealt either Entamoeba infestations and Closteridium food poisoning. They are both rarely fatal and are not as serious as a number of enteric conditions endemic in tropical countries and well represented in those days among Cuba's poor.

Some of the more spectacular achievements in medicine of the Havana Medical School made no impact at all among Cuban people. At the triumph of the revolution, Havana boasted one of the leading plastic surgery units in the western hemisphere. Moreover, the possible applicability of such a specialism in the Cuban context was not hard to find, for every sugar cane harvest witnessed thousands of crippling injuries among the poorly equipped and inadequately trained field workers. There was certainly plenty of scope for restorative plastics surgery in pre-Revolutionary Cuba! However, the centre in Havana specialised in cosmetic surgery. All of its clientele came from America - and paid heavily for the privilege. While many Cuban bread earners were rendered unable to earn a living through accidentally amputated limbs, etc, noses were being straightened in Havana.

Treatment in the Market Place

There is yet another side to this saga of the Havana Medical school before the revolution. It ran a number of medical-commercial enterprises which had been banned by American law as potentially unsafe , but which did not violate Cuban legal codes.

Advertisements for these somewhat dubious services (e.g. penis implants for men who could not please their wives, various weight reduction programmes etc) were advertised regularly in American newspapers and magazines. Nurses and ancillary staff hired to work in these special enterprises were required to be fluent in English, because the clientele were American. One of the most lucrative of these enterprises involved hormone treatments which, on the advice of the American Medical Association, had been prohibited in the US because empirical studies had yet to establish acceptable standards of safety. Ill-informed, but wealthy, clients desperate for such treatments, kept the operators in Havana well supplied with custom.

This sort of thing became such a lucrative source of income for those on the medical faculty involved in it, that they bought up (and in one case, even built) motel parks convenient to the medical school in order to put the patients up there.[30] The usual routine was for the patient to make the arrangements through a contact in Miami and to visit Cuba, ostensibly on a two or three week vacation. During the first few days, the patient would be examined by the doctor and prepared for whatever medical intervention was to be carried out. They could then remain in the salubrious confines of their motel accommodation until they had convalesced. Psychologically the patient was usually greatly disadvantaged in all of this. Usually he or she did not want the `folks back home' to know what they were up to and thus were not likely to fuss too much if things went wrong. But as well as that, in most cases they had to sign a legal undertaking to the effect that the doctors assumed no responsibility in the event of subsequent dissatisfaction on the patient's part.

With corruption at this level going on at the country's medical school, the question must arise as to what happened once the rebels had assumed power. It is common knowledge that Batista and his entourage were not the only people to flee for sanctuary in the US once the regime collapsed. In the first month of the revolutionary administration, a standing joke had it that Havana Airport was the most popular spot in Cuba. Long before the revolutionary administration had published details of exactly how it was going to remedy existing social injustices, large numbers of wealthy people saw the writing on the wall and left. Among them were all but five senior faculty members (out of 140) at the Havana Medical School. Also included in the exodus were at least two thirds of the ordinary doctors practising in Havana and Santiago. This happened, of course, at the very time that Castro was stating as one of the primary objectives of the revolution "universal access to medical treatment for all citizens".

---

[30]Personal correspondence with Dr Jorge S Pino Perez, Editor of the journal "Gencias Medicas", published by ECIMED in Havana January 1972

Initial Revolutionary Reforms

Fidel immediately put Julio Martinez Paez in charge of health, and this included establishment of health care priorities, provision of clinics and hospitals and training of medical and paramedical personnel. He was Fidel Castro's first appointment of Minister of Health and was not only an established revolutionary (having fought in the mountains) but had - and still has - a reputation for getting things done. He is presently Director of the Orthopaedic Hospital in Havana. Castro knew his man for, no sooner had the appointment been made, than a number of stop-gap measures were put into place. One of the most noteworthy in this regard was the retraining of prostitutes as paramedical staff. As mentioned by the author in a previous book[31], large numbers of former prostitutes also found themselves training as teachers. Laws prohibiting prostitution had been passed soon after the new regime took over, on the grounds that such activity "denigrated women and led to the exploitation of citizen by citizen." With Havana in particular, being a centre for American tourism up until the end of 1958, such legislation created a ready pool of unemployed women which could be drawn upon to meet the critical staff shortages in schools, hospitals and rural clinics.

The retraining programmes as such were not administered from Havana but were locally managed, so that levels of preparation, as well as being unavoidably inadequate, were also uneven. Some nurses that this author spoke to in 1961 had only been given a week's training, and equipped with a St Johns Ambulance first Aid Book (in English!- a huge unused supply had been found somewhere) before being sent individually and on their own to run rural health clinics where none had existed before. As one of them observed, prostitution had been much easier and more highly paid! All of those women subsequently enrolled for proper nursing training in 1960 because they found the work interesting. One can only speculate what impression they made on their first rural patients, or indeed, what unbelievable medical errors must have been

---

[31]Ibid. 1

perpetrated. Other ex-prostitutes found themselves assigned to hospitals where they took a six month emergency certificate course, involving half of each day on the ward directed by a fully qualified nurse and the other half of each day receiving classroom instruction. This represented the top' end of quality in these preliminary training programmes, but even here anomalies were not absent.

The dean of a nursing school in Cuba told me in 1986 that (in 1960) she found herself crammed in a hospital basement room "full of steam pressers" along with 90 other emergency nursing trainees. "Our course was to be three months long and then we would have to sit an exam to qualify for what they called a 'Temporary Nurse Status Certificate'. We were told that anyone who got an A+ on the exam would be allowed to enter the regular three year General Nurse training course without secondary school training. There were even a few on our course who couldn't read. Anyway, our lecturer was a medical student and in his lecture he said that the gall bladder was on the wrong side. One of the illiterate students argued with him. She said that her brother had a swollen gall bladder so everyone in the family knew where it was. The lecturer got mad and told her that if she knew so much, she should lecture about the spleen. He sarcastically gave her the chalk and told her to stand up front. I remember she was quite confident and told us about sickle cell anaemia and how it makes a child's spleen swell. I don't know where she got all the information, but it was good. After a minute or so the lecturer told her to write 'spleen' on the board. She told him it was not necessary because we knew what she was talking about. But he insisted. She hesitated for a few seconds and then handed him the chalk saying "Since you're so clever, you write it". She told us after that she had never been to school and could neither write nor read".

Help from Abroad

Despite all of the confusion, the revolution fortunately attracted a lot of goodwill around the world. Hundreds of doctors and nurses from the US had been cut off by legislation in that country, but by that time Cuba had already concluded treaties of medical aid from former East Germany and Poland.

Likewise, the medical school in Havana was staffed by volunteer professors, some of them extremely highly qualified and holding positions in universities in their own countries. The consequent linguistic confusions must have been frequent and, in looking through exam papers in Public Health from the year 1961-62, one runs across Spanish grammar errors in some of the questions. Most of them involved confusion between the two verbs of essence: Ser and Estar, and were obviously penned by someone for whom Spanish was a foreign language. Most such errors, of course, were picked up by clerical staff typing the question papers - but enough got through to keep the diligent archivist amused today!

Another major problem involved selection of students, a problem that was particularly acute from 1959 until 1963. Obviously the wealthy private schools were no longer in business and in September 1959 only 63 secondary school graduates applied for 40 first year places. A drop in the academic quality of the next cohort of medical students obviously threatened. However, even in this, the Selection Committee did not simply pick the forty with the highest grades. Instead they interviewed all 63 applicants and chose 38 on the basis of answers they gave to 'social issue' questions. This turned out to be a rather defective method of selection because by December of that same year, 14 of the 38 students so selected had requested to drop out as they found the course too strenuous.

In Chapter Five we shall discuss the resolution of these various problems. However, to give some idea of the magnitude of Cuba's achievements in health care generally, from the triumph of the revolution in 1959 until the present day, it is worth quoting some facts and figures produced in a new book by Jane Franklin.[32]

---

[32]Franklin, J. (1992), 'The Cuban Revolution and the United States: A Chronological History' Centre for Cuban Studies, Berkeley

Some Vital Statistics

Infant Mortality

In 1988 (October 19th) the 'Wall street Journal' - not renowned as a friend of Cuba! - published a table showing infant mortality rates in 20 industrialised countries, using the lowest figures available from each of the 20 countries in 1985,1986 and 1987. Japan had the lowest mortality - 5.2 deaths prior to one year of age for every 1000 live births.

The USA in 1987 ranked 20th, but had dropped back to 23rd place by 1991. In 1987, when it came 20th, its figure was 10.4 deaths per 1000 live births. In 1987, however, Cuba had an infant mortality rate of 13.3 - giving it by far the lowest figure for all of the underdeveloped world. In Latin America, the 1987 rates varied from 148 in Haiti to 18 in Costa Rica, and then even better, Cuba at 13.3. In the US the overall infant mortality rate was 10.1 for 1987, but for black people in the US it was 17.9! If nothing else, this certainly says something about the nexus between racism and health. Moreover, even greater variation can be found in the US figures, for the black average of 17.9 might well conceal the fact that in some US cities the black infant mortality rate exceeds 22 per 1000 live births. It is instructive to compare this with the 1987 figure for Cuba, which shows infant mortality down to 9.3 in one province, Cienfuegos, with a high of 13.8 in Las Tumas province.

The impact of changes in health care initiated by the revolutionary government in 1959 is shown in the following infant mortality figures for Cuba as whole [33] (Table 3.1):

---

[33] Ministry of Public Health - Cuba; statistical office.

51

Table 3.1: Infant Mortality Figures for Cuba from 1939-1987:

year	number of deaths per thousand live births	year	number of deaths per thousand live births
1959	60	1988	11.9
1969	46.7	1989	11.1
1983	16.8	1990	10.7
1984	15.0	1991	10.7
1987	13.3		

While we might expect figures to improve in succeeding years, this has not been the case with other Latin American countries and not even with all developed countries

Doctors

It has already been mentioned that by the mid eighties, Cuba had trained enough doctors to be able to provide one for every 700 people. What this has meant for some years now is that the relationship between doctor and patient in Cuba is rather different from that which prevails in other societies. A typical Cuban doctor in 1998, with only 300 or so people on his/her list, is in a position to routinely visit them all in their homes on a regular basis , rather like a priest making his parish rounds. One implication of this is that the doctor only rarely deals with serious ill health. Most of his/her visits take the form of rather avuncular health promotion exercises, e.g. "Hola Jorge! You know them cigarettes are no good for you, idiot". or "Hows's baby doing now since she had the shits. Hmm. Still a bit pale. I hope you're remembering to give her water and not orange juice". The author heard both of those comments from two different doctors in widely separated parts of Cuba simply by happening to be visiting the people concerned when the doctor called by on his bike, unannounced.

Such a doctor/patient ratio also guarantees a much less formal relationship and makes it much more likely that a person troubled by some problem, not necessarily medical, will discuss it with the doctor. In fact, it is only such a low ratio which makes the whole Cuban concept of `family medicine' possible. This will be discussed at greater length later on. But back in 1959 -1960, as the reader can imagine, the situation was chaotic as revolutionary rhetoric and promises confronted serious shortages of medical manpower.

At the time of the revolution, there were about 6000 doctors in Cuba. Over half of them left almost straight away and this virtually stripped Havana and Santiago of general practitioners. It was particularly the urban doctors, who had taken city practices with a view to making lots of money, who felt most threatened by the revolution. Or perhaps it was because those doctors who had taken up rural practices were less mobile. Now there are more than 40,000 doctors in Cuba. A good proportion of this book deals with the strategies employed to bring about this sea- change.

Improving Health

In 1959 trained nurses in Cuba were 800 in number. At present their numbers exceed 50,000. It is nurses, not doctors, who are more likely to be immediately instrumental in reducing infant mortality, especially in the rural areas of third world countries. Most such deaths, as the reader probably realises, are easily preventable - a litre of clean water with a teaspoonful of ordinary sugar dissolved in it (plus a pinch of salt if one really wants to be high-tech) usually being sufficient to arrest infant diarrhoea which would otherwise quickly lead to death through dehydration . This requires primary health care and a local source of insight into hygiene and public health. About 40,000 children die each day throughout the world and approximately two-thirds of those deaths are preventable.[34]

They do not occur in societies in which health promotion and primary care are regarded as priorities. Such a society is Cuba. Of those two-thirds elsewhere who need

---

[34]Zimbalist, Andrew (ed) Cuba's socialist Economy: Entering the 1990s Boulder, Colorado, Lynne Rienner, 1989

not die, about half (just under) die because of the lack of vaccines and they succumb to dehydration. Even rudimentary public health can insure a clean water supply and vaccination, the actual cost of which is trivial, but it presupposes easy access to a person qualified to administer it. These both presented peculiar difficulties in Cuba, with much of the rural population living in inaccessible areas. Neither clean water supplies nor adequate primary health care could be provided in such localities until a massive road-building programme had been carried out. Thus, in 1962, 4,157 Cubans died of acute diarrhoeic diseases in childhood. This constitutes a rate of 57.3 per 100,000. By 1989 the two figures were 385 deaths or 3.9 per 100,000[35]

Now let us look at vaccination. There are 6 potential killer diseases in children which can be eradicated by vaccination. They are: chicken pox, diphtheria, measles, polio, tetanus and tuberculosis. In the US in 1991, for instance, there were 25,000 cases of measles, resulting in 60 deaths. All of these could have been prevented by using a vaccination, each costing somewhere between 2 and 3 cents! In Cuba, they have been virtually eradicated. Of course, when it comes to vaccination, availability, although a necessary precondition, is not a sufficient pre-condition. Society has to be organised in such a way as to maximise parental co-operation in bringing their children forward for vaccination. This requires community support and community action. In Cuba, one of the main tasks of the CDR's (Committee for the Defence of the Revolution) is to insure that vaccination programmes in their areas reach the required targets.

Basic health is also an important pre-requisite to the elimination of disease. In the presence of the right bacteria, undernourished children will naturally fall victim to disease more readily than will well fed children. In Cuba, every child under 13 years of age was guaranteed a litre of milk a day. Because of the Blockade, this was reduced to age six in 1994. Likewise, maternal health is ineluctably linked to child health. The maternal mortality rate in Cuba in 1962 was 118.2 deaths per 100,000 live births. By 1983, this figure had dropped to 32.

---

[35]MINSAP figures

A comment in passing needs to be made here about maternal health and care in pregnancy. There is now considerable doubt expressed by some women's groups in the industrially advanced world about the need for a medically supervised pregnancy and delivery in hospital. People expressing this view point out that there is no statistical evidence that mothers- to-be who attend pre-natal clinic sessions are any less likely to experience problems with childbirth than are mothers-to-be who don't. The argument poses some interesting epidemiological anomalies, but that issue revolves around birthing practices in the developed world. Once one is in the context of the third world, home delivery carries much greater risks: the possibility of a sudden power cut, lack of available transport should something go wrong, uncertainty of water supply, inadequate sanitation within the home, etc. Cuba is energetic in its efforts to promote non-sexist attitudes to the delivery of babies, but it still has pushed hard for 100% hospital-based delivery. Even in the rural areas, the figure is now about 88%, whereas in 1959 almost no rural deliveries took place under hospital conditions. The figures as far back as 1991 suggest that, throughout Cuba, the average number of pre-natal clinic visits per pregnancy was 12.1.

Life Expectancy

Another commonly used epidemiological index to compare health standards from nation to nation, is the life expectancy at birth and at various stages beyond that. For instance, it is obvious that one's estimated life-span will be considerably lower if the estimate is made on the date of birth than it would be if the estimate were made when one commenced primary school. This is because, in all societies, the highest proportion of deaths are neonatal.

By 1970 life expectancy for men in Cuba was higher than it was for men in the US. In fact it was 7 years higher for men in Cuba than for Black American men. The figures are 68.5 years for Cuban men and 61.3 years for Black American men. In 1990, the Cuban life expectancies (all of these life expectancies were taken at birth) for ears and for men was 73 years.

ithout saying that life expectancy is also very much a function of the
... availability and quality of medical facilities. Table 3.2 reflects developments in Cuba in
this regard since the revolution.[36]

Table 3.2: Development of Cuban Health Care Institutions 1958-1994:

Medical Facilities in Cuba	1958	1984	1990	1994
Polyclinics	0	370	391	400
Hospitals	97	263	264	310
Rural Hospitals	1	54	60	65
Children's Hospitals	3	27	27	28
Dental Clinics	0	143	152	160
Blood Banks	1	24	24	24
Medical schools	1	15	16	28
Dental schools	1	4	7	8
Nursing schools	7	58	72	76
Teaching schools	4	99	100	104

Internationalism

Another singular aspect of the Cuban health system, probably its most interesting
feature to the world at large, is the fact that it has turned Cuba into an exporter of
medical know-how. Not only must this be regarded as remarkable, given that - when all
is said and done - Cuba is still a third world country and hence would not be expected
to be able to mount a sufficient scientific and technological base for such an
undertaking, but it reflects a pivotal aspect of revolutionary idealism. No other socialist
(communist) country has been able to match little Cuba in this respect. From the
beginning, the Cuban revolution identified with the third world and this was reflected

---

[36]MINSAP Figures

even in the slogans chanted by children in Cuban infant schools. Just as one sees American school children stand up at the start of each and say "I pledge allegiance to the flag...", Cuban children stand and say "Seremos como Che...Somos internacionalistas!" (We shall be like Che ..... We are internationalists).

From day one in school, Cuban children are taught that they have an obligation as a community, not just as individuals responding to moral prompting, to those less fortunate that themselves. Notice how they use the pronoun `we' in their pledge rather than 'I' and how the emphasis is on service outside of Cuba. This does have an impact. In Cuba people do not debate about the wisdom or otherside of extending foreign aid. It is taken as read. What they do debate about is how to mediate it most effectively. The author once attended a debate about foreign aid between a Canadian high school and a Cuban rural secondary school. Both sides produced refreshingly astute debaters, but on a number of occasions there was a complete breakdown of communications simply because the philosophical presuppositions underlying the teams' respective positions were so different.

This attitude toward internationalism is particularly evident in Cuba's allocation of its health resources and health priorities. Until 1992 they were forever sending `brigades' across to other developing countries in Africa, Asia and elsewhere. As observed earlier, when the Americans `restored order' in the tiny Caribbean island of Granada in 1984, they rounded up 1,100 Cubans most of whom turned out to be medical, dental and educational aid workers.

In fact, Cuba took about 4 years after the triumph of the revolution to set its own house in order - to mount a highly successful literacy campaign, build hospitals in the countryside, establish a technological and scientific base in secondary education, etc - and then it hit the international trail. Its own problems were by no means all solved and in fact many of had not yet been adequately identified. Cuba could have, as a matter of policy decided to turn inward and to worry about the rest of the world later. But, as a matter of policy, they did the complete reverse. They saw themselves as a beacon for other third world countries looking for a way forward out of the international debt trap. They were especially conscious of being closely watched by progressive elements in other Latin American countries. Voices like those of the celebrated Che Guevara won the day. The former Soviet Union, in its early history, reached a similar policy cross-roads, with the internationalist view argued by Leon Trotsky and the domestic side argued by Joseph Stalin. In that case, the outcome was opposite. It is important for the reader to keep that in mind because, even by many of those basically sympathetic to Cuban medical achievement, Cuba is often regarded as purely a soviet puppet, incapable of philosophical independence.

The first of Cuba's international brigades was sent to Algeria in 1963. It had a two-fold brief: public health education in the villages and the establishment of a literacy programme. By 1984, there were 2,000 Cuban health workers and 3,211 Cuban education workers scattered through 25 developing countries . By 1991, Cuba had more fully qualified doctors working abroad than did the entire World Health Organisation! In 1988, WHO conferred its `Health for All' Medal on Fidel Castro.

In this respect, it is also interesting to note that in 1960, UNESCO set basic standards for the development of national communications, arguing that primary health care would be an impossibility without such a basic communications network. Among the criteria set by UNESCO were: every country should have 100 newspaper copies, 50 radio receivers and 20 cinema seats for every 1,000 inhabitants. Cuba's medical aid programmes included large built-in educational components. Much more will be said about this in a chapter devoted to Cuban initiatives in the international health arenas.

Cuba compared with other countries

To close this chapter, it would be useful to look at some vital statistics from other Latin American countries to illustrate more clearly what Cuba has succeeded in accomplishing since those austere days of 1959. In 1975, the Inter-American Development Bank analysed Latin American economies and placed them in a 'socio-economic rating'. Cuba was not included in the countries analysed. In 1978, having ironed out some of the procedural difficulties attendant upon making such measures, the Bank widened its scope to include, not only Cuba, but a number of non Latin

American countries as well. Socio-economic Ranking is defined as an `average ranking' of Gross National Product, Health and Education per capita. This author has not seen the raw figures and is curious as to how the means were weighted to get `average rankings'. However, further information on that was not forthcoming when it was sought and thus, for these purposes, we must content ourselves with the figures as released by the Inter-American Development Bank[37]

Obviously, the lower the number, the higher the ranking. In table 3.3, only a few Latin American countries have been included for comparison with Cuba, although the original figures list 142 countries, comparing for each the 1979 and 1983 figures.

Table 3.3: Socio-economic Rating of Cuba and Some Other Central American Countries

Country	Socio-economic Ranking	
	1979	1983
Cuba	21	24
Costa Rica	52	65
El Salvador	82	89
Guatemala	86	90
Honduras	92	93
Nicaragua	86	75

Considering that both Cuba and the World Health Organisation, along with many other agencies, constantly stress the nexus between socio-economic measures and health care, it is of interest to compare these same nations in the same two years with respect to literacy rates.[38] See Table 3.4.

---

[37]Inter-American Development Bank (1984), Economic and Social Progress in Latin America.

[38]World Almanac (1990).

Rates in Cuba and other Central American Countries

Literacy Rate (%)

	1979	1983
~~Cuba~~	96.2	94.1
Costa Rica	93.0	93.0
El Salvador	63.0	66.0
Guatemala	50.0	54.1
Honduras	60.2	61.0
Nicaragua	50.0	88.0

The Inter-American Bank lists figures for public Expenditure on education, infant mortality under one year and public expenditure on health. In the two categories involving finance directly, they do not include Cuba. One can only assume that they could not gain access to accurate data. However, in a recent book by Holly Sklar, she includes figures for Cuban infant mortality, allowing the composite table (Table 3.5) to be drawn up.[39]

Table 3.5: Some Comparative Data

Country	Public Expenditure ($US) Education - per capita		Infant Mortality per 1000 live births			Public Expenditure ($US) Health - per capita	
	1979	1983	1979	1983	1990	1979	1983
Cuba			15.1	11.2	9.9		
Costa Rica	92	58	22	20	15.2	19	24
El Salvador	24	28	53	71	71	9	11
Guatemala	19	20	69	64	66	9	16
Honduras	20	28	103	81	73	10	11
Nicaragua	19	40	122	75	37	10	40

[39]Sklar, H. (1991), `Washington's War on Nicaragua`, South End Press, Boston.

One could make a number of interesting observations about these figures. For instance, they do not all improve over time, e.g. El Salvador's infant mortality figures. A major change occurred in Nicaragua between 1979 and 1983 and this change in social policy made a dramatic impact upon the vital statistics. But a major change has occurred again in that county with the eventual successful undermining of the Sandanista regime by US interests. Despite this, the Infant Mortality figures have continued to improve.

Having thus given an overview of what Cuba has achieved in the field of health between 1959 and the present, we shall devote the next chapter to personal accounts, with all of the subjectivity's that this implies, of three peoples' interaction with the Cuban health care system both before and after the revolution. While this chapter has given a broad overview of the sequence of events and structural changes in Cuba's health care system from 1959 until now, the issue of strategies used to bring this about is dealt with in chapter six.

References used in Chapter Three

1. Franklin, J. (1992). **The Cuba Revolution and the United States**: A Chronological History, Centre for Cuban studies. Berkley.

   With respect to the figures quoted, it is interesting that Franklin's figures differ slightly but not significantly - from MINSAP - figures, even though Franklin quotes UNESCO as his source, and UNESCO's figures are the same as MINSAP's. Thus, for example, Franklin put the impact mortality rate for 1969 at 46.7 while UNESCO and MINSAP place it at 47.9. Then, from 1988 to 1991, Franklin's figures all deviate to the right of the decimal point from MINSAP's but in each a very as to render the MINSAP figures lower that Franklin's! These difference cannot possibly be of any ideological significance's and must be due to clerical editorial errors.

   The book, as a whole, is a useful source because it is generally dispassionate.

2. Huberman, L:(1962): **Cuba - Anatomy of a Revolution**. Monthly Review Press, NewYork.

   As already observed, the Monthly Review Press is a purveyor of left-wing ideology and Leo Huberman's book is a well - written propaganda piece attributing no defects at all to the Cuba revolution! It does faithfully reflect the broadly liberal US concerns of the day, though, and this has definitely altered drastically since, to Cuba's disadvantage.

3. Inter American Development Bark (1984): "**Economic and Social Progress in Latin America**" Washington, D.C.

   This is an extremely useful source from which much of Cuba's achievement can be set in context with respect to other Latin and Central American Republics. Regrettably, it does not give detailed sources for some very specific figures. Even people I interviewed in MINSAP were unable to tell me how the IADP got its figures.

4.   Lomax, P. (1960): **Child Health in the Caribbean 1948-1958**. Forum - Journal of the American Paediatric Council vol.3. No.1. January 1960. Chicago

This is derived from a Ph.D. dissertation, submitted by Patrick Lomox to the medical school, University of Chicago, in 1959.

5.   MacDonald, T. (1996) **Schooling the Revolution.** London, Praxis Press

It is my view that basic to a proper understanding of any of Cuba's other social achievements must be a detailed insight into its sensitively tuned and structurally complex system of education from babyhood to, and including, adulthood. While the prevent book can be read independently of this one, certainly a better perspective is to be gained by reading them both. Other books have been written about aspects of Cuban schooling, but "Schooling the Revolution" embodies by far the most complete description of how the various components of the system inter-link.

6.   MacDonald, T. (1968) **Perspectives on Illiteracy**. Newcastle University Press, Newcastle.

In this small book I analyse "illiteracy" as a phenomenon, differentiating between incidental illiteracy (a one-off, highly idiosyncratic event in which, for various reasons, conventional schooling in a developed nation has failed to result in an individual learning to read) and institutional illiteracy of the type one finds in many third world societies. To address the latter by techniques appropriate to the former are psychologically doomed to failure and I discuss the reasons for this. I analyse the obvious success of the Cuban approach in terms of the way in which specific ideological features maximised certain social/psychological phenomena.

63

7. Sklar, H. (1991). **Washington's war in Nicaragua**, South End Press. Boston. Holly Sklar is a well-known commentator on social and medical issues related to central America and the Caribbean. While speaking from a left-wing perspective, her accounts are well researched and responsibly documented. In this instance, her health figures for Cuba are of value because they deal with the public expenditure aspect. MINSAP figures are very incomplete and tendentious on this aspect, while UNESCO gives no figures for it.

8. Williams, E. (1970), **From Columbus to Castro: The History of the Caribbean 1942-1** Andre Deutoch, London.
By no means pro-Cuba, this book is useful in delineating the social context out of which the whole region derived its separate public health and education policies. In the reference, Williams quotes Régis Debray and does underline the huge role that ideological commitment played in the establishment of a national health service provision.

9. **World Almanac** (1990):
Literacy rates are notoriously slippery and are often variously reported for the same time and place by different sources. The only consistent measures are based, rather unfortunately in my view, on the UNESCO 1960 definition of "functional Illiteracy - Level 1 ". The world Almanac from 1960 onward has been consistent in its reliance on those figures. A critique, in cognitive terms, of the UNESCO definition is given in my book, Perspectives on Illiteracy, but the UNESCO definition remains the only widely used one.

10. Zimbalist, A. (1989). **Cuba's socialist Economy: Entering the 1990's,** Boulder, Colorado: Lynne Rienner.
Andrew Zimbalist's account is strongly supportive of the regime and the publishers, as far as the author can establish, only publish leftwing materials and

books. However, the quote on worldwide figures for infant mortality is readily verifiable elsewhere.

CHAPTER FOUR

Poor and Rich in Pre-Revolutionary Cuba - Some personal Accounts

Variables Affecting Health Care

In every society, one runs across some discrepancy in the quality of health care offered in urban and rural settings respectively and, dare I say it, between treatment accorded rich and poor in either context. A workable, if somewhat imprecise, measure of social justice might well centre on the degree to which these structural discrepancies are mininalised. Until the revolution, Cuba's approach to health care was abruptly and charmingly free of ambiguity - if you were rich you received medical care when it was required (and sometimes even when it was not!), if you were poor you got whatever treatment happened to be available. In the case of city dwellers, that usually meant inadequate treatment, in the case of rural dwellers, that usually meant total neglect.

Silvia de Costa is now a department head in a government ministry. She never tires of telling people that she came, not only from an inordinately wealthy background but one that was known throughout Cuba as being opposed to any form of social justice at all. Her father, she says, even entertained the Dominican Republic dictator Trujillo on several occasions! Now 68, she was only 31 when Batista was overthrown and Fidel Castro came to power. All of her family prepared to flee to Florida and the assumption was that she would accompany them. She was personally a good friend of the family of the American Ambassador to Cuba. However, she had, unknown to her family "become involved with the Fidelistas in Havana" and decided to stay and throw in her lot with the Revolution.

She had married when she was 23, but her husband and two young children had been killed when the car he was driving ploughed into the back of a sugar cane lorry when they were on holiday in the summer of 1951. She had been extremely seriously injured and the only survivor in the car.

Taken into Mater Misericordia hospital in Havana, she was accorded the best

67

treatment money could buy. She says that her father paid out $34,000.00 in the first week, not including the hotel expenses demanded by the specialist American neurosurgeon who happened to be in Cuba on vacation at the time! Debate focused on whether she should not be flown to an American hospital in Florida, but it was eventually decided that her condition was too serious to allow it.

In the event it quickly became clear that the private facilities of the Mater were as good as anything in Florida and, indeed, a large proportion of the senior medical and surgical staff there were either American or American-trained. In those days the Havana Medical School students routinely sat the American medical registration examinations (the FMGEM - Foreign Medical Graduates Examination in Medicine) and passed it in sufficient numbers for the American Medical Association to recognise it as virtually equivalent to one of its own. More will be said about this later. Suffice to say, some subjects in the medical school were taught in English, especially ones that prepared students for various US Medical Board examinations. This imposed no real hardship on the student, as the medical students tended to be drawn almost exclusively from the higher socio-economic classes which were very tightly linked to the American community, American business interests and American values. Such people characteristically spent their holidays in places like Florida and had numerous commercial connections with the US. Fluency in English was almost to be taken for granted. Silvia was given a private room at the Mater, after spending 3 weeks in its state-of-the-art intensive care unit. She was allocated the services of a physiotherapist (trained at McGill University in Canada!) for 2 hours a day and an occupational therapist three times per week. Her diet was personally supervised by the Mater's resident nutritionist - available only to private patients!

Her treatment at the Mater alone involved a stay of over three months, followed by a year (or just under) spent convalescing - including 3 weekly visits by a physiotherapist, supervised exercise routines at outpatient's, daily swims in an artificially heated swimming pool (in Cuba!) and weekly sessions with a psychotherapist. As Silvia describes it, as she gradually recovered her own health and realised that Ricardo (her husband) and her two children (Leticia and Carlos) were dead, she was overwhelmed with a sense of deep and utter depression. "People were doing everything they could for me, but I could see no purpose. It seemed attractive just to die and, before I was mobile, I spent a lot of time working out how to kill myself. I wanted to talk about these things but the sisters would have been too offended if I mentioned it. Without the psychotherapist, I couldn't have pulled through".

I raised the question with her as to whether she ever contrasted her very favoured medical care with that accorded less wealthy Cubans. "Yes", she said thoughtfully, "but not until only a few days before I left the Mater. The women who cleaned the floors used to chatter to me about their children, family issues, etc., but always very deferentially. I was astonished at the number of 'personal disasters', like the deaths of children, etc., which seemed to pepper their conversation, but I was even more astonished by the obsequious way they used to apologise for mentioning their own problems! This was something that such employees had been strictly told not to do".

"One lady, in particular, Angela, had come to Havana from the country - somewhere on Matanzas. She wore a rosary with 7 little medals on it as she had had 7 children, everyone of whom had died in babyhood during the tiempo muerte. You know, I just didn't know that anyone could suffer that much and still live. I couldn't believe, at first, the stories this woman told me about kids growing up without proper food and schools."

"Then, just a few days before I left, Angela gave me a little statue of the Blessed Virgin and said to me; 'It is for luck. God loves you better than us, but a bit of luck always helps!'"

"I had never before thought of myself as different, you know. I never really knew any poor people and I never thought of them as being numerous or a separate group of people, but she opened my eyes. Suddenly, you know, I was angry at the way the cleaners and even some of the nurses used to curtsy and bow to us and smile, always smile. They could never cry. This was before anyone had heard of Fidel, but even before him, you know, we have a long history of writers who thought about those ideas. In 1953, when the revolutionaries attacked Moncada barracks and were defeated, I secretly admired them and hoped that one day they would show us how to live. An injury like I had gave me a lot of time to think. I became very religious, but I began to hate the Church. You know, it was a very reactionary outfit in those days, always on the side of the clean and the powerful and the rich."

Felipe's Account

If Silvia's tragic story shows us what the pre-Revolutionary medical service in Cuba could do when it gave its best, the account of Felipe, shows us what it could when it gave its worst. Felipe, aged 66, is retired from his post as a supervisor on the telegrams section of the Havana post office. He was born to a leather worker and his wife in the town of Cienfuegos. Poverty was a persisting theme throughout his childhood. When business was good, they ate, when it was bad, they didn't. As the children grew up, it became necessary for them to work to augment the family income. There could be no question of school. Felipe only attended for two years, his elder brother for five and his two younger sisters never. His father always said that it cost too much to send a girl to school!

Now let Felipe tell the story in his own words.

"I am a communist, not like that rat Gorbachev, and I will tell you why. Fidel keeps nothing for himself. The party don't keep anything for themselves. They serve the people. You believe me? - they serve the people. When I was 34, I had already worked on and off with unemployment for 25 years. My first job was when I was 9 to push the stems (sic. of the sugar cane) from underneath the slats into the mill. Some always missed the grabber chain. Man, that was work. You thought you would die with all the dust and bugs falling on your face and the sweat. But only children - and little ones at that - could do it because a man could not fit down there. I got a bit of food every day and ten cents a day for my father".

"After the revolution I learned to read. Now I read always. But when I was 34 I knew nothing. I thought only of useless thoughts like to go to Hollywood and be a millionaire. I didn't know that the reason people like me had only dreams and sweat to live on was because of American imperialism. Well, comrade, when I was 34 - my birthday - I got a full oil drum dropped from a loader on to me - Jesus! It was a mess! Some of the shift took me to the Mater on a double pallet trolley. I don't remember much about that. Accidents were common in that place and ambulances never came there - you had to go to them".

"A medical student said I would die and my friends should take me home. Then later, someone said that I needed plaster casts for both legs but it would cost 46 pesos. Could we raise 46 pesos? We could not, so they brought me home, but I did not die. [He has been wheel-chair bound ever since, though]. Well, the party was over for me after that. No more running around after the chicas! The doctor came. The factory sent him. But he said I would die and told my wife to keep me warm. For a month, I didn't get off the two pallets they brought me to hospital on. There was only one bed in the place where we lived and it wasn't straight enough and was too high". At this point Felipe laughed. "Incredible, but the boss never missed his two pallets!"

"I must have been built like iron! My wife was working as a maid at Hotel Havana so she was away a lot. She fed me soup and bread in the morning and soup and bread at night. I couldn't do anything - just shit and piss on the pallet and she cleaned me. There is no love stronger than that my comrade!"

"My arms and legs got so thin, just like sticks. One Sunday my friends said 'Today we sit Felipe up'. I thought it would be easy, but can I describe to you the pain? I shouted and cried like a baby! After some days of practice I could do it by pulling on a rope tied to the doorframe. At first my arms hurt so much whenever I tried to use them, but that went away. One of my friends said I should exercise my arms so he played arm wrestling with me. Everyday my wife did too. But my legs - no use. I tried to teach myself to walk and people would hold me and I would try to walk between them, but only my right one moved and it always went far over so I fell."

"I got a wheelchair. I can laugh now, but it wasn't funny then. Two of my friends - real companeros - went into the Mater Ambulance & Emergency section. One sat on the wheelchair and the other one wheeled him right the whole length of the hospital and out the door by the St Vincent de Paul society. It meant I could move around a lot, although there was something wrong with the right wheel frame and it was too narrow - as though it had been built for a child. Anyway, it worked and I used it without shame until it fell apart in 1962. Then the CDR (i.e. Revolutionary Neighbourhood committee) organised more treatment for me. Same hospital! The good old Mater! But this time the doctors said I had not been treated right and that if I had been I would be walking around and working. They tried to exercise my legs but after a few weeks they said it was no use. But I had a job. After the accident - no work for me until the revolution. Then I got a job distributing notices and letters in my district. I was in the post office until I retired and have worked in every department of it except Foreign".

"You ask me to compare health care before the revolution with now. Comrade, don't joke with me! Before the revolution the only people who got good service were the rich ones - the yo-yos we called them because come the weekend they go to Miami to do their shopping and back on the Sunday flight. Working people could get care for sickness, but not so much for accidents. There are still lots of cripples around who didn't have to be and lots of dead ones who could have lived if they had had money. The sick ones - well sometimes they could get into public wards where the treatment and food they say was worse than you would give horses, but only if there was room. If there was no room, you came to the clinic every day. If you could afford 5 pesos a time, the doctor could maybe come to where you lived. Only the rich did well in those days, comrade".

It is through accounts like these that one gains some sense of reality of the masses of pre- and post-revolutionary statistics, not because anecdotal reports are of more value than objective empiricism, but because the anecdotes tell one how people perceive their reality! It is the widespread perception of reality by Cuban people, by and large that will - if anything does - guarantee the survival of the Cuban revolution.

Juliana's Story

Juliana Ferra is a diminutive, and now lively Albanian girl with large, sparkling brown eyes. At six and a half years old, Juliana had been a life-long sufferer of a circulatory disorder that rendered normal physical activity impossible and, as well, she had hearing and speech impediments. This had been traced to a bout her mother had had with German measles during pregnancy.

Her father, Myrteza Ferra, is an automobile mechanic, who tried his best to seek out medical help for Juliana but - in conditions which then prevailed in Albania, was not able to do much. Limited in his own education, he had begun to accept what appeared to be the inevitable - namely that his lovely Juliana would struggle on for another year or so, but ultimately would die. He was even advised by the Albanian medical authorities, on Juliana's sixth birthday, that he should "leave everything in God's hands" for Juliana was beyond medical help.

However, one of his more widely read workmates advised him that he had read of similar cases being treated successfully in such centres as Paris, London, New York, Havana, etc. This energised him to further enquiries. He realised that America was out of the question for an Albanian citizen. People from whom he sought information were unable to find out anything about London, but he was put onto a couple of contacts in France. The necessary surgery could be done in Paris, yes, but the cost would come to more than 50 times his entire annual salary. More in desperation than hope, he looked to Cuba. None of his friends had contacts with that country, so he applied to his own country's Albanian Ministry of Health to see if they could initiate enquiries. At the Ministry of Health offices in Tirana, he was fobbed off with various bureaucratic excuses, until finally, in a dramatic gesture, he took little Juliana and marched with her into the Cuban Embassy in Tirana.

Somewhat startled, Cuban Embassy officials said that they would "make enquiries and let him know". Expecting another run-around, Ferra dejectedly returned home. However, only a week later he was asked to return to the Embassy. He took a half day off work and went immediately. Much to his surprise, he was introduced to two Cuban doctors who had been asked to call at the Embassy in Tirana on their way back from a medical conference. They were equally surprised that he had not brought his daughter with him! The doctors had no authority to leave the Embassy to give someone a medical examination in Albania, so Ferra had to return home and collect Juliana.

Back at the Embassy, the doctors carried out a preliminary examination. Making no promises, they told Ferra that they would recommend to Havana that the little girl be treated there, although Ferra would have to pay the necessary airfares. Only a fortnight later, Ferra was summoned yet again, only this time he was advised that it would not be necessary to bring Juliana along. Fearing the worst, he went. He was greeted with the news that, not only would a Cuban cardiac team agree to operate on Juliana but that the Libyan government had been approached and would pay the necessary ancillary expenses!

A month later, on May 4 1992, father and daughter were in Havana. There, the story of Juliana was reported for the Cuban daily "Granma" by Ulises Estrada Lescaidlle, one of that newspaper's international staff reporters. The result has been a massive volume of requests from all over the world of people who want to bring afflicted children to Cuba for cardiac care!

Ferra, when interviewed just before he returned to Albania, was overflowing with excitement. He described how, only a week after the operation, Juliana was already more active that she had ever been in her life. He is quoted as saying:

> **She used to get tired a lot, Her face had a purplish colour, her**
> **heart beat very fast, she looked awful and we were very worried.**
> **Now all those symptoms have disappeared and she looks very**
> **normal, thanks to the team of doctors that treated her, and mainly**
> **thanks to Dr Paulino, who operated on her.**

> **Here they didn't ask me what party I belonged to or what religion**
> **I professed; no one has spoken to me about politics, nor have I**

been asked to make any kind of commitment to the Cuban
Revolution.

The attention my daughter and I have received has been
meticulous, very humane, and we have received it all without
paying a cent. I hold the Cuban people in very high regard, for
we know the economic difficulties the country is going through
because of the United States' tightening of the economic blockade.
This is a people that is very determined about the path it has
taken".

Obviously more restrained and objective in his own comment about the case, Dr
Paulino Nunez Castanon, who led the surgical team, was clearly pleased with their
success. Back in 1988 he had been seconded from Cuba to do a two-and-a-half year
postgraduate course in cardiovascular surgery in Madrid and had performed several
similar operations back in Cuba before Juliana's case hit the headlines.

He quietly described how the rubella, suffered by Juliana's mother, had
prevented the normal foetal separation between the dorsal aorta and the pulmonary
artery to be completed. The condition, he pointed out can be life-threatening - as in
Juliana's case - and had it reached a more advanced stage before intervention, a lung
transplant would have also been necessary. He then went on to say:

"Here we operate for this illness as soon as it is diagnosed;
for us it is not a high-risk illness; while all the operations we do in
cardiovascular surgery involve a lot of risk, her condition is one
of the least complicated for us and we usually cure it before the
child is a year old, in order to avoid pulmonary hypertension. In
Juliana's case, due to her age, the duct was two centimetres in
diameter, plus the aortic arch, and we had to take special
measures during the operation to close the duct. We got
satisfactory results without any complications".

75

As Dr Castanon pointed out, surgical successes like that are not possible without a whole range of social attitudes and structures already in place. He expressed a reluctance for the achievement to be seen as a solo accomplishment of one person, but as an accomplishment of "so many people, institutions and ideas that they cannot really be singled out". "Even the actual work in the operating theatre should not be seen in terms of an individual star performer", he asserted. "It was a team effort; including another surgeon (Dr Felipe Cardenas), an anaesthetist (Israel Perez) and an intensive care paediatrician José Lambert). Moreover, none of those people would have been effective without the six resident nursing staff present".

CHAPTER FIVE

The Educational, Social and Political Context

Introduction

Obviously the specific and vocationally-driven training of Cuba's medical and paramedical personnel does not take place in a vacuum, but is closely integrated with the rest of the school system and, more generally, with the entire social fabric. It is therefore necessary to give a brief description of the schooling system, as it exists now, with some reference to its development and the social values it reflects and promotes. The Cuban system of education is an extraordinarily vast and complex enterprise, especially for a country so small and so economically disadvantaged, and in the brief description that follows, one can gain only a slight idea either of its essential flexibility or of the myriad changes it keeps undergoing. In a sense, this description has to be accepted by the reader as rather like a snap-shot of a ballet - the dancers are all there, the scenery and costumes make clear what is being performed and the staging renders its level of sophistication plain - but the vibrancy cannot be conveyed.

To gain some feeling for the whole sense of life and urgency of the Cuban system of education, and its peculiarly involved development, the reader is recommended to consult the author's book on the subject: "Making a New People".[40]

For present purposes, though, it is only necessary to delineate the main features of the schooling system and of the social context so that the reader can appreciate later reference to them in describing medical and paramedical training specifically.

---

[40]MacDonald, T.H. (1985): "Making a New People: Education in Revolutionary Cuba" New Star, Vancouver

77

Structure of the Cuban Educational System

Today, the system is divided into nine subsystems. They are

1. Day Care Centres.

2. Pre-School Education.

3. Genera Polytechnical & Labour Education.

4. Special Education.

5. Technical & Vocational Education.

6. Higher Education.

7. Training & Improvement of Teaching Personnel.

8. Adult Education.

9. Extra-Curricular Education.

In general, a child goes to a Day Care Centre from sometime in its first few months of life until the age of five years or so. Pre-School Education then takes over for a year before the child passes into the main body of the system - General Polytechnical and Labour Education. This includes primary and secondary schooling up to year 12. Higher Education then follows on from that. But the whole system is now so well integrated, and especially integrated with social welfare, that it is possible for a child to be moved (if such is deemed educationally justified) from, say, special Education to General Polytechnical and Labour Education. Again, Technical and Vocational Education can, and does, supply many of Cuba's vast army of medical, laboratory and paramedical technicians, sometimes on a basis of people entering the system through Adult Education of even via Extra-Curricular Education.

Since the more usual route involves the first three of the listed sub-divisions, it is important to look at them a little more closely.

Day-Care Centres

Until 1980 these were officially known as "circulos infantiles" and were run by the Cuban Federation of Women (FMC). This remarkable organisation is dealt with more fully in Chapter Seven. Basically, they were - originally - designed to free mothers from the burden of child-care so that they could join the labour force, and the "circulos" therefore took children of any age up to five or six years. There was immense variation in their scope and quality, from one part of the country to another, according to what the local FMC branch could scare up in the way of resources, volunteers, etc. Thus, urban areas tended to have circulos attached to every major industrial enterprise, as did even large blocks of flats or housing estates, whereas rural circulos were much less accessible and were not as well staffed or equipped.

Not only was great variation imposed on the circulos by such obvious exigencies as availability (or lack thereof) of personnel and equipment, but very few of the FMC members would have had a background in education of cognitive psychology and, on that account, there was no agreed-on philosophical structure guiding the way in which circulos were run. If a circulo was lucky enough to have more than two FMC volunteers running it, it tended to be subdivided into sections - one for babies in arms (say from birth up to two years) and the other for youngsters of two years and older. The first would be likely to be run rather like a baby-minding service, although examples also abound of highly innovative practices in some circulos with children in this category. The second group could be handled very unimaginatively - with the children released into a play area with a few toys and an adult or two to keep them from danger, but no programmed or progressive policy of intellectual and social stimulation. This tended to happen in the vast majority of circulos. But again, there were a few in which an energetic attempt was made to actively encourage cognitive and social development. Sometimes, if a particularly able or energetic FMC volunteer were available, this would even take the form of teaching the children, aged between two and five years, reading and numerical skills.

Circulos for All?

Although ideological statements made in the early years of the revolution, were somewhat ambiguous on this point, many people assumed that 'circulos infantiles' were an integral part of the socialist enterprise and that ultimately they would be universally available - if not compulsory - for all Cuban children between birth and five years of age. Much of the purist communist literature published in Cuban education journals between 1960 and 1968 suggest this quite unambiguously. The logical implication of such a belief was that, far from being a child-minding service available as a convenience to the mothers, the 'circulo' represented an integral stage in the ideological and intellectual preparation of Cuban children. It was also hotly argued that early child-health, an aspect on which Cuba prided itself enormously , could only be effectively mediated if the children of the appropriate age group attended regular institutional care. No doubt there is truth in this, but the Cubans have had to admit that they lack sufficient cash or resources to do it.

Thus, universal access to circulos did not come about. Provision of free and universally available primary education proved to be a large enough task for the revolution to set itself. Clearly, demarcation lines would have to be drawn, but for the period from 1962 (when the FMC was given charge of running and co-ordinating all the circulos) until 1980 (when that area of responsibility was taken over by the Ministry of Education), the circulos infantiles became increasingly varied and more numerous. They were certainly a distinct and endearing feature of Cuban life in those days and attracted immense international interest. Various early childhood education institutes in Europe, Britain and other parts of the developed world, sent observers and researchers to analyse the activities of the circulos.

The Poder Popular and the FMC

In the meantime, the FMC was active in a number of other fields relating to the interests and welfare of women. Inspired both by the feminist movement generally and by communist ideology in particular, it played a huge role in the development of more democratic institutions in Cuba. One of the these was the Poder Popular (people power) - the Cuban parliament.[41]

Until 1974, decisions relating to the administration of life in Cuba were made exclusively by the revolutionary council. This body, mainly of men but numbering some outstanding women in its ranks, never had been elected. Its size had never been officially set and membership of that body was a matter of appointment from within the council - often by Fidel Castro himself. The FMC, was no doubt aware that their interests more closely accorded with those of the Cuban masses, with its large proportion of exploited women, than it did with those of the revolutionary council! They were therefore dominant in pushing for the institution of an elected assembly. The inauguration of Poder Popular in 1974 crowned their efforts with success.

Only 14 months after it had been set up, and community representatives elected to it, poder popular passed its first really dramatic piece of social legislation - called La Codiga Familia. No other country has ever passed a piece of legislation like it (and certainly not in the same way) although China came close. The Family Code, in effect, brings relationships within the family into the ordinary legal arena and has popularised both its intent and its sanctions to the extent that even the way a family organises its household chores can become a discussion point at a weekly CDR (street committee) meeting.

If, for instance and as often happened in the early days of the legislation, it was reported by neighbours that a man was not pulling his weight in the domestic arena, the matter would be discussed at a normal CDR meeting. It should be pointed out that if

---

[41]Readers interested in how poder popular works should consult M. Harnecker, (1974) "Cuba: Dictatorship or Democracy", Lawrence Hill & Co. Westport, Conn.

the weather is agreeable (frequently the case in Cuba!) these meetings are often held out on the street, with local people casually bringing chairs and cushions from their homes and children running about, enlivening the proceedings. The element of embarrassment has often thus been used to good effect! But more than this might be involved. The CDR is free to let the revolutionary committee at the man's place of work know about his violations of the family code and persistent offenders can be brought to book more formally by loss of workplace privileges, etc.

It is all the sort of scenario that would make the heart of the average fellow in, say, Britain or in the US shrink with horror, but it must not be forgotten that the Cuban family code was designed to confront Latin American machismo. It has done so - to good effect.

When one understands not only what legislation like the Family Code entails, but how it is brought about , it is not hard to appreciate both the intimacy of the link between community and school, but also how medical students are as socially conditioned as they are to the requirements of the Cuban health care system. Let us therefore glance briefly at how Poder Popular works and then at how legislation is processed by Poder Popular, using La Codiga Familia as an example.

How Poder Popular Works

Poder Popular is strongly based on the grass-roots organisation of the CDR's - Committees for the Defence of the Revolution or, in practice, street committees in the urban context. These were initially set up immediately after the revolution came to power in 1959 and involve every citizen over 16 years of age. Originally, they were vigilante committees which watched out for, and reported, counter -revolutionary activities, etc, but by 1960 they had lost much of that function and become local pressure groups representing local needs, complaints, etc. They also acted as action points for policies enunciated by the Revolutionary Council, making sure that local children attended school, etc. They played a major role in making the Literacy

Campaign the success that it was.

Then in April 1961 the American-backed invasion of Cuba was mounted. As is well known, it was repelled within a week, the CDR taking a leading part in organising local defence and in maintaining morale. But the shock of that event did much to cause the CDR's to revert to their initial "a spy in every wormhole" mentality, an outlook which - given the normally generous Cuban attitude towards people - soon passed off, however.

By 1963 the CDR's had become what they still are today - a grass roots social interaction mechanism which argues the implications of government (and international) actions and elaborates a community response to it all. Each CDR elects a chairperson, usually only for two or three months at a time because the clerical work can interfere heavily with one's other commitments, especially since there is at least one meeting a month. That person becomes the spokesperson - in a loose sort of way - for the street, block or whatever that particular CDR represents. But more important than the chair, are the various small committees (usually only two or three people on each), such as the Health Committee, the Schools Committee, etc. The member of these committees act as liaison people to promote compliance with health initiatives, etc., being put forward by the ministry of public health. It is through the efforts of the CDR's, for example, that Cuba has such a good record in compliance with such public health activities as vaccination, children's medical and dental check-ups, etc.

When Poder Popular was organised, its members (delegates) were (and still are) elected first at the CDR level. Any one CDR could put up several Poder Popular candidates, but each must put up at least one, every two years. However, they do not all get into the National Assembly. A cluster of CDR's -anywhere from two to seven, depending on the total population involved in a cluster -then has to decide which one of those people will represent them. This can involve several ,mass meetings and run-offs. The delegate finally sent up to the National Assembly (Assemblea Nacional del Poder Popular) cannot relax at that point, however. Every three months each delegate has to return to his/her own CDR to "give an account" (Dar Cuenta) of his/her stewardship. These meetings are big and noisy and anyone from any of the other

CDR's in the cluster that elected the delegate can also attend. If people are not satisfied with a delegate's "Dar Cuenta", they recall him right there and then! It is not all that infrequent an event - a situation that would make British members of parliament or American congressmen rather glad that they are not involved in the Cuban system! Not only does the delegate face regular Dar Cuentas, but as the initiative of any CDR in his /her cluster, a motion can be put forward to demand an extra Dar Cuenta of him/her at any point between the regularly scheduled ones.

How legislation comes into being

Using the Family Code as an example, it is instructive to see how well articulated the system is and how ideological considerations are constantly honed on the practical and more immediate aspirations and feelings of people "in the street". The FMC, as well as organising the circulos infantales, had long been agitating at the CDR level for an equalisation of the burdens of family responsibility between men and women. Indeed, some FMC people I spoke to in 1980 actually expressed the view that the Revolutionary Council had handed responsibility for the circulos infantales over to the FMC in the hope that it would deflect them from their feminist goals!

As soon as the Poder Popular had been set up, its first delegates from the CDR's had been sent up, their ears ringing with imprecations about the "revolutionary equality of women". They, of course, were also mindful of the fact that their days as delegates were numbered unless they vigorously represented these feminist concerns - whatever their own private feelings might have been! The result was that the National Assembly drafted a Family Code that did not flinch from a detailed consideration of the domestic roles of man and wife.

However, the delegates to the National Assembly do not enact legislation at that stage. They only draft it. The draft is then reproduced and, section by section, is sent back to the CDR's to comment on it in open meetings, often with the delegate present to answer questions. The delegate reports back to the National Assembly on whether the draft section meets with CDR approval, whether it needs to be further simplified by re-wording, etc. Some sections of the Family Code went back and forth several times before they were rendered to CDR satisfaction. At that point - when all sections of the putative Act had been approved - the whole Family Code was enacted, on March 5, 1975.

Circulos Infantiles to Day Care Centres

If the FMC had been given charge over the circulos infantiles as a means of deflecting their concern for the more far-reaching issues of women's rights, it obviously didn't work. Also, by 1979, it was clear that any lingering ideological commitment to universal access to circulos infantiles could not be sustained. As well, they were of greatly uneven quality where they did exist and did not present any kind of ideological unity of purpose in their orientation.

The FMC were probably not at all sorry when, in 1980, the Ministry of Education assumed responsibility for the circulos , and changed their name to Day Care Centres. Although that has been the official name for them since 1980, they are still popularly referred to as circulos infantiles, even by government spokesmen!

Now that they are under the Ministry of Education, they are unified in philosophy and practice. The people running them (referred to as Educadoras) are given a three year training course, following on from Grade IX. It is now firm policy that the orientation of the Day Care Centres be "social" more than "cognitive". Although provision exists for the children in the two to five year old grouping to learn to recognise the numerals 0 to 10 and to know what they stand for in practical terms, and although they learn to recognise individual letters of the Spanish alphabet, they are no longer taught to read at that level.

The day care centre regimen is characterised by a warm and embracing atmosphere of acceptance with a strong emphasis on aesthetics (lots of listening to tapes of music with eyes shut), on the one hand, and social interaction on the other hand. Even at this level, the ministry of Education actively inculcates respect for the 'dignity of manual labour' by setting practical tasks - often in gardening - for each child to perform.

However, control of the Day Care Centres by the Ministry of Education does not guarantee either free or universal access to them. It is (regrettably) recognised that they cannot be set up in all parts of Cuba and that there will always be some areas not served by a Day Care Centre. Also, unlike the rest of the Cuban educational system, most parents pay some fees to send their children to the Day Care Centre, so it cannot be made obligatory. The scale of fees is a sliding one and the cost is ludicrously small by developed nation standards. This, coupled with the fact that all studies have shown that children who have attended the Day Care Centres, especially from 3-5 years of age, are considerably advantaged both intellectually and socially when they go to "real" school, makes parents anxious to send their children. Most Day Care Centres have long waiting lists!

Pre-school Education

This year-long preparation for regular primary school is virtually universally available, costs nothing for the parent and is compulsory for every child within reach of one.

In the pre-school, unlike the day care centre, there is a specific "skills module" which takes about eight weeks to impart and which is repeated four times during the course of the year. It consists of:- The Spanish alphabet - naming each letter, sounding each letter and printing each letter both in and out of sequence, on command.

All of the liaisons of letters in Spanish phonics, along with certain key words to exemplify them.

Listening skills - hearing a five-minute story and ensuring that the child be able to recount it in his/her own words.

Counting and putting numerals in ascending and descending order from 0 - 100.

Knowing how to use the RDA[42] apparatus to construct numbers and to do sums and differences up to 20.

Being able to identify sets, to name elements and subsets.

To specify whether pairs of sets are equivalent or not.

Being able to use such phrases as "more than", "less than", "diminished by", "augmented by", with respect to the cardinality of sets.

Giving an account of the sources of milk, bread, certain common foods, clean water supplies.

Knowing basic hygiene rules and having a knowledge of what bacteria are and do.

The lessons as such take place in four half-hour slots during the day. The rest of the day is spent in "constructive social interaction" and aesthetic development. In the pre-school a considerable body of rhymes and songs are memorised. The manual labour component is slightly increased over that in the day care centres. Garden plots are attended to and the children are given some responsibility for self-direction. Not every child is cycled through the skills module four times, for only a small group of children are processed at a time. This caters for children who enter the pre-school later in the year, of who need to repeat a module once or twice before they can use if effectively.

Voluminous notes are kept on each child, especially on his/her social development. These are treated seriously and follow the child all the way up through the schooling process. Access to these files is rather informal, and I was amazed at the free and easy way in which mothers were allowed to see the files on each others' children. They are also referred to openly at meeting of the pre-school council, which

---

[42] This is a set of plastic rods and other shapes which is used (under supervision) by children to gain some structured insights into mathematics. It is still called "RDA" maths because the kits used to be produced in East Germany (Republica Democratica Alemana).

are attended by people from the local CDR. If nothing else, the Cuban child soon learns that if he/she does wrong, the whole street will quickly know about it! Juvenile delinquency is rare in Cuba, but to what degree this is due to the cited lack of confidentiality is difficult to assess. Each primary school built after 1979 has a pre-school attached to it.

Primary School

Children enter primary school at five-and-a-half to six years of age. Here the academic skills are heavily stressed - with mathematics and science tending to dominate. Philosophically, the system enshrines three pivotal aspects of Marxist ideology:

1. The dignity of manual labour.
2. The necessity to keep balancing theory and practice.
3. Emulation, rather than competition, as an incentive.

Cuban children can be in no doubt about the officially approved attitude towards manual labour itself and toward manual workers as people. In operational terms, practice is based on the assumption that it is psychologically unhealthy, in a socialist society, for young children to grow up with the idea that they are exempt from the need to perform manual tasks. Every step, too, is taken to ensure that they don't acquire the habit of looking down on such work as somehow being less worthy than traditional academic or clerical activity. Every child in a Cuban primary school is given direct and continuing experience of what the schools call "socialist labour". Thus, even six year olds will be taught (by someone whose major occupation is in the field of work concerned) such routine skills as how to clean a floor, plant a tree, wash up dishes, etc.

The author once watched little ones, in clusters of nine or ten, each with a bucket of water in front of them and a small square of cotton cloth, being taught how to wash a patch of tile flooring. Moreover, the whole atmosphere of the lesson was cheerful and uplifting. The cleaner teaching them herself had not learned how to read until she was 28 years old and had had a very limited conventional education. But she seemed to know how to handle the chaotic situation in which almost every mishap that one might have anticipated when children, rags, detergent and water are combined did, in fact, occur! For her, it was only her second experience of providing such instruction - although she had been a school cleaner for four years.

Each of the children who had been involved would then be given a regular area of floor to clean once a week.

As the children grow up through the system, they are given more involved tasks and a greater variety of them - and not only in the school premises. The community is constantly stressed and by the time a child is eight or nine, he/she is probably working a two hour slot per week on some such activity as: reading to blind people, weeding gardens, etc. I once met one bright-eyed young nine year old rushing off to do his socialist Labour, carrying a tennis ball in his hand. His task was to play pitch and catch with a 90 year old stroke victim at the local old peoples' home for 8 fifteen minute sessions a week, on the recommendation of the community physiotherapist!

Socialist Labour persists right up through primary and secondary school and at tertiary level it can involve students, especially medical students, doing 3-6 months stints overseas in other third world countries. I must admit that I have yet to meet a student who did not feel that Socialist Labour conferred a sense of fulfilment. This is to be understood at a deeply psychological level which, if nothing else, certainly proves to the student that work is a necessary part of feeling fully human and is not merely a matter of necessity, at the level of having to work in order to earn money to live!

Emulation Vs Competition

The academic aspect of the primary school system in Cuba is, as mentioned before, the dominant one - and a "scientific attitude" is held to be paramount in mediating it. Even in the pre-schools, teachers are explicitly instructed to take a pro-active stand against "religious belief and superstition". Children, from the outset, are encouraged to think in

89

terms of cause and effect. However, more important - especially if one is trying to account for the extraordinary level of socially conscious commitment reflected in the health care system - than the curricular details is the official attitude toward competition in education. It raises interesting anomalies in the selection of students for medical school later on in the system!

Standards are high and excellence is both demanded and secured (by and large) but the children are left in no doubt about what the authorities think of competition. In their very first reading book, the children are asked to comment on the cartoon in fig. 5.1, underneath which is written "Asi pues, la cooperacion es mejor que la competicion". (Therefore, co-operation is better than competition).

Fig. 5.1. Competition Vs co-operation

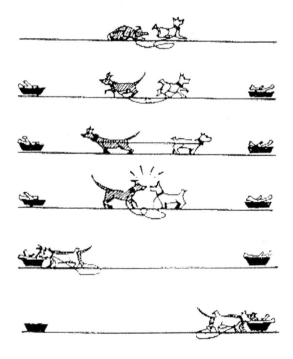

Educators have long realised that, although it certainly has its uses in some narrowly defined fields of human endeavour (for example, developing a single isolated skill), competition is neither an efficient nor practical method of stimulation in educational development. This is because educational development involves not only the mastery of isolated skills but their non-specific application, and the arousal of self-motivation and positive attitudes toward continuing one's education. It is with respect to these latter, less tangible aspects that competition is known to be so very destructive. For instance, competition for personal achievement tends to conflict with co-operation. A child engaged in preparing a social studies project in America, say, is not likely to share unusually relevant source materials with classmates if he knows that they will be graded. Instead, he/she is likely to keep it to himself. The "privatist" ethic and competition are intimately related and - in our societies - are enshrined and lauded as "individualism". This emphasis on personal development renders a positive, sharing set of social attitudes very unlikely to occur. There is also a negative aspect. Competition seeks excellence and exception, not a general raising of standards.

Thus, in a competitive situation children, and even adults for that matter, very quickly classify themselves as "winners", "possible contenders" or "failures". School systems try to structure things so as to encourage the bulk of children to see themselves as belonging to the middle group. But any number of studies have shown that this does not work; the middle ground is shunned and the great majority of a class in any subject regard themselves as having no strong commitment to their own development in the area concerned.

How relevant is competition?

Business and industry under Capitalism are often used (by educators) as examples of the benefits of competition and as a justification for emphasising it in school. But such a view does not stand up under scrutiny. Business and industry exemplify competition to some degree, but a much more obvious feature of those activities is co-operation and even the elaboration of rules and laws to prevent competition. Anyone who has ever worked for a large firm in an administrative capacity knows this. And it is a faithful reflection of a persistent characteristic of human societies. Historically speaking, raw individualism is a relatively new phenomenon, and can only be accommodated to a limited degree under social control. Its **reductio ad absurdem** would, of course, be chaos.

Mutual interdependence is a much more important social reality and competition in schooling tends to deny this.

Uses of Emulation

It is at this point that we must recognise a certain inconsistency, a sort of schizophrenia, in Cuban social values. On the one hand, socialism must promote co-operation and the collective good. On the other hand, the urge for technological autonomy must restrict choices and involve a winnowing of talent. How do the two co-exist?

Emulation is held to be the answer. Originally, emulation was held to be a group phenomenon, a striving after excellence in which everyone's standards were raised and new standards of achievement were made possible. Since 1980, however, this has changed dramatically. Now emulation's within one classroom are extremely common and all eyes unavoidably focus on the highest score, not so much as a pace-setter but as an anxiety - generator. In primary school, tests in the basic skills are held every week and the disclosure of the scores is referred to as an "emulation". An observer could be forgiven for confusing it with a competition!

Likewise, at the end of each of grades IV, V and VI in primary school, the students sit examinations in each subject except physical education and socialist labour (compulsory work experience). The scores in four general area are considered : mathematics, science, Spanish and social studies (including scores on "attitude"). Mathematics is weighted at 200, the others at 100 each. Hence the pressure is toward excellence in mathematics. In order to be promoted to the next grade, an average of 70% is required with not less than 60% in each of the four areas specified.

92

Repeating is not Failure

There are always a few "repeaters", as they are called. They are not referred to as failures, it being held that the speed with which the development of an individual occurs is less important than the fact that the development itself will probably occur! Repeating is not meant to bring disgrace on a child and, indeed, a repeater is invested with certain administrative and leadership responsibilities on his second time around. It was a consistently expressed view of the teachers that he finally succeed and that the number of attempts does not seem to relate in any way to the level of intellectual ability finally reached.

This seems to be borne out by the number of academically eminent people one meets in Cuban universities and research institutes who claim to have had to repeat one or more grades. One also runs across support for such a non-judgmental view in strange places. For instance, California has, since 1946, kept complete statistics on the licensing of drivers. These statistics include the number of lessons taken, number of times the test was failed before it was passed, distances driven and number of recorded traffic violations. The results show that ultimate driving ability has little to do with the length of time a person takes to learn or with the number of times a candidate fails the test before finally qualifying. How long a person takes to catch on to something is no predictor of his or her ability to use if effectively. Thus, in Cuba, children enter secondary school usually at age 11 or 12, but sometimes two or even three years later because of having had to repeat one or more grades.

Mediating the Academic Content

The curriculum in the primary school has been organised in two 'cycles' as a means of responding to these philosophical considerations without loss of rigour. The first cycle includes grades I through IV. Throughout that first cycle, the children have the same teacher and that teacher teaches every subject, thus the teacher that a Grade I child (say, at six years old) has in 1993, will follow the child up to Grade ll (when the child is seven years old) in 1994 and so on. This certainly assures that the teachers never get stuck in a rut!

It is claimed that this pastoral aspect to the first cycle has considerably reduced repetition rates because the teacher becomes thoroughly familiar with the difficulties of each pupil and can thus apply individualised teaching to help them overcome their difficulties in the course of four years, before they pass into the next cycle.

The second cycle, Grades V and Vl, begins developing the content of the subjects that will ultimately be included in the syllabi up to Grade Xll. Each subject is taught by a subject specialist. The only concession made to tenderness of years is that, in the second cycle of primary school, the children remain in their "home room" and the specialist comes around to them. In the secondary school, the children go to the teachers.

Secondary Education

General secondary education also comprises two cycles: lower secondary, which covers grades Vll, Vlll and IX, the students have attained the compulsory basis education necessary to continue general secondary education (equivalent to a senior high school certificate) or to begin studies in a technical and vocational centre, in a teacher-training school or in a day care teacher-training school. Before 1979 there was some variation in this, and children were admitted either earlier or later in different institutes. Now the procedure is standard.

Pre-university education (senior high school) enlarges and deepens previous knowledge and provides a complete general polytechnical secondary education. Grade Xll graduates having an adequate cultural background can continue higher studies in polytechnical institutes or at the university, or start working as mid-level technicians after taking a one-year specialisation course.

As far as its links with paramedical and medical education are concerned, the

94

transit points are as follows: Nurse trainees for specialised training in geriatric care and certain other areas, can leave the school system after Grade IX and be accepted into a three year training programme. Until 1986, medical laboratory technicians could also leave at Grade IX to embark on a four year training course. However, now Grade XII is usually required, followed by a three year pathology laboratory technician's course. Selection for these, and other, paramedical specialities involves the candidate indicating his/her interest in the work, followed by discussions with one of the Ministry of Education's youth Labour Counsellors. These people visit all secondary schools on a regular basis. Should a candidate decide, after this, to persist with his/her intention, an interview is arranged with one of the appropriate paramedical training colleges.

At that interview, the candidate faces a panel, one of the numbers of which is from the candidate's own CDR. Academic factors, including grades obtained on the externally validated Grade IX examinations, play an important role in reaching a decision, but evidence relating to social attitudes is also accorded some weight.

Before going on to consider the selection of medical students, it should be noted that most branches of nursing in Cuba now require a Grade XII (full pre-university education) followed by a four year course. This is also true of pharmacists and, in fact, each of these training's is held to be the equivalent of degree status in accepting students for postgraduate study and research training.

How Cuba Selects Medical Students

The selection of medical students constitutes a major problem anywhere in the world. The medical, course is of necessity, both long and expensive. Therefore there are sound fiscal, as well as educational and philosophical, incentives for making sure that the selection process is accurate. It is not sufficient, for instance, for the selection process to be such that all candidates (or the great majority) who begin the course in fact complete it, but that they then go ahead and practice medicine for a sufficient length of time to justify the outlay of state funds and resources in training them. The idea that anyone who completes a medical course may then decide not to practice medicine might strike the lay reader as too bizarre to consider, but it does happen and attempts are always being made to try to prevent it. Analysis of peoples' reasons for doing such a thing are apt to point up deficiencies in the initial selection process.

For instance, in a London suburb in 1989 a 31 year old GP of five years practice in the same surgery, suddenly gave it all up and took on work as a free-lance pop music pianist, playing in pubs, etc. Whereas in his role as a GP, he had always been harassed and worried, his appearance after he had dropped medicine and started palpating a synthesiser instead, was that of a man 10 years younger. When I questioned him about his remarkable volte face, his answer was that he had only gone into medicine to please his mother, As an only child from a single - parent family, he had always felt responsible for making his mother feel that she had "succeeded in bringing me up properly, even though she had everything against her". But then his mother died. He recalled: "I was grief stricken but also suddenly felt free. I always wanted to play pop music and I hated dealing directly with people. I quit medicine!"

People who work in medical schools know that this sort of scenario, although far from usual, is not uncommon. Not only is medicine poorly served by selecting students who fail the course, but it is poorly served by people who do succeed in getting through it but are in it for reasons (such as social prestige) which have nothing to do with people's health or some other aspect of the work itself.

Cuba's selection protocols try to avoid these pitfalls, as indeed do the selection protocols in the US and the UK. But because Cuba's schooling system has already oriented children toward an attitude of service to others, alignment with the practical, people-directed, requirements of medicine is more likely to occur.

A candidate's grades on his Grade XII examinations have to be high, but a long hard look is also taken at his/her CDR reference. The CDR's record of a person will show, for instance, to what extent a candidate's hobbies throughout his/her school life have been socially-oriented. They will show what sort of tasks a candidate had selected for his/her Socialist Labour projects, even in primary school. All of these factors, balanced with the academic, make a much more accurate assessment of a person's

96

commitment to medicine as a career possible.

Likewise 'potential earnings' is not the 'distracter' in Cuba that it represents in the US (and to some extent the UK) inducing people to decide on a medical career.

CHAPTER SIX

STRATEGIES EMPLOYED IN MAKING REFORMS

Personal Impressions of Pre-Revolutionary Cuba

As has been pointed out already, an effective health care system is itself interdependent on welfare services, especially child care and initiatives in public health. In accounting for how Cuba has made the spectacular gains in health care referred to in previous chapters, we shall first show how many of the advances came about through a preoccupation with the needs of child care. That is, the initiatives in public health made between 1959 and 1976 either were designed to meet objectives determined by the need for the Government to get involved in child care or were suggested directly by research being carried out to establish child care parameters themselves.

It is a truism that the first attribute of wretchedness which is noticed by someone from an industrially advanced country who visits a third world country is the conspicuousness of child poverty. Cuba was no exception in this before the revolution. In a visit the author made there in 1956, he was warned - before he got off the boat in Havana harbour - to watch out for the "thieving dogs". The phrase was new to me in Spanish, but it referred to children begging in the streets. They used to cluster close to you, holding onto your arms and legs, their hands seemingly everywhere, screeching: "pequeno perro" or "grande perros" (Little/Big dog - meaning nickels, which are 5 cent; or dimes, which are 10 cent coins). It is indeed true that unless one had eyes like a hawk, and reflexes to match, one would find oneself stripped of watch, wallet and even leather belt before one had even cleared the dock area. The children did make an immediate impact - visually, by violent body contact and also audibly. Their high, shrill, whining calls of entreaty to me, no doubt concealing their rapid exchanges of strategic information with one another, created a sense-numbing series of diversions.

I have experienced similar encounters with street children in many countries since, and have developed the necessary reflexes, but what remains indelible in my mind of that first encounter with Cuban children was the visible evidence of malnutrition and

skin diseases.

Although not a medical student at that time, I had seen black and white photographs of malnourished, disease-ridden children - and had associated such pictures with more distant places. To encounter it in the Caribbean, so close to my own home (Canada) came as a profound shock. This was especially so because Havana was a modern-looking city, with well-know business houses and shops on either side of the wide, clean streets. The Havana Branch of the Royal Bank of Canada, where I had to report first, was no different inside from its head office in Montreal. But immediately outside the door were the kids, who seemed to just materialise in their desperation, from nowhere.

Within a few days, I also realised that these groups of vociferous and grasping street children were not as young as I had at first thought. Conversations with them got me used to the idea that children I was taking to be 5 or 6 years old because of their size were, in fact, 9 or 10 - and much more sophisticated than any Canadian 9 or 10 year olds I had ever met!

On my first day in Havana I was solicited twice by young boys drumming up business for their sisters! It was a relief to conclude my modest financial affairs in Havana and head for the hills for a camping/hiking holiday. Rural life seemed much more idyllic - no raucous crowds of children and less visible discrepancy between wealth and poverty.

But this was an illusion, as I was soon to discover. Rural poverty, having very infrequent contact with tourism, was simply less ostentatious poverty. The sick and malnourished children were there alright, but hidden away in indescribably filthy conditions in bohíos. Quiet poverty or noisy poverty - the effects were still the same. Through encounters with Cuban peasants, whose open generosity of spirit never ceased to move me, I became familiar at first hand with the effect of many of the parasitic diseases I later studied at medical school. I experienced, by direct observation, the connection between poor health and economic exploitation, illiteracy and religious

100

superstition. It was all there.

Health Before 1958

Before the revolution, the health situation in Cuba was nothing short of appalling and yet, as shown previously, was better than in many other Latin American countries. The budget for public health was ridiculously low to begin with and then was the most often plundered (along with that for education) by the various corrupt politicians and government employees administering it. Even if a doctor declared a stay in hospital to be necessary, the patient could only secure a bed by gaining the recommendation of a politician. In turn, this could only be gained by bribing various intermediate officials. Once in hospital, bribery was necessary to secure food and drink and even adequate nursing attention. Clearly hospitalisation, whatever the need, was not an option lightly entered into and would not have been available to any but the relatively wealthy.

Doctors were concentrated in the capital, where, for 20 per cent of the population, there were 64 per cent of the available beds! Rural medicine was virtually non-existent. There were about 500 enterprises engaged in the production and distribution of pharmaceuticals, a business marked by high profits and frequent scandals. Big foreign firms, especially North American ones, controlled 70 per cent of the market and products were sold at many times their cost. There was no collection of health statistics. Thousands of people, especially children, died annually from diseases that could have been cured and generally such deaths were not recorded. Medical services represented yet another business to which the poorest sectors of the population had no access, and if they did, the services were of the worst quality.

Initial Revolutionary Reforms

The revolution, as we have said, carried out great transformations in this sector, and it has also achieved extraordinary successes. Top priority was given to the people's health and the resources and responsibility for this was concentrated in the ministry of public health by an act of the Revolutionary Government in February 1959.

The large scale exodus of medically trained personnel from Cuba on the accession to power of the rebels created immense problems, as did the lack of funds in the old Ministry of Health. But the new Government decided as a matter of policy to prioritise health and education. This meant that funds from other ministries, especially police and defence, were put at the disposal of the new Ministry of Public Health. That ministry also received funds sequestered (apparently 4.5 million dollars wrapped up in 25 shopping bags ready to be loaded into a plane bound for Miami with the owners which, in the rush, was left behind in a Casino pay office) from four Havana gambling casinos.

This cash was immediately put to use. The regime prior to that of Batista had received funding from various American government agencies to build several badly needed hospitals. In typical pre-Revolutionary fashion, building had started on these hospitals in 1949 and had then had been stopped when all the money had been spirited away by various corrupt activities. Building of these hospitals was now re-started and they were all complete within the year.

Improvisations in Staffing

Of course, buildings and other capital resources could not meet the demand for personnel. A number of Emergency Training Schemes, as described in a previous chapter were put into effect with two particularly acute needs in mind - a need for nursing staff (to run rural walk-in clinics being set up in remote areas and as ward staff in existing hospitals) and also a need for teachers to staff the multitude of primary schools which had been started up under all sorts of make-shift auspices (e.g. former jails and police stations, warehouses, etc) to meet the promise for universal access to primary education throughout Cuba by September 1959. Former prostitutes constituted a significant part of the intake into these emergency schemes. As well, all nurse trainees within a year of taking their final (third year) Qualifying Examinations were taken off their courses, and organised as Nurse-Teacher brigades to work in the hospitals alongside the large body of unskilled people pressed into nursing service. By mid 1960 it was realised, in any case, that the traditional high quality three year nurse training course, which had been successfully producing the "right sort" of people to wait on the wealthy classes in urban hospitals, was not particularly relevant to the needs of revolutionary Cuba.

What Cuba needed were people with a good grounding in emergency medical techniques, who could relate to those Cubans who were not known for their polish and sophistication and who could improvise with inadequate equipment stocks.

Along with the Emergency Training Scheme, which produced courses of varying length and intensity because they were not co-ordinated nationally, a three-year intermediate Nurse course was started in four technical colleges. These admitted girls who had successfully completed grade VI primary, who were 15 years old or over and who had expressed a desire to enter nursing. The three-year course, as well as touching on most aspects of conventional nurse training, with emphasis on practical work in the wards rather than on the sorts of theoretical issues focussed on by the existing Nursing Registration Board Examinations; also prepared the pupils in basic secondary school mathematics, science, Spanish grammar and composition.

The Rural Sector

Act 723 of the Revolutionary Government (January 23, 1960), which created the rural medical services, stipulated that, upon graduation, doctors were to serve in rural communities full time for a year, a period later extended to two years. It also formally stated that graduate nurses were public servants and could be sent anywhere in Cuba.

The construction of a network of 156 rural hospitals was quickly launched in 1961, which were added to the 118 dispensaries already set up in the interior. This was instrumental in wiping out the traditional sanitary neglect to which the rural population had been subject. Instead of the 161 First Aid Houses in precarious conditions that had existed in the urban zones, there were by 1976 also, 336 modern poly-clinics, with preventive as well as curative functions. By 1976 also, the total hospitals network consisted of 255 units, equipped with all the necessary facilities and, in many cases, with the most advanced instruments of medical science. The number of beds increased from 28,536 in 1959 to 45,402 in 1974. Medical care at home covered all big cities and a great part of the county's most important towns by 1963, with one doctor for each 1100 people.

Blood Services

Prior to the Revolution, there had been one blood bank - and that was in Havana. When approached in June 1959, the International Red Cross agreed to provide personnel from October 1 until December 30 to train Cuban nurses to run other blood banks to be set up all over Cuba. By 1974, 22 such blood banks were in operation. Drives were put on in factories, agricultural enterprises and even in the ministries to persuade people to donate blood freely. This campaign was much more successful than the most optimistic had dared to predict. However, since the AIDS scare in 1983 - 84, and especially since 1986, when AIDS was discussed more honestly and openly than had previously been the case in Cuba, there has been a marked fall-off of people willing to donate blood. More gimmicky, high pressure techniques have been brought to bear on potential donors.

Mental Health Care

Cuba had its first mental health hospital, the Mazorra Hospital in Havana, built in 1946!
That institution, widely known by a variety of uncomplimentary names and the butt of
sick jokes throughout Cuba, suffered more spectacularly from corruption in its
administration than possibly any other enterprise on the island.

Funds earmarked for patient care were routinely filched and found their way
into the pockets of doctors, politicians, police, etc. Under Cuban law, once a person
had been declared insane, both they and their relatives lost all rights with respect to
further review of the case. A patient's fate was entirely in the hands of the hospital staff
and/or of the Council for Public Safety, which had to issue the documentation
necessary to have someone sent there.

Stories were constantly being told of hair-raising scenes taking place there. A
number of patients, prior to 1959, are known to have died through starvation and
maltreatment. One director owned the funeral parlour which took on all of the
hospital's business in that department! In all respects, it was perceived as a Dante's
Inferno.

All of its senior staff, including several consultant psychiatrists, who had
lucrative practices outside of the hospital as well, fled the country in 1959 and Zamorra
had to restaffed from scratch. From 1959 through 1961, this was accomplished
through two Havana Psychiatrists and a succession of short-term residency volunteer
psychiatrists from other countries. Only in 1962 could it be said that staffing there had
become stable.

Expansion in the Mental Health Sector

But no sooner had that been accomplished when plans were put forward for the
establishment of five more mental hospitals throughout Cuba. The Cuban Economic
Plan envisaged that these would be operational by 1969. In the event, only one (in

Cienfuegos) opened its doors to patients in 1969. The others were not in operation until 1974. Since then, mental health has increased in profile in the health system generally, with Cuba having initiated some highly innovative treatment paradigms by which patients in residential care are able to work in the normal way outside of the caring unit. There is now a strong emphasis, in Cuban schools for instance, on promoting helpfulness, compassion and insight towards the mentally disabled and they are playing an increasing active role in public activities.

As the 1976 proceedings of the First Congress of the Communist Party of Cuba (Report of the Central Committee) somewhat unctuously stated:

> "Present psychiatric hospitals are scientifically-run institutions, where
> patients receive humane treatment, and which have a high efficiency
> and recovery index".

Of course, similar official comments were routinely made about USSR psychiatric hospitals before 1989 when such institutions were being used as punishment and brain-washing centres for political nonconformists. However, it must be said that Cuba has never been accused by Amnesty International of abusing its psychiatric hospitals in this way. Amnesty International has accused Cuba of other human rights violations, but never that one.

Establishment of Health Institutions 1958-1974

The physical provision of buildings to house new health institutions did not pose the problems for the Revolution that the sudden need for hundreds of schools had posed for the Ministry of Education. In the latter case, revolutionary authorities were obliged to use former police stations and local jails, of which the Batista regime had thoughtfully built many from 1954 onward in an attempt to counter growing revolutionary activity. Medical institutions were, by and large, housed in existing

106

buildings owned by the tourist trade, former night clubs, etc.[43] In 1966 the National
Institute of Microbiology still had the "Holiday Inn" logo on its walls and reams of
"Good Morning - Holiday Inn" memo pads in use!

Between 1958 and 1974, the following totally new initiatives were brought into
being: 96 dental and orthodontic hospitals, 47 maternity homes, 35 pathology labs (11
of them specifically related to community health), 4 microbiology units and 6
biomedical research institutes. The large number of local institutes devoted to
gastroenterology reflected a concern on the part of the Ministry of Public Health to
eradicate enteric disorders in the countryside as a matter of priority. By 1966 this
aspect of their original brief had largely been obviated and they found themselves
increasingly associated with the work of postgraduate, often foreign, medical workers
in public health epidemiology.

Maternity homes were very much a novel concept in 1958. A survey
conducted by Prof. Juan Batista Alvarez, an obstetrician and one of the very few
senior staff of the university of Havana Medical school who did not flee to Florida,
during the first 15 months of the new administration, persuaded him that a fundamental
prerequisite to improving child health in Cuba was to aim for the elimination of home
births. In May 1960, he suggested that this would require a minimum of 300 maternity
homes By 1974, he had 47 of them. As Cubans became increasingly educated to view
delivery under medical supervision in hospital as the "right" way to do things, the local
Maternity Home became an accepted part of community folklore and humour. They
are widely referred to as "Casa de las Trocas" (Houses of Tricks) on the grounds that
two walk in but three walk out!

This sort of thing reflects the essentially socially conservative value-orientation
of the Revolution. It strongly recognised, and has consistently been vigorous in its
advocacy of, traditional family values. This has sometimes led it into conflict with the

---

[43]Cuba's most eminent hospital, Hermanos Ameijeiras, - before the Revolution - the Havana
branch of the bank of America! It is now a national centre for research and treatment in a huge array of
medical specialities and is one of the crown jewels of Cuba's public health system.

107

more strident feminists of the FMC (Federacion de Mujeres Cubanas - Federation of Cuban Women) but, by and large, the effect has been to improve the quality of family life. As far as the maternity situation is concerned, husbands are strongly encouraged to participate with their wives in pre-natal classes and to be in attendance at labour and sometimes delivery.[44]

Selection for Medical Training

As has already been pointed doubt, there was only one medical school in 1958. By 1976 three more had been established - all at existing universities: Santiago, Oriente and Santa Clara. In order for a medical school to be regarded as viable, it had to admit at least 30 new students a year. The requirement of a science degree before entry to medical school was dropped and an extra year added onto the course. Students are admitted after Grade XII - which involves two years of highly academic "pre-university" study, ferociously examined, beyond the compulsory, and now universally accessible, Grade X standard.

The examinations that the students sit for Grade XII are about halfway, in level of rigour, between the old "O" level and "A" level standards in Britain. But Cubans must sit at least 10 of these papers! Selection of students for medical school was somewhat arbitrary immediately after the Revolution, but by 1963 had become more carefully organised.

In their first term of Grade XI, students indicate what professional training they are contemplating. Any who put who put down "Medicine" are asked to submit by the end of second term in Grade XI, a 3,000 word essay on their reasons for wanting to become a doctor. In 1986 the author ran across various comments to the effect that this was crooked because more fortunately placed parents could pay to have such an

[44]Some maternity hospitals, if they have not been purpose-built, do not allow husbands to be present during delivery on the grounds that they are not equipped to accommodate so many people in the sterile zone! This struck the author as somewhat of a rationalization.

essay produced. However, there was no evidence that this was anything more than the usual manifestation of parental resentment associated with any educational selection procedure. In any case, the essay would not be sufficient, for a "conditional selection" at the end of Grade Xl meant that the student had to score well in his Grade Xll examinations <u>and</u> satisfy the interview panel as well.

The interview panel would have before it two letters of reference about each candidate, one from his school head and one from his CDR. Heavy weight was placed on the CDR's evaluation. It was generally said, for instance, that if you had not - since your early teens - been involved in volunteer activities (either through Socialist Labour projects in school or the Young Pioneers) related to "helping people" who were ill, you would not be accepted.

A typical "acceptee", who this author met in 1984, had voluntarily spent two hours each Sunday afternoon reading to blind people since he had been 11 years old. Other commonly occurring patterns of "voluntary youth labour" looked on with favour by selection committees have been: unskilled orderly work in hospitals, individual non-medical services to patients in mental institutions, work in old people's homes, etc.

Academic Vs Social Criteria for Selection

In this way, candidates with the highest academic grades on their Grade Xll examinations are not necessarily selected. Weight is also placed on social attitudes. The industrialised nations of the world might well have something to learn from this. In Britain, for instance, selection for entry to medical school tends to rely heavily on one's scores on three "A" levels. What implications does this have?

For one thing, to gain very high "A" level scores requires a certain type of student. The sort who can discipline him/herself to aim for distant, rather than immediate, goals (delayed, rather than instant, gratification) is clearly favoured. Applied to passing written examinations (as opposed, say, to performing in an orchestra or being part of an athletic team) the sort of person who is ideally suited would tend to prefer solitary activities (such as reading texts and taking notes) to social ones. That might be why a common experience in British medical schools is that the selection procedure accurately predicts outcome in the first two years of the course, in which the programme is exam-oriented and based on the academic study of such disciplines as anatomy, physiology, biochemistry, bacteriology and the like. Then problems seem to arise in Year Three, when the course becomes more clinically oriented with the students having to relate to real patients. This business of having to relate closely to another person who, not only is a stranger, but who may smell or be socially objectionable in some other way and will likely fall well outside the student's own social and cultural class, can be extremely daunting for people who have been selected on the basis of quite different criteria!

Characteristically, there is a sizeable voluntary drop-out in Third Year in such medical courses. This is much more significant that drop-out phenomena in other courses. To get into medical school is very high status and is widely regarded as a sign of great intellectual potential. It is characteristically a matter of considerable family pride and social prestige and not something to be thrown away lightly. Also, we are talking about people who have already successfully survived the major academic hurdles. If one is going to actually fail medical school, it usually happens in the first two years. The prevailing wisdom is that if one gets to Third Year, it is only a matter of time before one would qualify, unless one decides not to!

Implicit Social-Class Discrimination in the Traditional System

But yet another aspect of the usual selection procedure to British medical school as opposed to Cuban ones, needs to be looked at. State run schools in the UK are at a severe disadvantage in preparing students to score high on "A" level examination. They are obliged to accept a huge social class range of pupils - and teachers. The atmosphere at many state schools is unavoidably not oriented to high academic achievement. Facilities are often limited, classes large and influences not entirely uplifting! Therefore, a disproportionately large number of high "A" level scorers (the sort who gain admission to medical school) have been prepared at the best fee-paying schools. Such schools are extremely expensive and, unless a pupil is there on scholarship, require that their students have wealthy parents.

In Britain, as in many other societies, it has been amply demonstrated statistically that there is a correlation between health and wealth. To put it crudely, most sick people (who would be attending NHS hospitals as patients) are not wealthy, while most medical students (who would be learning their practical doctoring skills on those same people) are wealthy. In other words, the system almost guarantees a social class mis-match.

The Cuban selection process tends to avoid that because they place so much emphasis on potential students' social attitudes, as expressed by their free-choice of voluntary activities. The CDR reference letter details these social attitudes in some depth.

The Training and Socialisation Process

By 1976, the four medical schools between them were graduating 1,000 general practitioners and 300 specialists a year. In 1974, Cuba was listed as having 10,000 physicians already. With figures such as these, it was possible to locate doctors strategically so that every part of Cuba was adequately served.

The structure of the medical course itself changed radically between 1962 and 1970. In 1962, the course was still being taught pretty well in the traditional sequence of subjects referred to as characteristic of British medical schools, with an emphasis in the first years on pre-clinical "academic" sciences and then moving in later years onto clinical work with real patients. Ideological factors, as much as pedagogical factors, forced a change. By 1965, the standard procedure was for students to start off on the wards. There they would learn the rudiments of interview techniques and the taking of the non-medical side of case histories. They would learn admission procedures and generally involve themselves in being helpful, under medical direction, to patients. At the theoretical level, they would listen to cases being discussed. As they sought to participate, they would be advised as to what they needed to know to understand particular cases. Bits of anatomical and physiological knowledge would be picked up in this way. Then, in the second term of First Year they would be attending routine academic lectures, but still spending at least two days per week on the wards.

This would serve to prevent the sudden culture shock occasioned by the abrupt shift from academic (solitary) to practical (patient contact) skills, which medical students tend to face elsewhere.

Nurse Training Programmes

As far as nurse training was concerned, it was recognised at the outset - as already discussed - that the need for an adequate nurse training programme was in some senses even more critical than the need for doctors. In 1959 there was only one nurse training school and it graduated a maximum of 80 nurses a year. Before the Revolution, nurses worked exclusively in hospitals - usually private ones. Nursing itself, before 1959, was regarded as a genteel occupation for girls from the middle classes who were not quite bright enough for a more exalted career. The selection process, in pre-Revolutionary times, tended to emphasise speed, manners and the social graces as much as intellectual and clinical potential.

The various programmes for Emergency Training became nationally co-ordinated by 1962 and by 1965 had evolved into a two year half-time course (the other half being spent working on the wards) for Assistant Nurses. Provision was made for people who had performed especially wall on the Assistant Nurse course to move, with some advanced standing, onto the Registered Nurse Training course.

As of 1975, 2,000 Assistant Nurse were being produced annually.

Alongside these developments, various training courses were started after 1962 for ancillary medical staff. These were people such as lab technicians, X-ray personnel,

112

dieticians, etc. Most of these training courses took place in provincial and regional teaching units. A report to the Central Committee of the Cuban Communist Party for 1976 put the figure for the number of ancillary workers trained since 1962 at over 56,000.

Public Health from 1958-1976

The reader can appreciate that, with such levels of activity in proliferating health workers of various levels as has been already described, Cuba was well placed in developing a comprehensive and responsive public health system. Running such an enterprise has not been without its costs and crises related to costs. On four separate occasions: 1960, 1961, 1967 and 1970 special re-allocations of funding, already earmarked for other areas in the economy, were undertaken, directing the money into the Ministry of Public Health.

Before the revolution, public health expenditure was listed as 20 million pesos. By 1957 it had become 400 million pasos, a 20-fold rise! A large part of the pre-Revolutionary public health budget had gone on medicines. Two American pharmaceutical houses dominated the Cuban market and they charged exorbitantly. With the new government came expropriation of the pharmaceutical industry. The production and distribution of medicines, in effect, passed into the nation's hands. This meant a radical lowering of prices and a great increase in production volume, as sectors in the community which had hitherto been unable to afford medical treatment became represented.

Instead of two pharmaceutical firms competing, the whole pharmacy enterprise was re-organised and modernised. By 1974, national production of medicines had increased in volume by 80% and in type by 300%. This has constituted one of the bedrocks of the general advance in public health. For instance, poliomyelitis which had been killing or crippling 300 children a year, was eradicated in 1963. Malaria, of which 300 people a year perished in 1958, was eliminated in 1968. Diphtheria, also a great child killer and which in 1958 claimed 600 victims, was gone by 1971.

A major impact of the revolution's emphasis on public health has been on enteric diseases, the greatest single killer of infants in pre-Revolutionary Cuba. For example, gastroenteritis, the main scourge of children in almost all underdeveloped countries, carried away 4,157 Cubans, even as late as 1962. Of these, 3,120 were children less than five years of age. In 1974 it had been so successfully controlled that only 761 Cubans died of it.

Similarly, cases of tetanus, tuberculosis, typhoid fever and various other infections, distressingly common in pre-Revolutionary days, had been reduced to statistically insignificant levels by 1976.

A major thrust of public health, as an effective social instrument, involves slow, patient education and the modification of deeply held attitudes and traditions. Nowhere has this been more radically evident than in the drive to create a 100% hospital delivery statistic, and the complete abolition of home delivery. Many readers may well disagree with such an aim, but -for better or worse (and in a tropical third world country, it is difficult to see how it could be for the worse) - it was an integral part of the public health programme and has now been largely accomplished.

By 1976, up to 97% of all Cuban births took place in hospitals and - even then - each expectant mother received an average of 8.5 antenatal clinical examinations. The figure now, of course, is considerably higher. Possibly these statistics relate to the spectacular drop in infant mortality rate which took place between 1958 and 1974 - from 60 per 1000 live births to 28.1 per 1000 live births.

Mother and Child Health

The emphasis, in public health, on mother and child welfare has been its principal preoccupation. This has not only led to the spectacular decline in infant mortality already alluded to, but has brought about a host of other measurable health changes as well. For instance, pre-school child mortality (children aged one to four years) dropped from 45 to 1.2 per 1000 inhabitants from 1958 to 1976. Over the same period of time, school age mortality (children aged five to 14 years) dropped from 40 to 0.5 per 1000 inhabitants. Obviously, maternal mortality figures have also been affected, moving from 21 in 1958 to 0.5 in 1976 per 1000 live births.

As has already been mentioned, life expectancy has increased dramatically. Even during the period under question, it had been moved from less than 55 years to 70 years.

That is, in only the first 18 years of the Cuban revolution, a free medical service had been established, featuring universal access to public health facilities and engaging the efforts of over 140,000 health-related workers. It had completely changed Cuba's health profile. Even by 1975, Cuba could no longer be regarded as a typical third world nation healthwise, although it certainly was (and is) by every objective economic measure.

It is not difficult to conclude that this has represented first and foremost a triumph of social organisation and has been the end product of a definite and coherent social philosophy and of policies stemming therefrom. However, serious problems lay ahead. Some of these were alluded to in the 1976 Report of the Central Committee of the Cuban Communist Party. Quoting from that document:

> **"Our country may be already compared with developed countries in health standards. The Ministry of Public Health and the mass organisations, CDR, FMC, ANAP, CTC, pooled their efforts to achieve all this. Had it not been for their contribution and their educational work, such extraordinary accomplishments with such limited resources could not have been achieved.**
>
> **The successes of the Revolution in the field of medicine have also been recognised and have evoked admiration in international health organisations.**
>
> **The generation of professionals trained in the new society and the older physicians who remained loyal to the revolution have**

developed an admirable spirit of solidarity, one of its features
being that of serving the people anywhere and in all conditions, as
required, both at home and abroad.

In the years of the revolution, 18 countries of America, Asia and
Africa have benefited from the internationalist, dedicated and
humane, sometimes even heroic work of our physicians and other
public health specialists.

But achievements in public health notwithstanding, there still
remain some difficulties.

In the next five-year period the results already attained have to be
consolidated and even surpassed.

In this period more then 100 new polyclinics and hospital units
will be built. The Public Health program also includes homes for
the aged and the disabled.

The indicators to be reached are one physician per approximately
750 inhabitants, one stomatologist per 3,000 and 55 intermediate
specialists per 10,000 inhabitants.

An intense effort will be mounted to reduce infant mortality to 25
per 1000 live births. The qualifications of medical personnel and
the quality of services will be further improved."

In succeeding chapters, it will become evident to what extent those Five-Year Plan
objectives were, in fact, superseded and how Cuba's public health system has been able
to respond flexibly to the most severe economic restraints imposed upon it. These

"periods of restraint" can be designated as from 1975-1979, from 1983-1987 and then from 1989 until now. All of them, of course, derive from the economic domination of Latin American economics -and of the western hemisphere generally - by the United States. It can be said that Cuba has really never had it easy, in its relationship with the U.S. since the revolution, but that these three periods have been particularly harsh.

Before considering those matters, though, the issues of child care in Cuba and its evolution from purely public health concerns to the larger role it now plays in health promotion in the broader sense must be addressed.

CHAPTER SEVEN

THE ROLE OF THE CUBAN FEDERATION OF WOMEN

Child Survival Pre-1959

When one reads the documentary material relating to government policies toward children in Batista's day, it quickly becomes evident that if children in government care did survive, it was more through luck than judgement. Had it not been for charities run by the Catholic Church, the situation would have been worse.

In 1958 there were 38 orphanages - 2 in Santiago, 31 in Havana and the rest scattered throughout Cuba. These institutions cared for about 1,600 Children between the ages of 1 and 6 years. More to the point, these institutions cost the Cuban government nothing. They were financed exclusively by various orders of nuns, of whom the Dominicans and the Sisters of Mercy were the principal administrators of these kinds of charity. Moreover, the orphanages were minimal in the extreme, the children in them receiving neither education nor medical care as a matter of routine. Whatever of either was offered was purely as a matter of individual good will. In 1960 and 1961, accounts began to come forward of bizarre and shocking treatment accorded some children behind the closed doors of at least two of the orphanages in Havana but, as far as this author knows, no systematic enquiries were made. Suffice to say, all 38 orphanages were closed down in 1959, Most of them re-opened as government schools. It goes without saying that the pre-Revolutionary government authorities had no inspection system in operation by which such institutions could be monitored. Any inspections which did take place were entirely in the hands of ecclesiastical authorities. Numerous gothic stories are also told about the infamous Casa de Beneficencia. This sombre and barrack-like building housed an institution run by the Marist Brothers as a "child refuge" for orphans and abandoned children. Once a child was in there, the state washed its hands of any further responsibility for him/her. The child stayed there until he/she was released at the age of 15 to survive as best he/she could. Not a great deal of information is now available about Casa de Beneficencia. Girls and boys were kept in separate houses. They slept in large, overcrowded dormitories with 20 beds along each wall and a narrow walkway down the middle. There was a written list of infractions and punishments. Among the infractions were counted bed-wetting, masturbation, being too friendly (!), refusal to eat, gluttony and various other peculiar categories. Corporal punishment, even for minor transgressions, reigned supreme. Possibly because the sexes were kept separate, the Casa administration seemed obsessively worried about homosexuality. That, apparently, was the reason that children were actively discouraged from showing affection for one another.

What such a regimen must have done to them psychologically can be left to the imagination!

There were limited facilities for teaching certain practical skills with which a person might earn a living on leaving, but there was no organised relationship with outside agencies by which children could routinely be prepared for jobs outside. The barrenness of life there can only be guessed at by comments made by former inmates, one of whom observed: " In the boys' house was a piano. It was only played by two of the brothers. No one else was allowed near it". and from another `graduate' of the place: "If you were over two-and-a-half years old, you were badly punished if you pissed the bed. They would make you kiss the wet patch, then beat you. Then you had to sit all day under the refectory table with your hands on your head and your arse bare on the stone floor. No one was allowed to talk to you. If you were under two, you would just get hit."

The Social Context

The fact that children could be "disposed of" so easily if they had no parents or if they had been abandoned, was a consequence of deep prejudices in pre-Revolutionary Cuba about marriage, the family, etc. It was a society which actively ostracised unmarried mothers (but not unmarried fathers!) and stigmatised their children.

In those days, working women had absolutely no state financial support - and previous little social moral support. This drove single mothers to attempt fearful strategies - such as tying very young children up before leaving for work in order to keep them from harm. It was routine for children, especially girls, of between 8 and 10 years of age to have to leave school in order to look after younger siblings or sometimes even an unemployed father! Under such circumstances, there were numerous fatal or near fatal accidents involving fire, boiling water, falls, etc.

The Federation of Cuban Women

On April 12,1959, the Federation of Cuban Women (FMC) was formed in Havana to "promote and protect the interests of women and their children, in revolutionary Cuba." However, it was not until March, 1960, that it was accorded statutory recognition by the Government. At that point it was assigned the task of establishing "institutions for the education and protection of workers' children."[45]

This brief clearly delineated the link between health and child welfare, but before developing that, something should be said about the character of the FMC itself. The women who initiated it were motivated by three things:

a.   Revolutionary idealism - Some of these women had actually fought with Fidel and saw the revolution as being dedicated to the eradication of all forms of oppression, including male dominance.

b.   A determination to counter the macho image of Cuban culture. Cuba, like all Latin American countries, was very much the home of macho attitudes. This was largely made possible by women acquiescing in it. The FMC members felt that this was largely a matter of education - and they were prepared to take on that role.

---

[45]Constitucion de la Federacion de las Mujeres Cubanas, 1962, Department of Social Welfare, Havana

c.   The awful plight of street children in Latin America, especially in the cities. Macho attitudes saw it as a necessity for a man to "have a chick for pleasure" - different girls different places, different times. When I was working at a hospital in Santo Domingo (in Republica Dominicana) in 1985 and was to work at the other side of the island for three months, one of the medical professors (a consultant in his field) casually offered to "fix you up with some chicks over there" since during week days I would not have my wife with me! This tacit assumption that that was the way to go on means that hundreds of children are fathered without any apparent claim to male parents. Many of them end up living (and dying) on the streets and are a common sight in all Latin American societies - except in Cuba.

Much of the credit for vigorously addressing such injustices in Cuba can be laid at the door of the FMC.

All three motivations bespeak feminism, but of a much broader variety than many of us are accustomed to in industrialised societies, where "feminism" is often perceived as "anti family."

The FMC were involved in so many aspects of Cuban life - for instance, they were one of the most stalwart mainstays of the Great Literacy Campaign of 1960-61 - that it would have been difficult to for them to assume too narrow, doctrinaire or ideological a point of view, even if they had wanted to. They had not been long addressing the task of "establishing institutions for educating and protecting children" when they realised that if they were to make any progress at all, new legislation would have to enacted.

Legislating for Domestic Justice

This eventually came to fruition in the form of the Family Law Code (La Codiga Familia), but it was massively resisted by powerful men, including some in the leadership. Many are the times that some of those revolutionary comrades must have wished that they had never given way to the FMC! But once it was implemented, the Family Law Code did much to systematise family health care and, at the same time, to make the whole community much more aware of the interface between the health of the individual and the good of the whole society. In other words, the FMC found themselves as advocates and organisers of health promotion.

The Family Law Code was not passed until 1974. Prior to that many health initiatives - such as organising vaccination drives - were left to the CDRs. Others were mediated through the primary school system. The 1974 legislation brought pre-primary, primary and secondary education into liaison with family access to medical care and public health education. It has represented a remarkable example of integration of government services under one piece of legislation and was largely the brain child of the FMC.

Institutionalisation of Child Care

Again, as an obvious part of its brief, the FMC took a serious look at the problem of institutional care of children below school age whose parents were both working. Attempts had been made to address this problem from early 1959 by establishing the "Circulos Infantiles", as discussed in Chapter Five, (which would take pre-school children of any age) in or near factories and other large enterprises. However, these were set up very much on an ad hoc basis, with no specific training required of people staffing them nor any specific requirements relating either to facilities used or to programme followed. The FMC moved into this administrative chaos in 1962 and first of all addressed the health issue. By working closely with people in the Ministry of

123

Public Health, they moved to make the Circulo Infantil an ideal home for the whole child - not simply a child-minding depot.

This involved the setting up of special classes to train "educadoras" (the Circulo Infantil teachers) and in gradually pushing for purpose-built facilities. They sought the advice of educational psychologists and others in the Ministry of Education about optimal conditions for infant cognitive development, etc.

By 1975 the Cuban Circulo Infantil had become an internationally recognised model of what pre-school centres should be. It was evident, from various educational research projects carried out in 1982-83, that children who for some reason stayed at home until they started school, had been intellectually, socially and physically disadvantaged by not having attended a Circulo Infantil. By 1965, there were 165 Circulo Infantiles catering for the 13,861 children. The movement then grew exponentially between 1965 and 1975. By 1976 there were Circulo Infantiles so widely available that only 3% of Cuban families did not have access to one.

In 1969 the training of educadoras was greatly extended, requiring four years full-time study after Grade X. Much of the training curriculum deals with health issues and educadoras are specifically trained to critically observe children's behaviour and to take note of anything which might suggest health problems - physical, mental or emotional. By this time the variety and levels of expertise required had become so involved that the Government set about creating a new body to mediate it and which could draw on the Ministries of Public Health, Social Welfare and Education.

This led in 1971 to the inauguration of the Institute for Childhood. It took over the management of the circulos infantiles, including all colleges training educadoras and as well, the paediatric psychiatric units. Its brief gave as its primary objective to provide scientifically-based child care for all Cuban children up to the age of 5 years. From then on, they have supervised the construction of all new circulos - with gardens, vegetable plots, health care facilities, wide halls, roomy class rooms, the finest hygienic conditions and stimulating surroundings.

Children Aged from 5 - 14 years

By 1976, many of Cuba's initiatives in health and education were beginning to be regarded as luxuries, for the country was feeling with particular severity, the effects of the American economic blockade. In force since the American-backed military attempt to overthrow the revolutionary government in April 1961, (some say since 1959) it has since increasingly cut Cuba off from a variety of medical and educational supplies and even from many visiting lecturers. For instance, a British lecturer in crystallography, a recent Cambridge graduate and with a brilliant scientific career open before her, had arranged to spend three months in Cuba, helping them to set up health-related research projects and lecturing at various universities and institutes. She knew that American citizens were not allowed to do this without having their passports confiscated, but being English, she felt perfectly safe. Then two months before she left, she was visited by two men from the American Embassy. She was the holder of a Fullbright Research Fellowship and had also applied for a research-teaching post at Cornell University in New York State. The gentlemen advised her that, if she visited Cuba, she would be barred from having an American visa should she subsequently want to visit the US. No young research worker in science can forsake any chance of visiting the US, where so many important advances in science are made and where so much better facilities exist for research than is the case anywhere else. As well, they pointed out that -under recent American legislation - she could not, while holding a US research grant (namely, the Fullbright award) visit Cuba. The grant would be withdrawn if she did. She reluctantly had to forego her trip to Cuba and the Cuban scientific community lost out as a result.

This sort of scenario was becoming more frequent during the late 70's and, during that same period, Soviet aid and trade were severely curtailed under a political rapprochement between the US and the USSR. The latter was also experiencing a protracted balance of payment problem.

Social Justice vs. Market Forces

The effect of these events on Cuba was to bring to the fore a group of people who - calling themselves pragmatists - felt that a retreat from revolutionary idealism was called for. Fidel Castro himself, and most of his ministers, were opposed to such ideas, but they did not automatically win every vote in the Cuban Legislative Assembly (called "Poder Popular" and in full operation since 1975). There was considerable pressure to compromise - to cut back on the high standards demanded by both the FMC and the Institute for childhood for the setting up and running of children's services. Health initiatives were particularly costly and were obviously a first target for people looking for ways of economising.

During these difficult years life did become tediously drab for many ordinary citizens. The punch and enthusiasm seemed to have gone out of the revolution and American government agencies were doing everything they could to foster unrest in Cuba. Two of Cuba's medical schools became the focus of anti-government activities, one of the more spectacular of which took the form of a putative Trotskyite movement. Discontent was strongly in the air, especially when it became necessary to re-introduce rationing of some goods.

But the Cuban revolution was not deflected on that occasion. Many commentators thought that its days were numbered, but they were proven wrong. Health and Education programmes continued in Cuba, although rates of growth of these were drastically cut. Cuban initiatives in health care in foreign countries were reduced in scope and in two cases abolished altogether. Child care won outright. In Cuba itself every child care initiative mentioned in the 1974 Five Year Plan was exceeded. Outside of Cuba, in foreign aid programmes, the two programmes that were stopped altogether were to do with adult health. In those countries in which Cuba had to reduce its total commitment, none of the child welfare programmes were trimmed.

Closing the Loop-holes

It was in this context that the Institute for childhood observed in a report, published in 1976, that many Cuban school-age children (5 years - 14 years) were slipping through the net - not being adequately cared for at home, truanting from school, missing out on eye and ear tests, not being nourished or protected in a way consistent with good health, etc. Their suggestion was that they too be included in a "unified" matrix of legislation as an extension of the Family Law Code. Because of the fears alluded to earlier, about the financial crisis facing Cuba, the enabling legislation almost went down to defeat in the Poder Popular in 1977. Fidel Castro cast the deciding vote.

This immediately brought both the FMC and the Institute for childhood into the schools. What was needed first was to establish and maintain continuous monitoring of children's activities and growth between teachers in the schools and parents at home. The FMC was represented on every CDR and used their influence to involve the CDRs in promoting school-parent dialogue. Parents who did not keep appointments at school, for instance, were brought to the attention of their CDRs and mention of it would be made at the monthly public meetings. It is amazing how attendance at parent-teacher sessions improved out of sight. The local GP was also involved. The author was once talking to a 17 year old youth in downtown Havana about juvenile delinquency in London. He listened almost wistfully and then said: "You know, that couldn't happen here. Too many people are watching you!"

Health in the Primary School Programme

Even in Circulo Infantil programmes, children talk about health, usually in the context of cleanliness and personal hygiene, but I have seen psychological health referred to and discussed. However, once children enter primary school, they encounter a fully set-out health and hygiene syllabus. I watched a class of 6 year olds grappling with the question: "How do you know if the person beside you is healthy?" Initial attempts to dispose of what appeared to be an easy question by a simple explicit answer, were enthusiastic: "Take him to a doctor", "Listen to his chest with one of those rubber pipes in your ears", "Find out if he went to the toilet", "Put your hand on his head", etc. As the subtlety of the issue became obvious, participation conspicuously waned. There was no quick way out of this one! But they listened to the teacher. She began to ask other questions: "Can you be healthy if you are unhappy?", "Is a blind person who is happy and is helping people (and here she mentioned some pop musician who was blind) healthy?", "To be healthy do you have to have perfect hearing, eyesight, etc.," "Can a crippled person be healthy?"

Gradually the discussion shifted to the social dimension and the link between the social and the psychological. I was amazed at the insights that some of the children were starting to come up with by now. "The person beside me is healthy if I am kind to him", "If I am healthy I can make other people healthy", etc. Out of the mouths of babes and sucklings!

The syllabus throughout primary school involves the children principally in "projects" rather than in importing detailed knowledge of physiology, etc. Even so, I was astonished at how much quite detailed knowledge was known about the body by Cuban primary children, as evidenced by the questions they asked me. The teachers often said to me that the children pick up a lot about health from the TV. They do learn the life cycles of important parasites, even learning the technical names for the various parts of the malaria and dengue fever cycles, the names of the species of mosquitoes involved, etc. Diet is discussed a great deal. Since 1981, smoking in areas designated as "non-smoking", has been better policed. But, in hospitals, Cuban doctors often themselves smoke and generally treat the health issues involved indulgently.

The children attend street theatre related to health and social issues and put on a good few such mini-dramas themselves. It always draws an appreciative crowd and one wonders why it is not done in British schools. Road safety is a constantly occurring theme and, indeed, it needed to be before the acute petrol shortages starting in 1995. Havana was not a safe place for pedestrians, even though the number of cars was restricted!

FMC Initiatives in Family Life

It was not long after the formation of the FMC - and well before it was directly charged with responsibilities relating to educating and protecting children - that it became involved in both monitoring and promoting ante-natal care clinics. In many respects this brought to the fore the traditional feminist objections to the medicalisation of women. The view quickly prevailed that, if this thing was going to be done, then they would have a controlling hand in it. The influence of the FMC in this respect has been beneficent in the extreme and this doctor has not seen more psychologically supportive ante-natal clinics anywhere.

They work closely with the CDR's at a general educational level, reminding women of the benefits of ante-natal care and of the importance of keeping every appointment. In the maternity units themselves they provide all, or many, of the creature comforts -congenial surroundings, informal and relaxing furniture and fittings - much of it originally selected from the vacated homes of those who fled with Batista! They are also represented in some way or other in most factories and government enterprises, where they provide ongoing commentary and education to men about the dignity of fatherhood, etc. In a country like Britain this kind of fervour would be regarded as distasteful, but in Cuba it is addressing generations of entrenched machismo.

However, it is when the mothers get home with their babies that the influence of the FMC really becomes pervasive in fulfilling the "protection of children" role assigned them by the government. To show how they do this, it is necessary to step back momentarily to the ante-natal situation.

129

Involving the Fathers

The expectant mother is not only expected to attend ante-natal clinics as such, usually held during the day and in a maternity unit itself, but also to attend ante-natal classes in the evening, characteristically run totally by the local branch of the FMC. These are usually held in CDR facilities or in local schools. Every effort is made to make sure that the fathers-to-be also attend. At the outset, they were only moderately successful in this, but now male participation is almost total.

At the classes, both parents are given lessons on the actual anatomical and physiological details of pregnancy and birth, and what to do in the event of various emergencies. At one such class this author attended in 1984, free copies of a Spanish edition of Dr Benjamin Spock's famous "Baby and Child care" were handed out! Assurances were given that this is not customary practice, however. In any case, more modest literary offerings produced locally are frequently given out and discussed - including poems written by participating parents-to-be. The whole atmosphere of these classes is warmly supportive and inviting. Their need was apparently amply illustrated in the early days when it was not uncommon to encounter astonishing levels of ignorance about sexual details among those attending. Some first-time pregnant women were not sure where the baby was to emerge, a common assumption being that it was removed surgically when the time came. The men, it seems, were characteristically even more poorly informed, believing a variety of myths such as that applying vaseline to the penis before intercourse would prevent conception!

Now, with sex education being a component part of the primary school health curriculum, and a course of study on its own in secondary school, levels of sophistication are much higher. The major contribution that these ante-natal classes make now are perceived to be largely in the social/psychological domain. It has led to a sea-change in the attitude of Cuban men, as is readily noticed if one spends a few days in, say, Mexico and then a few days in Cuba. In other parts of Latin America, one notices that fathers play highly stereotyped roles in public with their families. You do not often see a man looking after the more intimate and messy details of a young child's

130

eating or toileting needs. His role is to be present in such a way that there is no doubt in anyone's mind as to who he is, while his wife (the 'partner' idea produces a different scenario in the Latin American context) does the fiddly bits. In Cuba the difference is noticeable immediately, with fathers often seen alone with their tiny babies talking to other parents and doing what has to be done without any reticence. Partly this is because the parents are often involved in separate activities after working hours; meetings, evening classes, etc.

While the ante-natal evening classes are in session, the participants ate encouraged to get to know one another socially, to visit each other's homes, etc. Cards are typically exchanged as the babies are born and the FMC leader of each group then encourages continued contact between participants after they have had their babies and returned home. The new mothers 'compare notes', so to speak and, should one of them appear to be having problems - be they physical or emotional - this quickly gets back to the FMC who are then able to intervene.

Breast is Best - Throwing out the Powdered Milk

An interesting example of the effectiveness of the FMC in this role was the change of attitude that they have brought about with respect to breast feeding. Up until about 1960 in Cuba there appeared to be a strong reluctance to breast feed. Commercial baby milk was held to be more fashionable and many mothers felt that it was 'cheap', 'low class' somehow 'undignified' to forsake the bottle in favour of the breast. Initially motivated by difficulties in gaining supplies of Lactogen (the most popular commercial feeding formula) in 1961, the government ran a campaign along the 'Breast is best' variety. Even when supplies of Lactogen had been available, bottle feeding had presented problems common to all third would countries. Pure water supplies - required both to mix the formula and to clean the bottles and teats - was difficult to guarantee. Then, especially among the rural poor, attempts would sometimes be made to economise by using less powder or, worse, by mixing it with other powdery

131

substances that were more easily obtained. Much of the common infant diarrhoea/dehydration could be traced to that sort of thing.

The FMC accepted the challenge by first going into the birth units and advising the staff not to ask the new mothers whether they wanted to bottle feed or breast feed but to insist on breast feeding initially. In a study done by the FMC in two provincial centres in 1961, it was found that - whereas it was usual for 82% of mothers to opt for bottle feeding when given the choice at the outset, if they breast fed for 4 days first and then were given the choice only 26% chose the bottle. Thus, the first line of argument that the FMC used then, and still does now, was neither economic nor hygienic, but psychological. As one FMC teacher put it to the author: "suckling at the breast creates an even stronger love between the mother and the baby and, after a few times, she needs it because it makes her feel good just as much as the baby needs it for the milk".

Now it is commonplace knowledge, even among very young and inexperienced mothers, that no formula can be as accurate or as clean as the mother's own milk. Much of the previous attitude also stemmed from one of the more perverse influences of the Christian religion, especially in its Catholic form, in that the body was somehow regarded as 'carnal' and 'unclean'. The idea of a baby having to make close body contact to get its nourishment seemed much more unhygienic than getting it out of a sterilised bottle. This, in fact, might account for why breast feeding still has a low profile in other Latin American societies.

Thus it was that, by 1975, homeless children wandering the streets, orphanages and the Casa de Benficencia had been left far behind. Orphans were now hardly heard of, not because they don't occur but because the widespread attitude of affection and succouring of the young ensures that orphans are easily adopted. In fact, there is a constant demand for adoptive children with long waiting lists. As the 1974 Report of the Central Committee of Cuban Communist Party rather stiltedly put it:

> "Orphans are no longer a problem. With the broad and noble spirit of
> comradely solidarity that the Revolution has kindled in peoples'
> hearts, for every child that might have been left homeless and helpless,
> there are now dozens of families willing to welcome him as if he were

their own"   (Note the "he" and "him" - Author).

CHAPTER EIGHT

Developments in Public Health from 1976-1981

Platform for a Change in Strategy

Developments in Cuba's health care system from 1958 until 1976 can reasonably accurately be described as driven by three factors:

a.   The need to replace quickly the large loss of skilled health workers, including most of the country's doctors, occasioned by people fleeing Cuba when the revolutionaries gained power.

b.   Revolutionary idealism within Cuba, itself fed by the unexpectedly profound success of the Great Literacy Campaign and the implementation of such initiatives as the Family Law Code, Circulos Infantiles, etc.

c.   External expectations on the part of progressive forces in other third world countries which, observing Cuba's success in materially reversing the very negative statistics formerly pertaining to rural health, no longer could accept their own countries' appalling health figures as being purely an inevitable reflection of economic backwardness.

As we have seen, each of these factors were addressed by a combination of ideology and pragmatism that at times was so convoluted as to defy rational analysis and to mock attempts to describe them sufficiently objectively to make them immediately applicable to other new revolutionary situations. This was not through any lack of effort. Grenada, Nicaragua and Chile - to name but three examples close at hand - all tried to emulate the successes of the Cuban model, but to greater or lesser degree failed to do so. As Mao Tse Tung was once reported to have sagely commented: "Revolution does not export very well".

With respect to replacing man-power loss, Cuban attempts had more than succeeded by the mid-sixties, if not sooner. It was at first accomplished by "temporary" measures entirely: Giving perfunctorily brief instruction to unqualified people, accepting aid personnel from other countries and lowering admission standards to existing courses. But all of these strategies were only ad hoc and were modified as often as two or three times a year to accommodate the rapidly changing situation.

Social and Psychological Problems

As has occurred in every revolution we know about, once one gets past the generation of people who brought it into being, it becomes increasingly difficult to sustain the impetus - especially that psychological set of attitudes that allows one to suspend critical analysis - to believe implicitly in the nobility of the cause. Probably as an aspect of social evolution, the young tend to be cavalier about history. They want results and are not hindered in their judgements (or are less likely to be) by ideological constraints. Other revolutionary leaders have tried to address this problem in various ways.

Remember that the French produced the "busy guillotine" as the answer - keep the revolution alive by not letting people ever feel secure enough to institute anything! Robespierre even said that "The Revolution must keep cutting its own head off and, hydra-like producing new ones, if it is to survive". Mao Tse Tung set the Red Guards in motion when things became too inflexibly institutionalised. Stalin had to keep introducing purges, etc.

Cuba has relied on a curious mixing of pragmatic realism and ideology. The Cuban revolution is probably the most thoroughly documented in the world. This vast amount of documentary material - newspaper clippings, film footage, diaries, artefacts, etc - is constantly on public display. As well, the actions of large, industrialised societies, like the U.S. in trying to frustrate Cuban development, has rendered it unnecessary for the Cuban authorities themselves to "re-legitimise" the ideology. Generations of young people - and foreign visitors - have seen the film clips, read the newspaper accounts, looked at the artefacts and then listened to the American media! Ideology still carries a greater degree of moral clout in Cuba 40 years after the

136

revolution than it had done in any of the other major revolutions even 10 years on.

The Missionary Impulse

This has been especially true as far as public health is concerned. One senses it every time one interviews medical students, for instance. They talk like people selected for missionary training - and they mean it! But the role of foreign expectations - especially in Africa and Asia - both distorted and energised Cuban developments in public health. An Algerian delegation visiting Cuba in the early 60's was told how the Great Literacy Campaign had been used as a starting point in educating rural people as to how to cope with gastroenteritis in pre-school children. They were profoundly impressed and no sooner had they returned than the Cuban Ministry of Public Health was invited to send a "a group" of teacher-nurses to spend four months in rural Algeria teaching villagers the rudiments of hygiene. A humble beginning this was, indeed, to what, within two years, had unpredictably become one of Cuba's major export industries.

All three of these factors had become fully developed and integrated by 1976 and provided a platform for developments for the next five years. But, using that as a platform, the strategy changed.

Effects of the "First Noose"

One of the popular figures of speech in Cuba is to describe the U.S. embargo and the Economic Blockade as a noose which is always half strangling Cuban development but which from time to time, and for various external reasons over which Cuba has but limited control, is tightened even more severely. As observed already, the first of these attempts at total strangulation occurred in the middle and late 70's.

It caused economic strictures in Cuba's domestic affairs and very much exacerbated existing fiscal uncertainties occasioned in no small degree by Cuba's own rapid ideological shift with respect to sugar cane production. At the time of the triumph of the revolution, it was widely realised - both within Cuba and abroad - that one of the principal factors which made Cuba such an easy victim of imperialism was the tyranny of the "one crop economy". On the very first day of the new government assuming power - January 1, 1959 -Fidel Castro said in his victory speech that he would preside over a Cuba that "could feed itself with the full range of foodstuffs produced in Cuba and, export a wide variety of agricultural produce". `Diversification' was the propaganda 'in' word of the day, and the Cubans went at it with a vengeance. Che Guevara himself was one of the major architects of this line of propaganda.

Conflict Between Economics & Ideology

Without going into all of the technical economic arguments, problems soon appeared - and grew more insistent. Certainly Cuba could produce, say, enough citrus fruit for domestic consumption and thus not have to import it. But this would immediately create a tit-for-tat situation with respect to Cuban sugar, which at that point had dropped to its lowest price on the international markets for 35 years. In any case, Cuba did not have to import so many finished or semi-finished goods. These could be processed in Cuba. But by 1969, it had become abundantly clear that the cost of training Cubans to run these manufacturing processes and of importing and fuelling the necessary machinery would exceed the market value of the goods produced. In other words, Cuba had effectively curtailed its major export (sugar) when - because it had become cheaper - they should have been producing more of it, and had taken on manufacturing enterprises that had to be subsidised by the government.

When the author was in Hanoi in 1975, he met a French agricultural economist who had just returned from Cuba. We discussed the Cuban problems at some length until eventually I said : "I wonder how they came to make a mistake like that? " In reply he leaned forward and said : "Don't you know? It's because _true_ communists are insane!" In a very real sense, that response mirrored a growing despair in Cuba with ideology. One did not have to be counter-revolutionary to harbour such views - just

138

impatient.

Public Health and Education were the two ministries in Cuba at the time which were the most costly to run. Layouts had to be enormous and immediate, while returns were uncertain and long-term. There is no doubt in anyone's mind retrospectively , that the drop in morale occasioned in health circles by the lack of cash and resources, was exploited by such bodies as the CIA.

The Allure of America

Splinter political groups formed to the right and the left as centres of anti-government comment and sentiment. Cuba has always been troubled by small right-wing cliques forming every now and again. They are easy to account for and receive regular "nourishment" from Voice of America broadcasts and elsewhere. Florida is close by and the delights of consumerism - Levis, ghetto blasters, etc - exert a continuing fascination for the young. Testimony to this is provided by the popularity of places like Puerta Mariel, from which boats full of malcontents and thoughtless adolescents periodically "flee" Cuban communism for Floridean freedom. This all reached a height in the late 70's. The U.S. Government tacitly encouraged it by not requiring the customary proof of "political refugee" status that they ordinarily require of people seeking asylum from, say, Haiti. In a sense, the Cuban authorities also "encouraged" it by not being particularly vigilant with respect to it. The attitude seemed to be: "If they want to go , they'll only cause trouble here", in which case "flee" hardly seemed to be the appropriate verb to describe their departure.

In 1979, the exodus reached such numbers that some journalists became convinced that the Cuban authorities were simply dumping people at Puerta Mariel from Cuba's own mental institutions , remand centres, etc. - people they wanted to unload as a cost-cutting exercise - and letting them "escape". Florida newspapers ran a number of such accounts, but no comment about it either way was made in Cuba.

But if, by waiving the usual requirements for establishing refugee status where

139

Cuban nationals were concerned, the U.S. had hoped to attract Cuba's intelligentsia or a significant proportion of its technologically trained manpower, they gambled and lost. The stresses of 1974-79 showed clearly that the great bulk of Cuba's medical personnel - trained in the revolutionary context - put ideological and moral commitment ahead of consumerist comfort. Less than 1% were lost.

Emergence of Leftist Anti-Government Groups

More puzzling was the sudden appearance of two quite well organised groups on the left, one at Santa Clara University Medical School, calling themselves "Trotskyists". For about a month in September/October 1979 little packets of leaflets, 50 in a packet, would be dropped at strategic locations in secondary schools, nurse-training schools, hospital waiting rooms, etc. The leaflets were peculiar - replete with mistakes in Spanish suggesting that they had been produced outside of Cuba, and virulently anti-American, anti-USSR and anti-Castro. Many people claimed that they were printed in Peking, at the Foreign Language Press, but this was never proven. The Government did not publicise the matter and only one minor story appeared about it in an early January 1980 issue of "Granma" - Cuba's daily paper. School teachers and others were asked to watch out for such leaflets and to try to find out who was responsible for delivering them.

The leaflets, in effect, said that Fidel Castro had betrayed the revolution and had sent Che Guevara to his death because the latter knew "the truth". Formal "discussion groups" were convened at the two medical schools named to "analyse" the claims. Suspicion settled on the two institutions named because in a number of student rooms in both places, and - apparently - in some of the lecturers' offices - large unopened piles of the materials were found. Whatever the truth of the matter, any enquiries made about it met with closed lips and/or evasive disclaimers. What is certain is that a number of students and staff were dismissed from both medical schools.

One of the most conspicuous changes in public health triggered by these extraordinary developments was a re-alignment of courses along more orthodox lines and the time-tabling of a vast increase in "ideologically-oriented" instruction in the form of compulsory modules in "Marxism-Leninism", "Conflict between materialism and religion in the clinical sciences", "Marxist theory and praxis", etc. As well, many of the courses became more orthodox in the form of reverting to more lecture-exam format teaching in the first year, with much less open-ended clinical experience, less space on the time-table was accorded student seminars, etc.

The Enthronement of Preventive Medicine

At meetings relating to the promulgation of the five year plan (1974-79) it was explicitly pointed out that: "A peso's worth of preventive medicine equals 10 pesos worth of interventionist medicine. Keeping people from falling sick should cost only a tenth of treating them once they have become sick". In 1975 and 1976, compulsory first year modules in preventive medicine were instituted in all of the medical schools and nurse training schools. As well, these modules had to be designed to "undergird" at least one of the compulsory modules in each of the subsequent years of the course.

A new examination paper (3 hours) was also added to those already required for successful registration in the Cuban Medical Association when students reached their final year. This was a paper called "Community Health, Family and Preventive Medicine".

Intersectoral Education

In 1978 "common" professional modules were established between Nursing, Pharmacy, Public health licentiates, social workers and child care officers, so that as certain paramedical personnel were gaining their qualifications, they interacted with problems and issues raised by other professionals. Public health licentiates were community health workers who tended to be closely involved with school children's health - working with school nurses, circulo infantile educadoras and CDR immunisation committees. They first were created under that name in 1968 to put to effective use large numbers of Emergency Nursing trainee certificate holders who clearly had some aptitude for the work but could not score well enough on their final examinations to be allowed into the regular three year nursing course. Starting in 1971, long after there had been any Emergency certificate people being trained, a special two year course (based on Grade X) was started for licentiates at some nursing colleges. In other words, the licentiates had proven their worth and the Government needed more time.

By including licentiates in the common professional modules, recognition was accorded the immense improvement in academic standards they had reached since 1968. Among these common modules were: two in statistics (an introductory univariate analysis unit and a more advanced statistical inference unit), one in health promotion (only one year after WHO had suggested the need to establish such training!), one in epidemiology, one in nutrition and one in health, exercise and sport. As far as the more clinically oriented paramedical disciplines were concerned, this provided a refreshing social balance and a much more humanistic perspective.

Altogether, by 1980, around 21,000 health workers were working in a large number of public health and social welfare capacities. 15,200 of these were general practitioners, 3,600 dentists and 700 pharmacists. The schools of nursing had produced 14,000 registered nurses, 1,300 dental assistants and more than 13,000 "State Enrolled Nurses". These are people with two years training post grade IX, who are employed largely in old people's homes. In 1981, nursing was accorded university degree status and an extra year added to the training, making it now a four year course.

Table 8.1 below shows the increase in numbers of general practitioners and dentists graduated in three academic years over the interval 1959 -1980.

Table: 8.1 Number of Graduates in General Practice and Dentistry[46]

Academic year	General practice	Internal medicine
1959-60	190	55
1970-71	432	173
1979-80	764	215

In total, in the two decades spanned above, the various training institutions in Cuba had produced more than 70,500 technicians and auxiliary workers of various categories in health care. The graph below gives some indication of the rate at which these were produced. Note that in response to the desperate economic plight of Cuba from 1977-1980, occasioned largely by the U.S. blockade, these courses were drastically curtailed - but not decreased. See Fig. 8.1. below:

Fig. 8.1 Graph showing Rates of Increase in Numbers of Doctors and Dentists

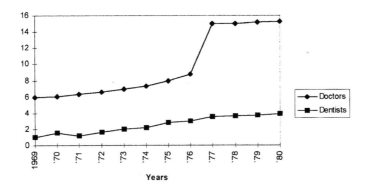

---

[46] All tables and Graphs in chapter eight derive from :Desarrollo Economico y Social Durante el Periodo 1958-1980, Comite Estatal de Estadisticas, Diciembre 1981. Also, see Appendix A

... was singled out for the "noose" treatment referred to earlier, it was
the only Latin American Country to have a nationally integrated system of public health
in which social legislation about its application was unified with the training
programmes of workers in it. In 1980, the number of Cubans per doctor had dropped
to 639, while in Peru, Chile and Columbia, the ratio had deteriorated - moving from an
average of 1,200 people per doctor in 1977 to more than 1,500 people per doctor in
1980. This represented a remarkable achievement!

One of the unique features of the development of Cuban health care has been
the extent to which, as conscious political and social policy, public health has been
integrated with social welfare - first with respect to children (up to 1976) and then
throughout the community (1976-1981). The effect of this is reflected in figures for
numbers of beds allocated to residents of health care institutions and social welfare
institutions. Table 8.2. illustrates this.

Table: 8.2. Beds provided for medical & social welfare services[47]

Year:	1958	1965	1980
medical welfare	28,536	42,412	44,380
social welfare	3,965	6,257	9,130
Totals	32,501	48,669	53,510

Particular Impact on The Rural Sector

With respect to these figures, one of the most notable features is the impact of health
and welfare services on the rural community. This began with the promulgation of
Law 723 (which in 1960 established postgraduate training health workers in social

---

[47]Ibid. 2 of Chapter VII

144

welfare issues) and thereby created a uniquely new conception of how community medicine and health insights might most effectively be mediated. In other words, the intersectoral approach in common professional education, was now being reflected in community health practice.

Without doubt, the rural sector, which in pre-Revolutionary times had been so badly deprived of corrupt officials, had (by 1980) benefited most spectacularly by these developments - with 151 medical posts and 53 rural hospitals established since 1959. Even from 1975-1980, there was an increase from 10 to 30 beds made available in rural health institutions, mainly for children. This was done to the accompaniment of a vigorous programme of community hygiene training, construction of safe privies, inspection and replacement of wells and pumps, vaccination schedules, local training in the detection of sources of infection, health promotion exercises and first aid.

Interventionist Vs Community Medicine

The 1976 Five Year Plan, as indicated earlier, specified the need to shift attention away from radical interventionist medical techniques to preventive medicine. At meetings held in the Ministry of Public Health in October 1975, it was said that some rural family doctors felt that most of their time was taken up with taking samples of blood, urine and phlegm from sick people, sending these samples off to one of the Government pathology labs and then waiting for the results before being able to advise the patient. By the 1976 edict, the doctor was to become much more pro-active in actually involving him/herself in community decisions which had health and welfare implications. In this they were organised in collaboration with the CDR's and such bodies as the FMC.

Smoking - Community Health Problems and an Economic Paradox

In 1981, a poster in a rural post office in Havana province itself declaimed: "If your doctor sees you smoking in the street and admonishes you, don't tell him to mind his own business. He is". Cuba occupies a quixotic position with respect to cigarette smoking. Even now tobacco is still one of its main foreign currency generating crops. Despite the thorough training in hygiene, given in both primary and secondary schools, little was said prior to 1975 about smoking and drinking. Then, in 1974, Cuba suffered an epidemic of "tobacco mozaic", a viral infection that kills off tobacco plants. The tobacco harvest was threatened. In order not to compromise its export requirements, the Government severely decreased the domestic tobacco ration. The hygiene books in secondary schools started to include extensive treatment of the hazards of smoking. An anti-smoking ban was launched. Posters appeared on the large outdoor hoardings and in Government offices, urging a non-smoking lifestyle.

One of the best of these shows a harassed-looking public servant sitting at a ministry desk, surrounded by paperwork and two telephones. Beside him is an ashtray full of butts, some still smoking. He has a cigarette in his mouth and is surrounded by clouds of tobacco smoke. Above the man's head is written: "If you smoke because you've got problems...', then underneath is written, '... then you have yet another problem!'

Family Planning and Child Health

Advice on family planning is also freely available, and condoms and contraception pills, not only from doctors but from a whole range of ancillary health workers, are ludicrously cheap. In fact, as has already been discussed, the revolution has always regarded child welfare as one of its major priority areas. Especially during the two periods: 1959-1974 and 1974-1979, it aimed to reduce the rural infant mortality rate, to bring it into line with that of the most technologically advanced nations. That they

146

succeeded in doing this has already been demonstrated. However, the graph below shows just how spectacularly effective this campaign was. Again, in 1979 there was a dramatic cut-off of funding for the programme, but existing services were not compromised. See Appendix A for a fuller appreciation of this. These phenomena are clearly shown in Fig 8.2., below:

Fig 8.2 Graph showing Change in Infant Mortality per 1000 live Births from 1970 through 1980

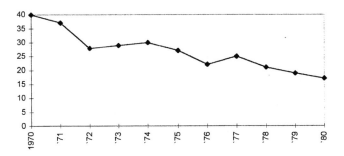

The Changing Childbirth Scene

By 1981, as has been noted elsewhere, almost all deliveries were taking place in hospitals, especially in the city, and this was associated with increasing rates of maternal acquiescence in attending pre-natal clinic check ups. From 1978-1981 there was an enormous increase in paternal participation in pre-natal classes. Along with this, and up until the present day, there has been a much greater awareness, among both parents-to-be and health workers, of the huge importance of psychological factors in pregnancy and family life generally.

This has been attributed, not unnaturally, to the formation of a new social consciousness, a general increase in the appreciation of human dignity and a sensitivity to the needs of other people. One cannot help but feel that such an evaluation is largely to the point. It is so evident, when one is talking to Cubans, that they take an almost ecstatic pride in the extent to which Cuba has occupied such a high international profile in its willingness to collaborate so freely with other third world people in the arena of public health. Even in casual conversations in the street, at bus stops, etc., ordinary Cubans reflect an awareness of their country's extensive international involvement with respect to mother and child health.

Medical Consultations and the Family Health Practitioners 1958-1981

Although the emphasis shifted dramatically in 1976 from interventionist medicine to preventive medicine, this did not bring about a decline in the number of patient-doctor visits, but rather the reverse. Government critics, with an eye on costs alone, who may have felt that the edict to promote 'prevention' rather than 'cure', was largely a fiscal rationalisation manoeuvre, would not have been impressed with such figures. However, in many ways this mirrors the early history of the National Health Service in Britain. Health care, if it is administered according to canons of social justice, can never be cheap. But it can be cheaper and more efficient than if it is not perceived as a community responsibility! An increase in public awareness about health issues, and more especially, about all the social factors and community issues involved in being healthy, cannot help but make people more astute in their own assessment of health needs. Given this, an increase in doctor visits should have been anticipated, but these visits are different in character to what they were before.

People who have been made aware of hygiene and public health, and who are sensible to their own responsibility in maintaining the health of the community, will go to see their doctor as a participant in the health enterprise. Under the old system, the doctor was seen as an authority figure with access to arcane knowledge outside of the patient's grasp. The patient perceived his/her own health as being largely outside of

148

his/her own intellectual and moral jurisdiction. "Going to the doctor" meant receiving oracular wisdom. Now, as studies of doctor's attitudes to the new working conditions indicate, they see themselves more and more as helping patients help themselves that all might benefit.

Table 8.3. indicates how the figures for doctor/patient visits have changed over the time-period concerned. In this table, only specific interactions requested by a patient are counted. This clearly makes a great difference when we are discussing patients visited at home.

Table: 8.3. Medical Consultations between 1965-1980 (in millions)[48]

Year	1965	1970	1980
visits to surgery	12.2	21.5	30.0
visits to patient at home	5.0	7.9	15.2
Totals	**17.7**	**29.3**	**45.2**

What the figures do reveal is that the increase has not been as great over the 10 year period between 1970 and 1980 as over the five year period from 1965 to 1970 for surgery visits, but it has been very much greater over the later time interval for home visits. Clearly this is a reflection, not of increase in need, but of increase in doctor availability. It is also a reflection of a material change in doctors' attitudes.

The "new" family doctor sees him/herself as a social worker as much as a medical/technical expert. For instance, the spectacular improvement in child health, insofar as it related to vaccination programmes, was not entirely due to the availability of vaccines in sufficient quantities and of medical personnel to administer them. Rather, as doctors became accepted as living "with" and "in" the community (rather than "off" it, as was the case of private doctors), their opinions on health issues were recognised as carrying more weight. Vaccination education met with great resistance in the early years, but as the number of doctors increased and as their roles as community agents,

---

[48] Ibid. Also see Appendix A

149

od of the neighbourhood, became more fully appreciated, people

.ing their children forward and to accept advice on such subtle

..sues as herd immunity.

Table 8.4. shows the dramatic impact this has made on contagious illnesses. 'Duplex' refers, of course, to Whooping Cough and Diphtheria and 'Triple' to polio as well.

Table 8.4. Populations Immunised (thousands) in the Vaccination Drives of 1964 and 1980[49]

Vaccination	1964	1980
BCG	290.0	373.4
Triple	236.4	302.6
Duplex	180.3	305.2
Tetanus	694.6	1,582.4
Typhoid	481.6	765.8
Smallpox	66.7	13.2
Polio	2,450.4	3,342.6

In other words, the health situation in Cuba by 1980, was that its health care system, including community health, preventive care and health promotion, ranked it with the most advanced countries in the world. Subsequent chapters will show how, despite two more extremely severe tightenings of the "noose" of the U.S. Economic Blockade, the revolution has so far been able to continue to respond flexibly and creatively to preserve the extraordinary gains it had made up until 1981.

---

[49]Ibid. 2. Also see Appendix A.

150

CHAPTER NINE

The Cuban Health Scene 1981 to The Present

The Second Noose

Fidel Castro's comment about his country still being ahead of all other Latin American countries in the field of health, even if Cuba stopped and made no further advances for five years (quoted in Chapter One) was true, even as far back as 1974. As we saw in Chapter Eight, advances made in Cuba - in the face of extreme economic difficulties - between 1974 and 1981, actually brought Cuba's health care system up to a level which compared favourably with that of the industrially advanced nations.

Since then, Cuba has faced two more "tightenings of the noose". Starting in 1982, the Reagan administration in the U.S. tightened the Economic Blockade through a series of steps re-interpreting the promulgation (way back in 1909) of a piece of legislation known as the "Trading with the Enemy" Act [50]. Until that had become enforced with respect to Cuba, the Americans could not prevent Cuba from gaining access to textbooks, equipment, etc., pertaining to the health sciences. Even an ordinary economic blockade is not intended to stem the flow of educational or humanitarian goods and services! But the new legislation of 1982 went considerably further as shown in greater detail in Chapter Sixteen. It not only banned any trade with Cuba, it made it illegal for any foreign nation to export goods and equipment to Cuba of which any part or process in its manufacture had been mediated by American firms or individuals. An obvious example of this draconian piece of legislation in action affected a shipment of tractor motors from a Birmingham firm in England to Cuba. The shipment was prevented because two of the parts of the motors concerned were American made.

---

[50] The trading with the Enemy Act was originally intended to apply to any nation that was an imminent military threat to the U.S. Reagan was able to interpret it in such a way as to include Cuba by reference to the "Evil Empire" of states held to be "clients" of the former Soviet Union.

But the implications were much more negative than that. The Trading with the Enemy Act, as thus interpreted, included any activity, even by a third country with which the Americans had trade agreements, which could be construed as amounting to "aid or comfort" to the enemy. Thus, for instance, books or lectures written about Cuba could not be published in the US or on any printing presses elsewhere if those machines were being serviced under American contracts, if the sale of such publications was going to generate money for Cuba in any way whatever. It became illegal for, say, "Scientific American", to honour subscriptions of it from Cuban individuals or institutions. Standard health and medical journals were cut off, etc. The previous economic blockade had been bad enough, but there had always been people in America and elsewhere who had been positively disposed toward Cuba and helped to keep it supplied with educational and public health materials. Now energetic attempts were being made to cut off these links. As we have already seen, the "trading with the enemy" legislation could even be used to curtail the scholarly activities of non-American academics wishing to visit Cuba.

Cuba Emphasises Self-Sufficiency

As Ho Chi Minh once observed in 1953, with respect to Vietnam: "Nothing makes a people more resourceful than any attempt by a larger power to thwart them."[51] Cuba was no exception in this respect. For instance, it addressed the shortage of paper by researching techniques for using sugar-cane husks, of which huge quantities were normally consigned each year to the flames, for making a pulp from which paper could be manufactured. Initially the result was a greyish-brown rough textured material unattractive to look at, easily damaged and difficult to print on. Within a year, methods had been found of bleaching it considerably and it became used for all Government publications in schools, etc.

---

[51]Minh, Ho Chi (1968): Step-by Step to an Independent Vietnam. Foreign Language Press, Hanoi.

In the field of pharmaceuticals, the lack of access to high tech developments has had serious consequences, but now at least many standard vaccines can be produced with Cuban materials and labour on Cuban soil. With regard to the wider ambit of public health, Cuba has had to design machinery for manufacturing sewer piping - which it used to import - to replace damaged sections and to extend the network of sewered areas. The fiscal overhead required as an initial capital outflow to finance the production of such machinery is so great that this has caused severe dislocation in other parts of the economy. Even if Cuba were to succeed in setting up the necessary machinery, its own modest needs could never account for the total amount of piping produced. But the trade embargo effectively prevented other developing nations from buying the surplus or from shipping it out of Cuba once it had been purchased.

Goals for The 80's

In 1984, the Cuban authorities, while acknowledging that the U.S. embargo was damaging their system of public health and hygiene, announced that they would cut back on some programmes, but that three areas would remain sacrosanct. These were: maintenance of general health indices (e.g. Life Expectancy, Infant mortality Rate, etc); Distribution of human resources in the public health service (e.g. Transplant surgery, Laser surgery, etc) and Medical Aid to other countries.

Actually, although that was the plan and those the goals, much more was accomplished. Instead of simply maintaining 1984 levels of each of the three criteria, Cuba had exceeded every one of them by 1989 and, with respect to high technology, her success has confounded even the most optimistic Government expectations. In fact, as we shall see, as a result of work in that arena, Cuban specialists found themselves engaged at the frontiers of medical research. Some statistical data will objectify much of this commentary. Appendix A contains Cuba's national health statistics up until 1988. The next such document is due in 1998, but in the meantime Cuban Ministry of Public Health Officers have given the author permission to publish them in full. A decline set in during 1994 (see Chapter Sixteen) due to the stringency of the U.S. Blockade and, of course, this is not reflected in the figures in Appendix A.

Child Health Care

Infant mortality as of 1991 had been reduced to 9.7 deaths per 1000 live births. This refers of course, to neonatal deaths - within the first year of life, but it does include all live births in contra-distinction to many Latin American countries in which a death within 24 hours of partem is not counted! What this meant is that, even then, Cuba ranked 18th in the world with respect to national infant mortality figures. As we have seen, the background to these remarkable figures involved first a two -pronged attack on vaccination against the six most common infant killers plus programmes designed to reduce death by dehydration. Those two fronts alone reduced the infant mortality rate dramatically, but further reduction continued throughout the 80's through research on infant influenza's and pneumonia's and public health education on sepsis. Most Cuban medical authorities also regard the campaign to achieve 100% hospital birth deliveries as having played a major role in this triumph.

Figures for 1998 now put at 99.8% (including both rural and urban)the proportion of Cuban births taking place under medical supervision in hospital conditions. In many rural areas, since 1985, it has even become routine practice for expectant mothers to enter hospital some weeks prior to delivery. This is for two reasons. Many rural homes are still inaccessible and one cannot always count on the availability of easy transport to the community hospital just when it is needed. Also, most rural homes, although now electrified and no longer earthen-floored bohíos, are not as well equipped with sanitary provisions as are their average urban counterparts.

Close co-ordination of the work of the FMC, the CDR's and the Ministry of Public Health also ensures an exceptionally high standard of infant and mother care. On average, each baby born in 1990 in Cuba received 11.2 puerculture examinations - an extraordinarily high figure, even by British or American standards.

154

Other Pharmacological Initiatives

By persistent community education, not to say popular propaganda, throughout the 80's, vaccination is now virtually universal. In April 1991, the Ministry of Public Health quoted a figure of 93%, but even this is regarded as conservative and other agencies, including WHO, have placed it higher. Those April 1991 Ministry of Health figures also claimed that all Cubans below the age of 20 years had been immunised against Meningococcic Meningitis type B. If those figures are accurate, that would place Cuba top of the league in that respect internationally. One of the more rewarding, and in some ways unexpected, breakthroughs in child health that has arisen as a result of this intense emphasis on neonatal health care, is the decrease in deaths due to hypoxia and also of hyaline membrane diseases. The former bespeaks the existence of an exceptionally thorough perinatology programme generally and figures relating to hypoxia rate decrease first became statistically evident in 1986.

The latter, relating to hyaline membrane disease, certainly could not have been achieved without the concern for neonatal safety as such, but as well reflects a triumph for Cuban medical research. Hyaline membrane disease arises through a deficiency of lipoproteic substances and is associated with developmental lung immaturity. But in 1988, Cuban biochemists, working at the medical school in Havana University, succeeded in synthesising the compound Surfacen, which increases the respiratory efficiency of the alveolar lining cells in the lungs. This has proven singularly effective in preventing death by hyaline membrane disease. Moreover, the RDS (Respiratory Disorder Syndrome) in premature babies responds well to Surfacen.

The Cuban experience with Surfacen, in the context of a socialist system which renders access to medical treatment universal and free at point of delivery, is all the more remarkable when one compares it with the situation in the developed world. In Japan, the United States, Germany, Sweden and Britain drugs similar to Surfacen are used. But each 100 miligrammes (as of 1998) costs U.S. $1250 and every patient needing it requires 100 miligrammes per kg of body weight!

Abortion and its Social Context

Of course, abortion is available upon a woman's demand in Cuba, although commonly quoted propaganda to the effect that Cuban School girls are encouraged to use abortion as contraception have no basis in fact. The only restriction is that the woman concerned must sign the request in the presence of two other witnesses - often nurses on duty at the time - and it is generally not recommended after thirty weeks of pregnancy. This is tied in with a programme for Prenatal Diagnosis, for which every ante-natal clinic is equipped. Its main purpose is to detect congenital disorders of the neural tube and other embryonic malformations and this allows the mother to interrupt the pregnancy if she so desires.

With respect to ante-natal care, the compliance of women in attending is almost total. This might seem remarkable when contrasted with the situation in the developed nations, but the CDR (and the FMC) are active in promoting it. Each CDR knows which women on the street are due to attend ante-natal clinics and the pressures brought to bear on them to do so are not so subtle! The aim is for every pregnant woman to give birth at her local maternity hospital, and not at any other outlet, such as the polyclinic. The latter are equipped to handle delivery in an emergency, but the emphasis is so much on getting all deliveries done at the maternity hospital that each pregnant woman attending the ante-natal clinics is given at least one ultrasound scan. If an anomaly is suspected, further such scans are carried out. She can be advised to terminate the pregnancy, but cannot be compelled to do so. Such a high level of ante-natal care in a third world country has to be seen as remarkable.

Paediatric Cardiac Care

Along with all of this, the 1980's witnessed immense developments in paediatric heart care. By 1988, three paediatric hospitals in Cuba could boast a cardiocentre - one in Havana, one in Villa Clara and the other in Santiago. These centres are institutions specialised in heart diseases. They include full facilities for cardiovascular surgery to be performed on children below the age of three years. They were originally brought into being as part of a more modest programme, started in 1980, to facilitate premature detection of cardiac disease in children, but like so many health initiatives in Cuba, they have vastly superseded their original brief. They render assistance to about 8 - 10 babies, out of each 1000 live births, who suffer from congenital cardiopathies of one type of another.

Needless to say, the successful mediation of such a comprehensive service in childhood public health, requires highly flexible and conscientious medical experts. These are now provided by the new family doctors, which have been trained since 1984.

The New Family Doctors

By 1981, there were various indications that, although Cuban advances in medicine were largely meeting the needs of people, some disarticulation was being occasioned by radical breakthroughs in the research front of considerable practical potential, and many working G.P's were unable to apply the fruits of such work to the family members whose health they were charged with guarding. Meetings of medical educators from the various medical schools were convened in 1982 and 1983 to ascertain how best to address this problem.

In July 1983, a plan was put forward by which every medical graduate who either volunteered or was assigned to community general practice could be given a three year part-time course in family medicine that would then make him/her a recognised specialist in that area. Especially in the context of the serious attempts being made from outside of Cuba to destabilise it economically, it was decided that such a proposal would be impossibly expensive to mount. Instead, an alternative proposal was put forward, and accepted in 1984 by Poder Popular, by which Family Medicine would be accorded speciality status and that an objective would be for at least 20% of Cuba's general practitioners to qualify in that speciality by 1989. The extra qualification would require at least 3 years study in the context of work experience as a general practitioner.

General practitioners were asked to apply for selection for the training. So many applied that an extra condition was then imposed : only GP's with 5 or more years of experience would be accepted onto the strenuous part-time training programme. Again, Government plans were superseded and, as of 1989, in excess of 50% of Cuba's population had family medicine specialists as their regular doctors.

Equality of Access to Family Doctors

No effort has been spared in trying to make equitable the distribution of these specialists. They are now found in both urban and rural areas, mountainous communities with notoriously difficult access, educational institutions, industries, merchant and fishing fleets, nursing homes for the elderly, the armed forces and in the Ministry of the Interior.

The philosophy behind this development is that the doctor must be perceived as an integral part of his/her own community. A family medicine specialist who has to commute, say from a teaching hospital, to see people in a distant urban area, would be regarded as contrary to this basic idea. Within a community, he/she not only sees patients in the ordinary way, making regular calls on homes, schools and workplaces in his/her district, but also must be involved in such community health activities as local food safety, hygiene committees, sheltered workshop provision, etc. Such a specialist is expected to occupy a high profile in the elimination of environmental problems, addressing sources of community stress (such as bad housing and bad social habits within families). He/she is to be seen as an agent for health promotion and as an advocate for preventive and prophylactic projects and other enterprises aimed at improving community health.

Often by innovatory means, such as participating in street theatre or fairs and

158

carnival occasions, the family doctor attempts to modify poor dietary l
behaviour patterns (such as a sedentary life style), inappropriate child
etc. In the 1984 enabling legislation, specific reference was made to t
Family Doctor should make an impact on the incidence of ischaemic c
number one cause of death among Cubans, as it also is in the U.S. and Britain. The
preconditions for these conditions are said to reside chiefly in life-style modalities,
especially the eating of the wrong types of food and of sedentary habits. It is at this
level that the 1984 legislation envisioned the army of Family Health specialists acting.

They also find themselves working to prevent premature pregnancies,
supporting family planning and fighting against smoking and alcoholism. In industry,
they are seen as guardians of worker health. For instance, in a number of workplaces
they have reported increasing rates of hypertension and this has led to a major research
initiative, sponsored by the Ministry of Public Health and begun in 1991. Another
research initiative organised by Family Health doctors has centred on the fact that
certain areas seem to have a higher than average incidence of congenital malformations
and/or medical retardation.

An outstanding account of the role of these specialists was published in 1992
by MINSAP (The Cuban Ministry of Public Health). It is strongly recommended that
interested readers consult that account.[52] A full account of the organisation and
philosophy of the Family Doctor programme is given in Chapter Eleven.

Life-Expectancy Rates

The World Health Organisation recognises Life Expectancy at Birth as one of the
fundamental health indices on the basis of which empirical comparisons between
societies and nations can be made. The Cuban average, including male and female, life
expectancy at birth was measured at 75.2 in April 1991 -78.1 for women and 73.0 for

---

[52]MINSAP (together with UNICEF, UNFDA, OPS and OMS), 1992: Cuba's Family Doctor
Programme (English translation by Cynthis Slade) ISBN 92/806/0999/8.

men. That places it in the top 5 of the world's nations and far beyond any of the other third world nations. How have such impressive figures been brought about?

The answer is to be found in analysis of Cuban epidemiological data, especially over the past two decades. The big killers of older people in most of the advanced industrial nations - Britain, the U.S. Canada, etc. - are related to hypothermia. In heavy winter conditions, even when people over 70 years of age are living in centrally heated accommodation and are adequately fed and clothed, it can sometimes only take a brief exposure to cruelly low temperatures combined with wind (say, while waiting at a bus stop or standing at one's own door trying to fish out a latchkey) to initiate a terminal decline in health. It goes without saying that, if that is true of the well looked after, it applies with even greater force to the homeless, of which we see increasing numbers in the major industrialised countries.

When we come to Cuba, hypothermia is not a problem, nor is homelessness. The Cuban climate is such that one could sleep on the streets and remain healthy, but the fact is that no-one does. Epidemiological figures in the metropolitan countries next list common contagious diseases as the major triggers to geriatric ill-health. In Cuba these were, until 1984, first on the list. Relentlessly, the vaccination programmes eroded this source of death until finally, by 1984, the major causes of adult death appeared on the lists as heart disease of various types and cancers. Even the non-medical reader can gain a far better appreciation of these phenomena by carefully looking through the date in Appendix A.

Thus it was principally the success of the Cuban vaccination programmes of the 70's and early 80's, that made such an impact on life expectancy. Also, it must be remarked that it is in infancy and pre-school childhood that most deaths characteristically occur. Once death rates were reduced among children under five years of age, and large numbers of ages less than five were no longer averaged in, the mean length of life rose greatly.

The Cuban national health system is a complex enterprise and it is, on that account, often difficult to ascertain the antecedents of various epidemiological details . With 35 specialist medical services (as in 1991) available to every Cuban, a doctor for every 305 inhabitants, 5.7 hospital beds for every 1000 Cubans, 264 hospitals, 421 polyclinics, 113 nursing homes for the elderly, 23 blood banks and 12 medical research institutes - any attempt to state categorically what accounts for Cuba's good lifespan figures poses problems ! But there are certain features of the Cuban health service that are unique and these may well have a bearing on the issue .

There is, for instance, a particularly aggressive programme for the premature detection of both cervical and breast cancer. Likewise, Cuba is one of the only countries in the world with an organised plan for the prevention of renal failure. Again, researchers have shown an immense amount of interest in allergy-related phenomena in Cuba . Apparently something in excess of 12% of the population suffers from it - especially asthma and eczema. Since 1989, doubtless as a result of early detection and prevention, the figures for asthma among school children had declined by 1991. It has apparently risen again since 1994 (See Chapter Sixteen) as direct result of the Blockade. This, in time, is bound to have a positive impact on life-expectancy. This is particularly interesting, as asthma incident among school children in Europe and North America actually rose over the same period.

Smoking, though, needs to be much more aggressively addressed as the health hazard that it is before much further progress in countering cardiac and respiratory illness can be made.

The Struggle Against AIDS

When one speaks of the flexibility of the Cuban system of public health, it would be difficult indeed to find a better example of it than has been reflected in its complete turn around with respect to the question of AIDS. When the author was in Cuba in 1984, The official attitude towards AIDS was replete with all of the worst features of an ideology based on sexism, homophobia and moral intolerance. When questioned back then about the incidence of AIDS in Cuba, an official of the ministry of public health made several points:

a. AIDS is spread by homosexual contact. As will be shown in Chapter Ten, even this turned out not to be as true in Cuba as is the case in the U.S.

  b. Homosexuality is a reflection of defective social development and a
      symptom of capitalist attitudes.

  c. Homosexuality hardly exists in socialist Cuba!

  d. Any victims of AIDS in Cuba had either been misbehaving abroad or with
      other Cubans who had been abroad.

I would not have believed it possible that in only 15 years such a change in attitude has been effected as has been. Even in primary school, children are taught about AIDS in a context of compassion for the victims. Homosexuality is no longer denigrated nor denied. It is probably true to say that Cuba is now perhaps the most socially enlightened of all the Latin American/Caribbean nations with respect to tolerant acceptance of homosexual life-styles.

Started in 1987, a fully rational approach to the AIDS problem was initiated, in co-operation with the ministries of : Defence, Public Health, Education and Social Welfare. By 1990, Dr Jonathon Mann, Director of WHO's 'Global Programme Against AIDS' was able to say:

"The Cuban programme of struggle against AIDS deserves special
recognition. It is effective because it is guided entirely by
epidemiological data and the objective analysis of it".

He went on to say how profoundly he had been impressed by:

"the compassion shown sufferers, the quality of diagnosis, the uses of
the mass media to educate the population on matters of sanitation and
sex education for students."

As of 1991, Cuba was absolutely the only country on earth that imposed compulsory examinations for HIV+ infection and of AIDS on the whole population of people aged 12 years and over. As well, sanatoria have been set up for treatment of any victims.

WHO, in 1991, listed Cuba as having one of the lowest incidents of HIV+ infection and of AIDS.

By August 1990, over 75% of the sexually active population had been tested. Of these, 479 HIV+ people were identified, after 8,530,000 tests had been carried out. The figures as of January 1993 were said to be 800 people HIV+ and 90 with active AIDS.[53] By February 1998, with over 85% of the sexually active population tested, about 1300 people were recorded HIV+ and 230 with active AIDS. The HIV+/AIDS issue is of such wide interest, and Cuba's approach to it so honest and reflective of revolutionary values that an entire chapter has been devoted to it. See Chapter Ten. An excellently written account of the phenomenon (up until June 1993) is to be found in "Aids in Cuba".[54]

Cuba's Assault on Hepatitis B

It may startle readers to realise that, as of 1992, Hepatitis B is considered to be the most widespread contagious disease in the world, including AIDS. It especially menaces children born to infected mothers and it is at this health front that Cuban medicine has notched up yet another victory.

Hepatitis B is transmitted via the bloodstream and commonly is passed on during sexual relations and in the `perinatal period'. This latter is the technical term given the interval of time just prior to, during and just after delivery of a baby. As shall be made clear, Cuba has made gigantic strides in both genetic engineering and medical biotechnology. One fruit of this activity has been the production of a Hepatitis B vaccine. A measure of its potential applicability is given by the grim statistic that about 300 million people worldwide carry the disease!

---

[53]Quoting Dr Joaquin Percy Labrador, Vice - Director of Medical Social Assistance for province of Pinar del Rio, in an interview granted April 4, 1993.

[54] Waller, J; Adams, L; Lyms, B; Redgrave, P and Schatzberger, P. (1993) AIDS in Cuba - A Portrait of Prevention. Cuba Solidarity Committee, London.

The programme to vaccinate the children of hepatitis B carriers during the perinatal period began as a pilot project two years ago in Pinar del Rio, City of Havana, Matanzas and Santiago de Cuba, and it has now spread throughout the whole country.

At the beginning of a pregnancy's first trimester, expecting mothers are given a blood test to localise the superficial antigen of Hepatitis B, which indicates infection by the virus.

In the maternity wards themselves, the children of mothers who carry the virus are already given a first dose of the vaccine. The vaccination plan is completed with two more doses when the baby is one month, then again when two months old. Another injection is given at the end of a year.

Children who acquire the virus in the perinatal stage run a 90 percent risk of developing a chronic infection .

Dr Graciela Delgado, head of MINSAP's Hepatitis Control Programme, indicated that vaccination has also begun for high-risk groups, such as the health care workers who attend to the country's nephrology services and patients who undergo dialysis or hemodialysis or are awaiting transplant. Early protection via active vaccination is recognised as the only effective way to prevent the state of carrier, serious and chronic infections and the long-term consequences of Hepatitis.

CHAPTER TEN

HOW CUBA DEALS WITH HIV+ / AIDS

From Reaction to Action

As mentioned in Chapter Nine, Cuba moved quickly on the HIV+/AIDS issue from a position of homophobia (resonant of the Latin American macho tradition) and ideological intolerance (reminiscent of Stalinism) to a position reflecting a higher level of social insight and community responsibility than found almost anywhere else in the world. The strategy guiding its 1984 programme was five-fold:

1. Introduction of HIV screening of all adults in an attempt to locate infected people.
2. Development of residential facilities (called 'sanatoria') for isolating infected people, with a view to offering treatment if and when they developed AIDS.
3. Testing of the blood supply to prevent HIV contamination.
4. Initiation of high profile research programmes to treat either people with full-blown AIDS and even those who only tested HIV+.
5. Targeting youngsters, high-risk groups and the population generally - but in terms of identifiable groupings, such as by gender or age-group - with accurate and non-moralistic educational programmes about the AIDS risk.

Obviously such an undertaking carried enormous cost implications but the Poder Popular was readily persuaded by dispassionate argument that this would save money in the long run and serve to enhance the social integrity of the nation.

The HIV/AIDS Situation in Cuba as of 1985

As pointed out in Waller, et.al (1992), the epidemiolgy of HIV+/AIDS in Cuba tended to be different from that experienced in most other countries. For one thing, it was not most conspicuous among the poor, but among Cubans who had spent time overseas (such as returned servicemen or medical volunteers). Also the condition in Cuba was not so dominantly associated with the gay community as had been the case in San Francisco. From 1986 onwards, anyone returning from service abroad was tested on return and then again six months later.

It is also a positive reflection on Cuban values that the use of drugs is not the problem that it is here and the almost all HIV infection is spread by sexual contact alone rather than by shared needles. Young people, therefore, are the main risk group because of their proclivity for unsafe sexual activity. This does represent a bit of a sticking point not only because condom use tended at first to be resisted by the Cuban men (a Latin American phenomenon generally) but because the US Blockade has meant that access to condoms has not been as easy to facilitate in Cuba as in other countries.

Up until July 1998, approximately 35 million blood tests had been made for HIV infection. By now the Cuban population, especially the adult population, must have all been tested and most more than once. By 1992 new-borns were also being routinely screened. On top of all this, HIV+ people are of particular interest to the health authorities and any partners they may have are tested routinely. Even a routine sexual partner is tested three or four times (once every three months) after the initial contact.

Isolating Infection

When Cuba first set out, in 1986, to isolate HIV+ people, the programme became the focus for suspicion in Cuba itself among some, but was a target for intensely hostile propaganda outside of Cuba. The US press, in particular, was full of stories

166

about concentration camp-like establishments in which people were held under harshly punitive conditions against their will. The truth of the matter is much less sanguine and does not fit the totalitarian image that Cuba demonizers would prefer. People are not grabbed off the streets and arbitrarily slammed into sanatoria. Instead, once a person has been identified as HIV+, he/she is offered the opportunity to enter a sanatorium. Many, in fact, accept rather readily as the sanatoria have a reputation in Cuba as pleasant places indeed, but obviously an even larger number are reluctant to do so. All sorts of pressures are gradually applied, beginning with the strong advice of the family doctor and then of CDR members, etc. The matter is discussed openly and in most cases the person finally acquiesces. Under Cuban law - but only as a last resort - a person can be compelled to enter a sanatorium.

The institution themselves are well appointed and most are purpose-built. The one which the present author visited in 1996 (Los Cocos in Havana) had been built a decade earlier - and like many institutions in Cuba reflected the usual need of repainting - but was far removed from the holding fortress image projected in the US media. Instead it was more similar to a family holiday camp, with inviting ground, swimming pool, etc. There was certainly no evidence of barbed wire fencing, guards or other prison-like features. Los Cocos is pretty well self-contained with its own library, cinema, sports and crafts facilities, a drama and music workshop, etc. Moreover, the residents routinely integrate - under supervision- with the larger community outside, with trips to the shops, beaches, etc.

Living quarters are motel-like apartments for singles or couples, equipped with the usual facilities such as TV, kitchenette, etc. Meals are provided in a central dining hall and, of course, medical care is accessible on site. In all, life in a sanatorium has much to recommend it and it generally does not take much to persuade a person to take up residence.

Once a person has entered a sanatorium, their social rights remain intact. For instance, their income continues and, wherever possible, they are encouraged to continue with the same kind of work they had been doing outside. They all participate in the day-to-day administration of the facility. Much emphasis is placed on the psychological impact on both the individual and of his/her community of HIV+ infection. In the sanatorium itself, the stress is on the development of an optimistic outlook and positive self-esteem, while back in the person's neighbourhood, the affected family is given positive support by the local CDR. Neighbourhood education programmes are featured, emphasising tolerance and acceptance.

Enforcement of Quarantine

As stated earlier, while it is true that residence in a sanatorium is not to be equated with a custodial sentence and that arbitrary arrest and detention are not the vade mecum for entry, their purpose is to protect the community and there consequently has to be ultimate authority to consign someone to one against their will. An even greater problem arises as far as holding people there once they have taken up residence. Treatment can seem long to a person who is anxious to re-establish family and community links and hence the temptation to abscond is often great.

Generally speaking, such "runners" have returned within days, either because their contacts outside (family, etc.) persuade them of the wisdom of going back or because they themselves voluntarily do so. In the cases of a few really intransigent cases, tougher measures are called into play. The person is apprehended and held by the authorities while a psychological counsellor has one to one sessions with the person. If this fails, the person is usually sent to another sanatorium.

These sanatoria are administered in such a way as to reduce the risk of unauthorised departure. For the first six months, supervision of a resident is close. Although he (or she) is consulted in planning his/her daily activities, a schedule is drawn up for each person within two days of arrival, and each new person is assigned an 'adviser' (another, but more experienced inmate) who insures that the schedule is observed. Visits by relatives and friends are allowed, usually in the afternoons. Once that initial six months has passed, however, the regime becomes much more friendly. For instance, many (somewhat in access of 80% in 1998) residents are allowed out on three day weekends, unaccompanied, and on an honour system under which they agree only to have sex with one regular partner.

Of course, critics of anything Cuban have been quick to point out that it is highly totalitarian to run a system of incarceration (however pleasant conditions may be) in which authorities other than the police and/or the courts decide whether or not a person should lose his freedom. But such commentary is fatuous. In freedom-loving Britain, people can be 'sectioned' under the Mental Health Act and - as Waller et al pointed out in their 1992 book[55], many American states force tubercular patients to spend a year in sanatoria against their will.

Medical Treatment

The sanatoria, of course, are not merely holding centres - like old-style leper colonies - to protect the broader community. Medical treatment, which despite the Blockade, is constantly being updated, is provided and to the degree that the patient wishes. That is, whether a person accepts any medical treatment at all, is a matter of their choice. But even once treatment is agreed to, the actual conduct and extent of the treatment is carefully discussed with, and subject to the approval of, the patient at each step in its development.

On entry, the vast majority of patients have no symptoms of illness, but have tested HIV-positive. Therefore, with them the first priority is to build up their general health. To this end they are given a highly nutritious diet, comprising in excess of 5000 calories daily, and supplemented with the RDA's of all vitamins. Physical fitness is promoted and, of course, facilities for doing so are much better in the sanatoria, in many cases, than in the patients own community.

---

[55] Waller, J et al. (1992) - ibid. Chapter Nine.

As AIDS symptomology manifests itself, the medical treatment becomes much more specifically focused. There is considerable variation in this, from one patient to another, but broadly the pharmacological regime is virtually the same as it is in the industrialised nations. Death at the sanatoria is largely avoided by transferring patients to the Institute for Tropical Medicine just prior to the onset of terminal illness.

While it has already been commented that Cuba's health care system is certainly the most advanced of any third world country, its record with respect to HIV/AIDS is even more startling. Most third world nations cannot afford the necessary pharmaceuticals, let alone provide the psychological and social infrastructure that are part and parcel of the Cuban system. AZT and Interferon are both extremely expensive and what is more, the U.S. is making every effort - under Bill Clinton's administration - to try to cut off supplies of AZT to Cuba using Embargo legislation. Interferon is now manufactured in Cuba.

Epidemiology of HIV+/AIDS in Cuba

Table 10.1 shows the incidence - as of May 1, 1998 - of HIV+/AIDS in Cuba.

Table 10.1: Incidence and Mortality of HIV+/AIDS in Cuba (May

Year	HIV+ People	AIDS Cases	AIDS Dea
1986	99	14	2
1987	75	17	4
1988	94	20	6
1989	120	22	5
1990	137	21	24
1991	180	23	22
1992	146	21	17
1993	195	24	24
1994	238	39	31
1995	273	53	39
1996	308	65	31
1997	316	86	47
1998	344	104	49
TOTAL	**2525**	**441**	**305**

To give some idea of how these figures compare with other Caribbean countries, one has only to look at, say, the Dominican Republic and Jamaica. The Dominican Republic has a population of just over 4 million. Its 1996 figures for HIV+ people, AIDS cases and AIDS deaths were: 810, 280 and 158.[56] Cuba had nearly three times the population of the Dominican Republic in 1996 yet its figures for all of these categories were far lower. Jamaica in 1998, had a population of only 2 million, yet its figures for these three categories were also higher than Cuba's for 1998, being: 449, 250 and 122 respectively.[57] While the Cuban figures suggest that rates of infection gradually increased from 1986 up to 1993, it has since - equally gradually - slowed down to some degree, the figures in the other third

---

[56] WHO (1997) Report 'Health Profile of the Dominican Republic for 1996'. Geneva.

[57] Private Correspondence : Infectious Diseases Centre, UWI Hospital, Mona, 1998

171

world countries reflect spectacular increases and no sign of it being brought under control.

Of course, Cuba's good statistics not only reflect the impact of the specific measures described in this chapter, but probably owe much to the excellent levels of basic health enjoyed by Cubans since the revolution. As well, one must not forget social and psychological factors. Not only do all Cubans have easy access to medical care but they have an extraordinarily high level of social responsibility, as nurtured by such institutions as the CDR's, schools, etc. and are used to co-operating with the implementation of health measures in the community.

In the excellent 1993 account by John Waller and colleagues, already referred to, there occurs a wonderful excerpt of a letter to the New York Times (16/2/1993) written by some Cuban citizens infected with HIV who were, at the time, all active in AIDS prevention. It is quoted, as follows:

> The US can learn from Cuba's AIDS programme
> "Cuba has the same population as New York City. Visiting and exchanging experiences with AIDS care providers in your city….we learned that New York has had 42,737 reported cases of….AIDS. Cuba has 159.
>
> Your Center for Disease Control, which has no official figure of AIDS deaths, says that two-thirds of reported cases of AIDS can be assumed to have died. That means that…at least 28,000 New Yorkers have died. In Cuba, where records are kept, the number who have died of AIDS is 84.
>
> Nobody knows how many New Yorkers are carrying the virus; the estimates vary from 5 to 10 times the number of…AIDS cases. In Cuba, after massive routine (not mandatory) testing, fewer than 900 have tested positive…..
>
> Even more heartbreaking are the figures relating to children. New York City has 987 reported cases of pediatric AIDS; more babies are born with HIV every day and children are dying or left orphans at a frightening rate. In Cuba only one child has died of AIDS; three are carrying the virus….
>
> To those who say that we Cubans who are HIV positive are deprived of our rights, or that our health benefits come at too high

172

a price, we ask:

Aren't the people who are dying of AIDS without proper medical care, often without jobs, food or housing, aren't those infected because of lack of adequate education, too little money for research, too much indifference and too much rampant individualism, paying too high a price?"

What can possibly impede such wonderful progress? Apparently, the U.S. Embargo on Cuba has the potential to do so. As discussed in Chapter Sixteen, not only is Cuba now artificially prevented from gaining access to otherwise internationally available new modalities for treating HIV and/or AIDS, it is even constrained in the degree to which it can continue with traditional AZT and Interferon treatments and even with the running of their sanatoria.

CHAPTER ELEVEN

THE FAMILY DOCTOR PROGRAMME

The Need Arises

As already indicated (Chapter 9) Cuba introduced yet another innovation in 1984 to its already versatile and complex national system of health care - namely the Family Doctor Programme. This has been fully described already in another publication[58] and the reader in search of more detailed information, would find perusal of that account of great interest.

Study of the morbidity figures in Appendix A will show the reader that during the 70's, the incidence of acute disease had declined in importance. The Cuban medical system was increasingly being faced with the needs and demands of the chronically ill. In that respect, we can say that Cuba - as a society - made the extraordinary paradigm shift in health status from a third world to a first world society. While in all naturally measured economic parameters Cuba ranks with the poor undeveloped nations, she faces the medical and educational problems of industrialised societies. Cuban epidemiology has less in common with, say, Jamaica than it does with the US!

It is beyond question that credit for this state of affairs must reside, not only in Cuba's broader social philosophy, but in the way in which Dr Julio Martinez Paez actually organised aid planned for the Public Health system back in 1959.

As we saw in Chapter Six, the linchpin of Martinez' system was to be the polyclinics. It was the polyclinics which successfully mediated all of the primary health care initiatives, such as immunisations, ante-natal and neonatal care, school health, etc. which in turn led to Cuba's spectacular successes in disease control and then prevention.

---

[58]UNICEF (with UNFPA, OPS-OMS, MINSAP), 1992: "Cuba's Family Doctor Programme!, Havana.(English translation: Cynthia Selde)

In trying to address an appropriate response to these changes from, say, 1973 onward, MINSAP declared primary health care and community health promotion to be the priority targets. Four medical specialities were held to be pivotal in promoting these two aims:

1.   Child health (Paediatrics)
2.   Maternal health (Obstetrics and Gynaecology)
3.   Internal medicine (especially enteric disorders)
4.   Dentistry.

Moreover, it was quickly realised that a team approach to such a range of health activities would be necessary and that it would have to satisfy the following criteria.

1.   Integrated health care.
2.   Inter-sectoral co-ordination.
3.   Accessibility throughout each region.
4.   A nationwide network allowing for continuity of care and access to specialist facilities as required.

This, of course, is what is now known as the Family Doctor Programme, but when it was first piloted, it had not yet been graced with that title. The Lawton Polyclinic in Havana was selected as the focus of this first pilot project in 1984. Many of the ideas brought forward by the professionals involved reflected the new community health models emergent since Lalonde's pioneering work in health promotion in Canada.[59] The emphasis was to be based less on response to individual illnesses than on response to health issues arising in the context of family and community relationships. The major change, and the one predicted at the time to cause the most difficulties, hinged on communication between various levels of the medical establishment. It was recognised that this would have to involve devoting less attention to the hierarchical

---

[59]Lalonde M (1975): A New Perspective on the Health of Canadians: Ottawa: Information Canada.

communication pathways - very characteristic of the existing system - and much more attention to means of expediting lateral lines of communication.

This was the beginning of Cuba's Family Doctor Programme, so called within six months of the Lawton Polyclinic trial run. Before 1984 had run its course, it was realised that not only would doctors in the programme have to be rotated through various sectors in the network of health related enterprises, but that GP's themselves would require specialist training in the relevant community medicine fields - to say nothing of psychology and sociology. In fact, the very reason that the Lawton Polyclinic had been selected as the trial flagship of the programme was that, included in its staff, were a number of former WHO delegates, community health workers and the like and it itself was linked to the University of Havana Medical School's Department of Social and Preventative Medicine.

Training The New Family Doctors

The success of the Lawton Clinic - and its wide popular support -showed MINSAP that they were onto a good thing. By September 1984, similar programmes had been negotiated in 19 other polyclinics. Obviously these other polyclinics did not have the trained staff that the Lawton institution had and, once again, further training became the order of the day. The University of Havana, together with some of Lawton's teaching staff, drew up twelve study units, rather like modules, which GP's could take by correspondence. Teaching staff travelled about, holding monthly 3 hour residential tutorial sessions on these materials at each of the 19 polyclinics participating. The idea was that each GP worked three full days a week at the polyclinic as a "Family Doctor in Training" and devoted the rest of the week to study.

Those people took four years to complete the units and to take the examinations required. But, by 1986, each of Cuba's medical schools was offering three year (full time study) post graduate diplomas for people wishing to qualify as Family Doctors. Medical graduates cannot enter the course immediately upon qualifying as a GP, but must have relevant hospital experience first. Until 1990, each province tended to have its own regulations regarding exactly how much on-ward hospital experience was prerequisite to entering training as a Family Doctor. But in 1991 it was standardised at two years.

The Network and Its Gatekeepers

As things stood in 1998, there was one family Doctor and ancillary nurse to every 100 - 110 families in Cuba. But these two work in a social matrix comprising a combination of voluntary and professional individuals from other agencies. For instance, every CDR has links with the network in its own district, as does the FMC. The latter, in fact, have organised "Health Brigades" in each district, which encourage and advise individuals in complying with medical care and preventative measures. It is largely because of the work of these health brigades that the average Cuban is now so knowledgeable about health matters. This author was impressed, in talking with some of these voluntary agents of the health network, at how many of them referred to the American Medical Association as providing effective models for lay education in community health matters.

Often a patient's initial contact, when troubled by a health-related issue, will be at a CDR meeting or in some other informal context. He/she is them visited by the Family Doctor and/or nurse. It is the Family Doctor who acts as the gatekeeper should the issue transcend his/her skill or resources. On the whole, the inter-sectoral communication is impressively smooth, even to the point of organising any necessary transport to other centres or the acquisition of documentation from other government ministries. As has already been said, it is as a response to chronic health problems, that the Family Health Programme was largely called into being, and this - rather than incidents of acute illness - provide most of its work.

As MINSAP itself states:

"The family doctor, then is the cornerstone of Cuba's primary health care system. As a result of the implementation of the Family Doctor

178

Programme, the organization and operation of the Polyclinics - which had been in operation prior to the institution of the Family Doctor Programme - were modified. Following the institution of the Family Doctor Programme, the Polyclinics took on a predominantly co-ordinative role, as well as that of training medical personnel and carrying out research. Another important function of the Polyclinics is that of facilitating inter-disciplinary consultations amongst different specialists regarding problems identified by family physicians. The Polyclinics also provided auxiliary diagnostic services, and it is in the Polyclinics where the family physicians receive their initial and continuous professional training.

Family physicians work closely with the Polyclinics and with other secondary and tertiary health care institutions. It is in this manner in which the specific needs of the entire population are served. This form of organization has enabled the Cuban health sector to offer prolonged attention to patients suffering from chronic illnesses, provide health education programmes and ensure immunization coverage to the entire population. It has been through this form of organization that Cuban health authorities have been able to identify and control health hazards, and control environmental risks as well.

In addition to working directly with families, in their homes, the Family Doctor Programme is implemented in workplaces, schools, day care centres, the merchant marine fleet and agricultural co-operatives, serving individuals at their places of work or study. In these cases, (see Table 1.), the physician's work is determined by the specific health situation found to prevail in each institution. For example, a physician working with children at a day care centre must address the health needs characteristic of pre-school children, including the surveillance of the children's growth and development, the prevention of accidents, the treatment of outbreaks of infectious childhood diseases, actions aimed at ensuring adequate nutrition, and other risk factors common to children of this age.

Family doctors carry out actions aimed at promoting the adoption of adequate health practices, the prevention of disease, the timely diagnosis of health problems and their treatment, and the rehabilitation of those afflicted with disease. These actions constitute an important part of the course of specialization in integral general medicine. The implementation of the Family Doctor Programme throughout the Cuban population at large has enabled the health sector to dramatically increase the timeliness of detection of disease and the referral of patients with health problems to the appropriate levels of health care and treatment. This programme has also permitted the application of a more effective direct consultation (ambulatory or out-patient) system of health care, and a programme of postoperative patient care in the home. More generally speaking, the Family Doctor Programme provides suitable conditions for conserving the population's physical and mental health, by means of practical health education and the promotion of appropriate health practices.

Health Promotion and Health Education

Children in schools, workers in factories and farms, groups gathered at CDR meetings, etc., are now all thoroughly used to seeing their local Family Health team - Doctor and Nurse - usually involved in some kind of health education activity. It is they who head up drives on sex education, family planning, classes on living with the elderly, etc. They advise teenagers on contraception and sexual life-styles, abortion and AIDS, etc. All of the Family doctors to whom this author spoke felt that these issues constituted the lion's share of their work.

A common response was to regard responses to particular questions from troubled adolescents as "health education", while regarding regular programmes which the ran in the community - even in school - as "health promotion".
MINSAP states[60]:

> The chief objective of the Family Doctor Programme is to improve the state of health of the Cuban population in its entirety, through the implementation of integral, broadly-based health programmes aimed at serving the needs of families, communities, and the physical environment in a dynamically interrelated fashion. The normative documents for this programme set forth the following specific objectives:
>
> i)   The promotion of health by disseminating relevant and

---

[60]Work Plan for the Family Doctor Programme, Polyclinic and Hospital, Republic of Cuba, MINSAP March 1988.

useful health information and the adoption of
appropriate health and hygiene habits on the part of
individuals and the community at large.

ii)   The prevention of the outbreak of disease and damage
        to the health of the population.

iii)   Guarantee the timely diagnosis and integral treatment
        of disease through the system of direct consultation and
        hospital health care.

iv)   Provide community-based rehabilitation (CBR) for
        physically and mentally ill community members.

The Smoking Issue

As previous chapters have indicated, and as the data in Appendix A also attests, this
combination of health education and health promotion, mediated through the smoothly
articulated network of Cuba's Family Doctor Programme, has so far been outstandingly
successful in most respects. One area stands out as not having been as successfully
addressed, and that is the area of respiratory illness. Cuba's response to such illness has
been both vigorous and resourceful in terms of treatment and diagnosis. It is at the
level of prevention that fault can be found.

It is now a truism in medical circles in the developed countries that the largest
single risk factor in respiratory health - if not to health generally - is the smoking of
tobacco. But Cuba's stand on this has been ambiguous at best until now it is at least 25
years behind the developed nations with respect to community attitudes to, and
knowledge of, the health risks of tobacco. For instance, only since 1987 have Cuban
manufactured tobacco products for domestic use carried the health warnings used in
the UK and the US since the 1960's. A common-enough attitude, even among many
educated people, is that: "In theory it's bad for you, but so is too much of anything" -
rather like the indulgent, semi-humorous comment a Londoner might make about
taking sugar in his tea. Most hospital doctors I met in Cuba were themselves smokers
and admitted that, even when dealing with asthmatic patients, smoking was something

181

they rarely advised against. "After all, everyone enjoys a fag now and then and it would be a bit hypocritical for me to say anything about it!"

In a secondary school in Pinar del Rio, I asked a class of 16 - 17 year olds what they thought was the single greatest easily preventable cause of death in Cuba. They came up with all sorts of things, some of them not at all easy to prevent, including AIDS and air disasters! When I mentioned cigarette smoking, they all laughed and looked out of the louvered windows leading into the corridor. There, only slightly embarrassed, stood their teacher having a smoke! Obviously smoking in classrooms and hallways of Cuban schools is prohibited, as it is any other country, but it is frequently done and blind eyes are courteously turned. The same holds true in many of the hospitals and polyclinics this author visited.

The reason for Cuba's reluctance to act more decisively on such a comparatively simple matter is not hard to find. Cuba produces some of the world's finest tobacco products. Cigar-makers are regarded as craftsmen of a very high status and introduce themselves with great pride. Some I spoke to were not even aware that it had been definitively established that tobacco was a killer and thought of it as a passing preoccupation, rather like cranberries and stomach cancer. One cigar-maker I spoke to at length in Cienfuegos, proudly told me that he was apprenticed to a cigar-maker at age 9 and had been at it steadily for 57 years! When I asked for his view about the health implications, he said: "Well, you can always find something wrong with anything - even sex. If the scientists think that smoking cigarettes is harmful, it might be the paper causing the problem, not the tobacco. Nobody says that smoking cigars is bad!"

Responsible authorities in MINSAP know the truth and have, since 1974, periodically initiated campaigns against smoking tobacco. Some of these have been extremely imaginative and forceful, but never sustained or total. When tobacco mosaic destroyed a huge percentage of Cuba's tobacco crop in the 70's (an epidemic widely attributed to CIA activity at the time), drastic reductions in the domestic tobacco ration were invoked. This was backed up by the inclusion of strong anti-smoking components in school hygiene syllabi. But once that particular economic crisis was

182

circumvented, and the standard tobacco ration was back in place, the anti-smoking message was no longer emphasised. This author's impression is that, at the community level, people tend to regard the smoking and health issue as one of those things that the authorities periodically get excited about for political or economic reasons.

Broader Social Effects

An interesting, if partially predictable, impact of the Family Doctor Programme has been on general social consciousness and on popular insight into social structures. Cubans, unlike British or North American people, had had 25 years of communist indoctrination before the health care system became formally organised along the health promotion lines enshrined in the Family Doctor Programme. They had already grown accustomed to interacting with social policy matters through the CDR's, for instance, and were (by 1984) much more alert to issues relating to community ethics and social responsibility than were most of their counterparts in the first world nations. Therefore, linking into the newly fashioned national health network, with the local family doctor and nurse as gatekeepers, in a sense simply reinforced and validated many attitudes that had already become almost instinctive.

Through increasing public awareness of general health and nutritional matters, for instance, mediated through lay discussion in such venues as CDR and FMC meetings or in work collectives, the Family Doctor Programme enhanced neighbourhood participatory and advocacy skills. Such skills soon transcended purely medical matters, linking with matters relating to transport, domestic and industrial rights, schooling, etc.

This broader impact of the programme is reflected in the essentially sociological perceptive of many of the articles now appearing in the Cuban Review of Integrated Health care[61]. This journal is published monthly by MINSAP and is made up of contributions sent in by family doctors themselves, reporting and reflecting on various

---

[61]Revista Cubana de Salud Integral.

aspects of their work. It is one medical journal which most Cuban doctors actually read and, since it is available in the waiting rooms of many family doctor clinics, not a few lay people also dip into it.

Action Points of the Programme

As the reader will gather from the account given so far, the major focus (or "point of action" as MINSAP call it) of the programme is between doctor and family at the clinic. In fact, this accounts for about 72% of the service commitment of the family physicians. The other 28% are divided between factory and workplace clinics (about 6%), schools and colleges (about 8%), polyclinics (about 1% and all other outlets (13%). This latter includes the armed forces, epidemiological research units, prisons, etc. But, as well as these "fixed" commitments, there is a fair bit of interflow between these action points. For instance, although a particular polyclinic may have 1% of the region's family physicians on its regular staff, each other family physician in the district is rostered for duties there, so that the doctor at the family clinic is perfectly aware of what the situation at the local polyclinic is when he/she sends a patient there.

Fig. 11.1 shows the situation as it prevailed in 1990. The actual percentages of point allocation have not changed much between 1990 and now, nor are they likely to.

Fig 11.1. Cuba: Share of Total Population Served by Family Doctor Programme, by Province, 1990

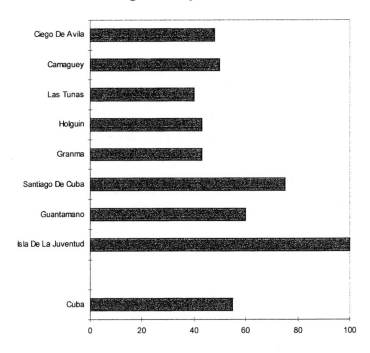

Moving from the family clinic action point to the Polyclinic, we find that the basic medical staff consists of about 20 doctors, each paired with a nurse. But they are augmented by such specialists as professors of internal medicine, obstetricians, clinical psychologists, social workers, etc. This augmented team is, of course, supported by a variegated service staff - from typists to technicians to cleaners. One of the articulating functions of the polyclinic is to co-ordinate the participation of specialists from the regional hospital in areas such as: dermatology, psychiatry, orthopaedics, surgery, immunology, ophthalmology, etc. Much of this activity is given further focus by epidemiological reports on small communities sent in by the family doctors.

185

An Example of Integrated Medicine in Action

Probably the best way to illustrate both the simplicity and the complexity of the programme is to show how it articulates around a specific medical problem. MINSAP's own publication[62] does this with respect to chronic kidney disease (CKD) and it is from this publication that we now quote:

> "Between 100 and 120 people per million inhabitants die each year in Cuba of chronic kidney disease (CKD). The rate of infant mortality attributable to this cause ranges from 7.4 to 7.6 per million children. Cuba's annual morbidity rate for kidney disease is over 30 per 100,000 inhabitants. This disease is detected, in over sixty percent of the cases, in advanced stages of development. The treatment of chronic cases must be referred to secondary levels of health care. Early detection of the disease and control of risk factors are essential in abating the incidence and severity of the disease. Such activities are carried out by the family doctor.

All of the above is indicated schematically in Fig. 11.2 below.

---

[62]Ibid 1, p 23.

Fig 11.2. Cuba: Ties Between Family Doctors and Higher Levels of Health Care*

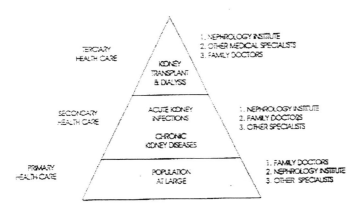

* This example corresponds to the care of chronic kidney disease.

Achievements so far

When the Family Doctor Programme was pioneered back in 1984 in Havana, the basic idea was that the service should not be perceived as purely a reactive, emergency, interventionary response to illness; but that it be regarded as a community resource for healthful living in the widest possible sense. It was intended to reflect the best of a personal, human, warm relationship based on trust and honesty. In the intervening years, the programme has wholly justified itself along these lines, but also at the purely statistical level, it has shown itself capable of addressing close to 95% of all health problems on a direct consultational basis.

This is reflected in tables 11.1, 11.2 and 11.3 derived from MINSAP's account of the programme[63]

[63] Ibid 1 pages 26, 28 and 29 respectively.

Table 11.1: Rates of Detection Per 1000 people of Hypertension in General Population Compared with Population Served by Family Doctor Programme 1988.

Provinces	Amongst general population	Population served by Family Doctor Prog.
Pinar del Rio	23.0	55.0
Havana	36.6	77.5
Havana City	59.9	74.7
Matanzas	68.7	71.0
Villa Clara	30.0	57.4
Cienfuegos	36.0	69.0
Sancti Spiritus	23.9	33.9
Ciego de Avila	14.0	70.9
Camaguey	20.8	50.4
Las Tunas	17.2	43.2
Holquin	34.0	71.1
Granma	12.1	22.4
Santiago de Cuba	29.7	35.6
Guantanamo	25.2	46.1
Isla de las Juventud	19.7	93.3
TOTAL	**37.0**	**60.0**

Table 11.2: Rates of Detection Per 1000 People of Asthma in the General Population Compared with Population Served by Family Doctor Programme.

Provinces	Amongst general population	Population served by Family Doctor Prog.
Pinar del Rio	13.4	40.4
Havana	24.6	62.6
Havana City	33.3	50.7
Matanzas	13.7	40.3
Villa Clara	15.2	24.3
Cienfuegos	16.2	29.3
Sancti Spiritus	11.5	24.2
Ciego de Avila	13.4	55.5
Camaguey	12.4	40.1
Las Tunas	12.8	39.2
Holguin	21.6	51.9
Granma	8.1	16.8
Santiago de Cuba	20.6	31.7
Guantanamo	12.3	39.1
Isla de las Juventud	14.3	80.4
TOTAL	**20.5**	**41.1**

Table 11.3: Rates of Detection Per 1000 People of Diabetes in the General Population compared with Population Served by Family Data Programme.

Provinces	Amongst general population	Population served by Family Doctor Prog.
Pinar del Rio	11.8	22.0
Havana	18.0	27.4
Havana City	21.8	23.7
Matanzas	26.3	17.2
Villa Clara	15.7	17.0
Cienfuegos	11.8	17.6
Sancti Spiritus	10.4	10.1
Ciego de Avila	8.7	20.8
Camaguey	8.2	14.9
Las Tunas	6.9	7.7
Holquin	15.7	31.4
Granma	5.2	5.8
Santiago de Cuba	12.5	8.6
Guantanamo	8.6	8.7
Isla de las Juventud	5.8	27.3
TOTAL	**15.1**	**18.8**

At the health promotion level, we have seen that the programme was designed to bring about changes in life-style, as much as anything else. With respect to smoking, the impact has been muted - although MINSAP's publication[64] stoutly denies this. But it has been spectacularly successful in other areas - such as sedentary life-styles and even

---

[64] ibid 1, p 27

190

alcohol consumption. As well, the programme - by encouraging open-ended community participation - has generated some remarkably innovatory initiatives. One of these is the Grandparents' Circles. These are comprised of community members of 60 years or over who meet daily for exercise routines and less obviously gross muscular recreations. In these groups, great emphasis is placed on addressing issues of loneliness and marginalization - intimidating aspects of old age anywhere in the world. Just as one often feels that Cuba might well be the "society of choice" for a young child, it would also be a much better place to live when retired than many other consumer-oriented societies which spring to mind!

Coming back to the general issue of life-style education, though, the impact of the programme on local communities since 1984 has been particularly notable in the areas of:

1. Women's health - especially prenatal and peri-natal education and care.
2. Care and socialisation of neonates.
3. Parent education.
4. Childhood growth and development - both physical and psychological.
5. Aggressive promotion of the "breast is best" concept.
6. Immunisations.
7. Inculcation of a broader sense of community responsibility for young people, including adolescents.
8. Family Planning.
9. Sex education in schools.
10. Reducing hospitalisation by emphasising the normality of consultations about health rather than only in response to illness.

With respect to this latter point the author once more most gratefully acknowledges MINSAP's publication[65] in the following direct quote.

---

[65]Ibid 1, page 39.

The Family Doctors Role In Reducing The Rate of Hospitalisation: The Case of Pinar Del Rio.

The Provincial Training Paediatric Hospital in Pinar del Rio Province provides advanced paediatric care for the entire province. This hospital has a 415 bed capacity. Recent figures related to the hospitalisation rates for specific diseases suggest that the Family Doctor Programme has helped cut hospitalisation rates, and thus relieve pressures on these institutions for increasing their capacities. A close analysis of information for 1985 and 1990 show the following trends and results:

The total number of patients hospitalised dropped from 90,738 patients in 1985 to 74,495 in 1090. This is a significant drop considering that no patient requiring hospitalisation is denied this service.

The number of beds for treating patients with respiratory ailments (390 beds) remained constant during the two years under consideration. These diseases constitute the principal cause of hospitalisation, and among this group of illnesses, bronchial asthma is the most important.

In 1985, a total of 51 beds were used for treating patients with clinical ailments in general. Of course, the most important causes for hospitalisation were intestinal parasites, chronic diarrhoea, acute intoxication's, acute indigestion, urinary tract infections, acute convulsions, anaemia, and other infectious diseases. In 1990, with the same number of beds, the hospital was able to create areas of specialised care, such as Dermatology, Neuro-psychiatry, Endocrinology, Cardiology, Haematology, Nutrition and Nephrology. Each of these specialities allocate approximately 30 percent of their resources to offering patient care.

The number of beds used in the areas of intensive of Intermediate Care increased form 14 to 16. It is worth noting here that in 1985, the majority of patients receiving intensive or intermediate care were transferred directly from the emergencies section, due to the severity of their condition upon arrival at the hospital. In 1990, however, approximately 75% of the patients receiving intensive or intermediate care came from other areas of hospitalisation. This has been due to the adoption on the part of the hospital of a more efficient method for monitoring the evolution of patients, in order to move them to intensive or intermediate care with the first sign of deterioration.

192

Previously, the majority of patients were hospitalised due to acute respiratory or diarrhoeal diseases. Today, however, the greatest number of patients receiving hospital care are there awaiting surgery, and amongst these cases, the majority have experienced multiple traumas, or suffer from neuro-infectious problems.

A total of 25 beds are used for neo-natal cases. No change was observed in this number in the two years under consideration. The conditions in which neo-natal patients arrive at the hospital have improved significantly in recent years, as a result of the increased awareness of the adverse effects that a poor system of transportation may have on a patient's health and on that of the infant as well.

As regards the number of beds used to treat surgical patients (64 beds), this number has not been modified, either. Access to specialised health care in this area, however, has improved, as a result of the incorporation of several specialists on the hospital staff. In addition, the number of paediatric patients hospitalised in this section due to acute paediatric health problems has declined, as mentioned above, which has allowed an increase in the number of surgical operations performed from 1896 major surgical interventions and 1816 minor interventions in 1985, to 2503 major operations and 2490 minor interventions in 1990.

Another improvement which should be noted as regards the Family Doctor Programme's positive influence in this hospital's provision of surgical care, has been an increase in outpatient paediatric surgery. Prior to any such intervention, the hospital's surgical staff meets with the family physician attending the case, in order to decide if the patient in question is eligible for receiving this type of care. In the event that the patient is deemed eligible for out-patient surgical care, the family physician is charged with closely monitoring the patient's post-operatory condition in his or her home.

The Programme in the Total Health Context

As of 1998, the Family doctor Programme consumed about 5% of Cuba's GNP. MINSAP's total budget accounts for about 8% of the Cuban GNP. From this one can gain some insight into the primacy with which Cuban Society invests health promotion and community medicine. This needs to be said in order to place Cuba's ostentatious preoccupation with "heroic" surgical techniques, high-tech diagnosis and such status initiatives as genetic engineering, in perspective. These latter issues are dealt with in Chapter Twelve, and, as already suggested in the Foreword, can easily represent a basis for some criticism of Cuba's health policy generally.

The manner in which the Family Doctor Programme articulates with MINSAP's activities in total is shown in Fig. 11.3, kindly provided to the author during an interview on April 13th, 1994, by Dr Jose N Mendez Rodriguez, National Epidemiological Assessor of the Cuban National Institute for Medical Information in Havana.

Fig. 11.3 Administrative and Territorial Structure of Cuba's National Health System, Including Levels of Medical Attention

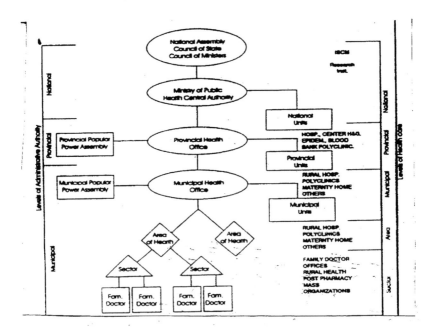

CHAPTER TWELVE

HIGH TECHNOLOGY IN CUBAN MEDICINE

Cuba's Background in Commercial Medicine

One ordinarily associates the wonders of high technology medicine with the most advanced and privileged nations. But paradoxically Cuba has flirted with it almost from the first days of the revolution. Partly this was because the University of Havana Medical School ran a number of research programmes in such up-front specialities (back in 1958) as dialysis, lipid liquefaction/extraction and endocrinology. As well, as have been mentioned previously, some of the more market forces-minded specialists ran commercial health concerns on the side, drawing their clientele almost exclusively from America and offering treatments not available in the U.S. because they were regarded by the American Medical Association as having been inadequately validated for safety.

Most of these latter involved at least minor surgery and a short stay in hospital and were often procedures of a `personal' nature that the client would not necessarily wish his/her family and friends to know were being undertaken. Such is the nature of human vanity that some people will take the most extraordinary risks, and pay large sums of money for the privilege (!), in order to look "better", whatever discomfort it might entail. Clients such as these are ideal when it comes to questionable health treatments because if things go wrong, they do not often wish to draw attention to themselves by engaging in litigation.

Have Penis, Will Travel!

One of the most bizarre of these clinics ran a service for men who had marital problems due to inability to sustain an erection. This is not an uncommon problem, especially in highly pressured competitive societies, and is widely recognised as being largely

195

psychogenic in origin, rather than being due to, say, an endocrine deficiency. As such, the best approach would involve some sort of psychotherapeutic counselling. But this takes a long time, has no guaranteed outcome and involves telling too many people - the very thing that a victim who feels disgraced by the condition is not likely to do. For many people, of course, even those whose basic problem may be psychological, Viagra provides a quicker solution than does any kind of psychotherapy!

But in the instance referred to above, a Dr Hervé Lasco set up a cosmetic surgery clinic in 1955 in Havana to address the problem by mechanical means. His solution involved opening the penis by a "stem-to-stern" dorsal incision, implanting a vinyl rod of appropriate length and resuturing the cut. The client ended up with a permanently erect penis which, as long as the rod stayed in place, wouldn't deflate on him at the height of his love-making activities. But possession of such an implant occasioned some embarrassing problems of its own. Because it held the penis erect all the time, the owner would have to - for the rest of his life! - keep re-adjusting its position by hand in order to keep the circulation to the region from being interfered with. Just how he would do this surreptitiously, say, while at a long executive meeting beggars the imagination.

Also, although rarely occurring, the implant sometimes didn't stay put, but retracted inward ending up in the man's coelomic cavity, from which it would have to be surgically removed. Again, how would he account for its presence, without giving his secret away is best left to the reader's conjecture. The critical feature is, though, that the client had to sign an undertaking with Lasco prior to surgery absolving the latter of any responsibility should anything go wrong. As such, the good surgeon was not doing anything contrary to law - either Cuban or American. He was making a huge fortune (put at $US. 3 million between 1955 and 1959, when he up and fled) out of men's vanity, but so do many people and in occupations other than medicine. He had sought permission from the AMA to carry out such medical procedures in the US., but permission was refused on the grounds that the procedure was not yet regarded as having been adequately researched. It is interesting to know that such research has now been done, and in a modified form, using a shorter rod which serves as an aid only to an existing erection, the procedure has been declared valid. Under certain, more stringent, conditions than applied in 1959 in Cuba, a man can now have such a procedure carried out in any developed country, but again Viagra has largely obviated the demand for such surgical approaches.

Cutting The Fat

Another procedure, now well-known in the U.S. and Britain, but pioneered in Cuba before it became so acceptable elsewhere, is one which involves surgical weight loss. The overweight person who has the two attributes of being unable to keep to a diet and/or an exercise regime and also of being extremely wealthy, would present to the clinic concerned - not Lasco's in this case! - to have his/her excess weight melted away. In strict market-force philosophy the charge for the service was pegged (in 1959), when the revolution inconsiderately brought the whole enterprise to a grinding halt), at $50 U.S. per pound!

The client would be measured up and weighed and the areas of his/her body where the more obvious fat deposits closest to the outside were located were determined. The procedure would then be carefully explained to the client. He/she would be placed under general anaesthetic. Subcutaneous injections of fat dissolving enzyme would be made into the various targeted fat deposits. These areas would then be carefully massaged, gradually reducing the fat to a viscous liquid. This would then be drawn off. The amount drawn off would be carefully measured to correspond to what the client wanted to pay. Medical ethics were observed, in that no one was allowed to have more drawn off than was consistent with what their body weight should have been.

Selling Health For Dollars

Those were but two of the avenues in which Cuba was marketing its medical technology in pre-revolutionary days, but it seems to have established a tradition! By 1969, Cuba was feeling a desperate need for hard currency, and U.S. dollars were especially prized. It was not long before some people in the Ministry of Public Health came up with the "Specialist Medical Clinics for Foreigners" idea. It occasioned three years of heated debate in both medical and political circles in Cuba - the purists being against it on the grounds of "revolutionary morality" and the pragmatists being for it. By 1972 the Government gave the go-ahead - provided that certain conditions were strictly observed. Among these were : that no resources were to be withdrawn from use in the public health sector to meet the needs of this new private health initiative, it was to be available only to foreigners paying in hard currency (so clients from the Eastern European communist bloc would not have been welcomed!) and, most importantly from the point of view of Cuba's good foreign relations, no procedure undertaken must violate the health laws of the client's own country.

With these, and the more mundane, restrictions in place, a variety of clinics again hit the open market in Havana (and elsewhere in Cuba), and advertised their services in the capitalist press. It brought out the best in Cuban medical/technical ingenuity and no doubt had a positive feedback to domestic surgical and medical practice. Although the fees charged were high enough to bring in a good supply of hard currency they were still far lower than would have been charged in the countries from which the clients came. A brisk business was thus ensured. This, among other things, allowed the Cubans to purchase sophisticated and expensive equipment which was then also made available to its own public health system.

Benefits to Cuba's Public Health System

Among the many medical initiatives thus engendered, and now available to all Cubans are the following:

In 1970, before the Cubans had started on the commercial marketing of its medical expertise, a team of physiology researchers at the Havana Medical School had set up a CID-201 mini computer to analyse neuro-physiological phenomena. Shortage of funds had, by 1973, brought their research almost to a standstill. However, by renting out their CID-201 facility to a group of psychologists who had started a commercial clinic on "biofeedback training", they were able to generate enough income to maintain their own project. It progressed admirably, giving way to the current MEDICID systems, which have produced important results in neuronic, cardiocid and other research areas.

As a result Cuba is now at the forefront of medical research in automization of encephalograms, analysis and diagnosis of certain neurological disorders and automatic intraoperatory monitoring of brain surgery. Its position, though, is now more serious than ever threatened by the Blockade, as explained in Chapter Sixteen.

Similarly, Cuba has now achieved international standing in computerisation and laser technology for physiotherapy, acupuncture surgery and the pharmaceutical industry. Ultrasound technology is now firmly established in Cuba, having had its humble origins as a commercial service to pregnant American women, who could not afford routine ultrasound services back home. It has had a spin off in such area as the production of nebulizers for asthmatics and foetal detectors. Now routine in third world Cuba are systems for processing images for cardiology and large -scale automization of computerised axial tomography.

International recognition has already been accorded the Ultra Micro Analytical System (UMAS) developed by Cuba. This is a computerised and automated electronic device capable of detecting, and assessing the severity of congenital hyperthyroidism and other thyroid gland disorders. It can also be applied to ascertaining predisposition to allergies, foetal malformations and other dysfunction's associated with pregnancy.

It is currently being used in the front-line of medical research on: antibodies against AIDS, surface antigens in Hepatitis B toxoplasmosis, Chaga's disease, simple herpes, sitomegalovirus and hyperlipoproteinaemias.

Through the commercial use of much of this medical know-how, the Ministry of Public Health has been able to purchase such high tech apparatus as Nuclear Magnetic Resonators and a Linear (electron) Accelerator System - used in radiotherapy.

For the medical export market, Cuba was (as of 1991) producing such items as: surgery furniture, electro - chemical stabilisers for the treatment of pigmentary retinosis, ultrasound nebulizers, sound detectors, cardiac arrhythmia stabilisers, intensive care apparatus, complete dental units, etc.

Cuba in the Vanguard of Surgical Technique

Long before the revolution, Cubans as individuals seemed to manifest a particular talent for surgery. Not only was their own medical school highly regarded in this area, but Cubans themselves were often found in leading surgical units all over the developed world. As a national tradition of which to be proud, this has certainly been cultivated and nurtured by the revolutionary government.

When it was still a reasonably novel procedure in the more advanced countries, Cuban cardiac patients in the early 60's were being fitted with pacemakers in the surgical unit at Havana medical school. In 1985, Cuba carried out its first heart-transplant - the only third world nation to ever to have done so. Then in 1985, a heart-lung transplant was successfully accomplished. Cuba then actually pioneered in the elaboration of a technique called cardiomyoplasty, by which the energy released by the long dorsal muscles on either side of the spine, can be used to support heart contractions.

Another significant achievement in the field of cardiology has been the creation (in 1989) of two models of the Cuban Mechanical Heart - CORAMEC. These are linked to a patient whose own heart has been arrested for surgical reasons or for transplant purposes. The Hermanos Amejeiras hospital can accommodate four or these operations simultaneously.

Also Cuba occupies a dominant position in the field of renal transplants. Of these, 1438 had been carried out in Cuba by 1991. On Havana Radio in 1992 a Cuban who had had a kidney transplant in 1970 was interviewed! Things like this do not occur in other third world countries. Every Cuban province now has nephrological and dialysis services and in each of Havana, Santiago and Camaguey there are seven kidney transplant facilities!

Microsurgery is another area in which Cuba has excelled. It is applied largely to the replacement of fingers and toes and, since 1977, to ophthalmologic procedures. These latter will be discussed in greater detail under a separate heading as they have attracted such international commentary. Suffice to say, though, Cuba has pioneered in the efficient treatment of pigmentary retinosis under the leadership of Professor Orfilio Petaez.

Since 1985, bone and liver transplants in Cuba have been almost routine. As indicated previously , Cuban surgeons have a history of innovatory approaches to cosmetic surgery, most recently applied in a reconstructive procedure known as Colgajo Mio and used in cancer of the mouth surgery, greatly easing the patients psychological recovery and social re-integration.

A Cuban first in transplant surgery was achieved in June 1992 with the transplantation of the internal knee meniscus to counter a sports injury. The operation, which was entirely successful, had never been tried elsewhere and involved subtle endoscopic techniques.

Another unexpected Cuban success story was the opening, in 1990, of the Iberian and Latin American centre for Nervous System Transplant and Regeneration. Here they carry out surgical procedures and clinical treatments for such degenerative conditions as Parkinson's Disease, Huntingdon's Chorea, heredoataxias and Alzheimer's Disease. Also included in their sphere of activities now, although such a proliferation of activities was not envisioned when they opened, are: treatment of bone marrow and

201

craniocerebral traumas, eclusive craniovascular diseases and neuroendocrine disorders. The huge variety of ancillary techniques they have developed to mediate these advances include : suprarenal marrow self-transplantation, foetal brain tissue transplantation, and many others.

Advances in Pharmacology

In 1959, of course, Cuba was totally dependent on American pharmaceutical firms for all of its needs in that field. Because of the exorbitant profits these firms were generating for their stockholders back home, the cost to the Cuban public health departments were such as to preclude anything approaching universal access to treatment. If revolutionary deeds were at all to match revolutionary rhetoric in the new Ministry of Public Health, some way had to be found of gaining cheaper access to important pharmaceuticals.

As has already been described, Cuba developed its own pharmaceutical production system, relying in the interim period on aid from other countries. The U.S. Trade Embargo and Economic Blockade, especially as modified by President Reagan in 1982, rendered it virtually impossible for Cuba to gain much value at all from the international pharmaceutical trade and thus, from 1983 onward, it was forced even more completely to rely on its own talents to meet the need. Again, it surpassed its own expectations in this regard and has even gained international standing in its own right as a result of some of its more innovative initiatives in pharmacology.

In 1990, it was asserted by the Ministry of Public Health that 80% of Cuba's drug needs are being met by domestic production. However, much of that has required use of imported materials, some from former Soviet Bloc nations. The loss of that source alone now poses immense difficulties for Cuba's development of a domestic pharmaceutical output. This has forced Cuban pharmaceutical scientists back to lines of production that can be sustained by Cuban research and materials.

By 1991, new haemoderivatives had been obtained, such as specific and

202

polyvalent immunoglobulins. As well, they have successfully synthesised
against Hepatitis B and several preparations that breakdown cholesterol i
This latter is obviously important in a country with cardiovascular disease listed as its
number one killer. Other successful products listed in the July 1992 report of the
Cuban Ministry of Public Health - but about which other information was not given
are: Epidemic Growth Factor, Nervous Growth Factor, Melagenine for the treatment
of vitiligo, a cream effective against psoriasis but not yet named and various other
drugs tailor-made for specific high tech research projects. Perhaps the most notable of
all these, in terms both of its wide applicability and the international acclaim accorded
it, is the Hepatitis B vaccine. It means that Cuba is the only country in the world that
produces a meningococci vaccine type B.

What is also evident is that these most recent developments suggest the
emergence of a new level of scientific research infrastructure in the third world scene -
and one in which Cuba is certainly leading the way. The emergence, in Cuba, of the
Genetic Engineering and Biotechnology Centre (and about which more will be said in
the next section) has all by itself created a demand for such an infrastructure, merely to
support ongoing research. Also the Immunoassay Centre and the Haemoderivatives
Plant will make similar demands.

These centres will complement, or be complemented by, others that are still
being built, such as the National Centre for Bio-preparations and the Therapeutic
Steroids Plant. Also nearing completion is the Carlos J. Finlay Production Centre and a
series of smaller factories dedicated to vaccine production.

Lifeline Over the Blockade: Biotechnology

In world terms, biotechnology has marked the opening of a totally new era for
mankind, so much so that many now speak of a "biorevolution". In Cuban terms, the
significance of its own contribution to this revolution is of less exalted significance - it
has given Cuba something to sell which the trading with the enemy legislation can't

touch and therefore constitutes, finally, a hard-currency lifeline across the U.S. blockade. The wider, scientific, significance of course is that man can now synthesise products superior to those derived from nature. Together with genetic engineering, surely biotechnology, must be seen as an even bigger conquest for man than the production of atomic energy.

The President of the Latin American Association of Biotechnology and Bioengineering, Professor Oscar P. Gomez, asserted in 1998 that the "levels of development attained by the Republic of Cuba in these fields gave it, even as early as 1992, not only a pre-eminent position in our continent, but in the world a vanguard place!"

It was in July 1986 that the Genetic Engineering and Biotechnology centre (GIBC) was inaugurated in Havana. The building itself does not in any way reflect its third world origins but is equivalent to such facilities in the U.S., U.K. or anywhere else in the industrialised nations. It embraces research and production units in clonage, DNA mapping, gene transfer, etc. As well it includes the necessary facilities for the evaluation of products involved in the relevant biological systems - including means for the large-scale production of monoclonal antibodies, micropropagation of vegetal cells, etc.

Designed to address specific problems in biotechnology, not all of which derive from considerations of pure research, its working lines embrace proteins and hormones for obtaining products applicable to both human and veterinary medicine through various recombining processes. It is also concerned with implications for the use of vaccines against diseases, both in Cuba and elsewhere in the tropics. One of these investigations considers the possibility of cloning proteins from the surface of viruses, parasites or bacteria. This ties in with monoclonal antibodies developments. Some of the practical outcomes of this type of activity have already been felt in Cuban agriculture - such as the use of policlonal antibodies and DNA probes.

Of greater important, or potentially so, moment has been work on this modification of antibodies. In one instance, the genes of four antibodies have been obtained and used in oncology studies to prevent rejection of liver and renal transplants

(IORT -3) and in another instance for the treatment of cutaneous lymphomas (IORT-1). Cutaneous lymphomas, of course, are becoming a preoccupation in the tropics and are likely to in other regions as well, as a result of the holes in the ozone layer.

Other examples of the sort of outcome of this interface between theoretical research and practical application abound in the field of nitrogen fixing in fertilisers and other applications to food production. It also includes investigations in the sphere of genetics of higher organisms, aimed principally at the clonage of genes, the production of proteins, the obtaining of biological reactives, etc.

In 1998, the GIBC created, 291 products, 20 of them synthesised in their entirety by genetic engineering techniques. No other third world country has ever made strides of this magnitude in this field. The Cuban Institute of Research into Sugar Cane Production is now totally dependent on GIBC for much research supporting its activities. Such research formerly was carried out in the USSR and the DDR.

But just as noteworthy as the high tech enterprises themselves has been the creativity with which revolutionary Cuba has been able to develop a basis and infrastructure to support them. For instance, it is widely known that seaweed of various types is rich in many nutrients, and since it is so quickly replaced by mitosis, even in colder waters - but much more quickly in warm - it may eventually serve as a world food resource. While this has been known for some time, it had not been substantially acted upon until Cuba addressed the practical implications in 1990 in Santiago province. The aim had been to derive commercial quantities of Sodium Alginate from dark marine algae. A cubic tonne of this species, removed from the tropic waters off the coast is replaced by normal mitotic division in 24 hours!

Sodium alginate, in the meantime, is vital to biotechnology and to the textile food and pharmaceuticals industries. Now large-scale cultivation of these algae has been initiated at a special marine farm located in the waters near Cayo Libertad, in Cardenas Bay, Matanzas province, about 240 km east of Havana. Prior even to this research development, however, similar studies on Sargasso algae had been underway for over ten years at Oriente University.

It is said that Sodium Alginate has in excess of 5000 applications, including as a thickener in purees, Pasta, desserts, ice cream, cheese, toothpaste, creams for medical use, etc.

Cuba Fills The Breach

The Chernobyl disaster in the Ukraine has been so overshadowed by other events that many of us in the advanced nations have forgotten about it. But its effects are still to be found among thousands of people living within a 100 mile radius of Chernobyl itself. The world as a whole, will not be able to even begin to assess the extent of this disaster for decades to come, but in the meantime real people are still suffering and few nations have stepped into the breach with the vigour and generosity of spirit shown by Cuba.

Some 10,000 Children affected by Chernobyl were, in 1991 and 1992, being treated at special facilities in Tarara, east of Havana. A Cuban medical team whose brief it was to ascertain the extent of the victims' radiation dose (called the "dosimetry" group) were formed to cope with that influx. In 1993, their skills had been immediately applied in addressing the needs of a newly arrived contingent of 6700 children from Brazil. These were victims of the Gioana nuclear plant disaster, which occurred in September 1987. To make this possible, President Fidel Castro and Leonel Brejole, Governor of Rio de Janeiro, signed a scientific co-operation agreement with regard to treatment of the victims of that disaster.

Cuba Gives Hope A Chance

In closing this chapter, the author would like to return to the remarkable story of Dr Orfilio Palaeg and his work on retinitis pigmetosa, to which passing reference was made earlier.

Retinitis pigmentosa was, until Palaeg showed otherwise, an illness producing incurable blindness. It generally strikes in childhood, and a conservative estimate places the number of sufferers at about 20,000. At a conference in August 1991 (Inter American Ophthalmologic Congress), Orfilio Palaeg, a professor of Ophthalmic surgery and a consultant in the Ministry of Public Health, gave a paper in which he described a technique involving laser therapy and which he claimed held out promise for victims of retinitis. A Costa Rican doctor was present. He explained to Palaeg that he had a ten year old patient, Jonatan Gonzalez Diaz, who had already lost the sight of his left eye totally and only had 10% vision in his right eye. Could doctor Palaeg see him?

Jonatan, who came from a farming family more than 60 km from Costa Rica's capital, San Jose, had never before been more than 5 km from home. However, with Pelaeg as their only hope, his parents sent him off to Cuba with only his older brother to accompany him! To cut a long and dramatic story short, the laser surgery was a resounding success, and caught the attention of scientists all over the world.

At the request of Costa Rican authorities, both Orfilio Pelaeg and the Cuban Ministry of Public Health, sent Costa Rica full details of the treatment. Because of the U.S. blockade, now in the "third noose" stage, as a result of the collapse of support from the former Soviet Union and its allies, thousands of Latin American children with retinosa are not free to visit Cuba for treatment. Their governments could not dare jeopardise the delicate trade relations they have with America. But nothing, it is hoped, will stop them from going to Costa Rica to receive treatment.

It is stories such as this that convey the real significance of Cuba's achievements in health. We are not only talking about one country which happened to strike it lucky. We are talking about a small ostensibly backward people who discovered, in their own way, the meaning of socialism and who have been inspired to build it. That it has made an impact on their development of public health is not remarkable. It is to be expected, for socialism is about embracing communities and enhancing human dignity. Anything that speaks of the dignity and oneness of man - be it great music or great science in the service of people - should be a natural product of socialism. It is also not remarkable that Cuba should circumvent a blockade erected to keep socialism out of the rest of Latin America by giving freely of its public health treasures. It always has, because it is socialist.

Therefore, this author would argue that the wonderful thing about Cuba is not only what it has done for Cuba, but what it has done for all of us. It has given the third world hope in the face of its exploitation. But one can look for the day, and work towards it, when that hope will also extend to the whole world - that wherever people live and work, they may do so for the good of all.

This spirit of internationalism is shown not only in these spectacular, and emotionally satisfying, rescue efforts, however, but in the extent to which Cuba has offered its expertise through setting up training programmes for students from other countries. The only barrier to continued progress in this area is the U.S. Blockade.

The Isle of Pines, home of one of the most notorious prisons in Latin America during Batista's regime, and from which the imprisoned Fidel Castro smuggled out his now famous "History Will Absolve Me" statement on scraps of paper, used to be called "Hope's Graveyard". However, soon after the revolution triumphed, the old prison was converted into a series of residential training centres and island was renamed "Isle of Youth". Over the years, more and more facilities were added to it, until it was hosting students from many countries doing a range of courses, from practical agricultural training to post-graduate medical research.

Since 1961, and especially since 1985 - as far as health related courses are concerned - the former "Hope's Graveyard" has become "Hope's Rebirth"

More than 3,500 foreign students have completed their studies there (and also in other Cuban training institutions) and have returned to their own countries empowered a thousand fold to address the many conditions holding such societies back. These include 2,681 graduates from the technical and professional teaching programme, as well as 831 graduates at postgraduate level. These latter include 400 clinical teachers and 97 fully trained doctors and nurses. More than 2,200 of these students came from Africa, especially Angola and Zimbabwe, with 967 and 300 graduates respectively.

CHAPTER THIRTEEN

A MEDICAL VOLUNTEER'S ACCOUNT

Putting Voluntary Service in Context

As anyone familiar with the Cuban schooling system is no doubt aware, strong emphasis - even with children in pre-school and day care centres - is laid on 'co-operation' as a moral imperative. A logical extension of this is the frequently stated attitude that the more fortunate must come to the aid of the less fortunate. Even though Cuba is technically a poor third world country, its citizens (especially its school children) do not have to look far to realise that, compared with the rest of Latin America, they indeed belong to the 'more fortunate' category.

In this context, the theme of 'internationalism' is stressed daily in pre-schools and primary schools where children as part of their morning assembly ritually intone: "Seremos como Che, somos internacionalistas".[66] Such 'Pledges of Allegiance' (not dissimilar to the ritual which begins the school day for American children) must have some long term impact. One is struck, for instance, on any visit to the United States, by how much stronger patriotic sentiments are there than, say, in Britain. In the Cuban situation, the whole protocol of classroom practice and school administration is designed to underline and reinforce that type of idealism. As the author relates in a previous book[67], if a child performs well on a school test, he/she is expected to help the child seated beside him or her to do well also.

Therefore, it is not entirely surprising that most medical students in Cuba seem to feel that their reason for taking that particular course of studies is to prepare themselves to help people. Likewise, the international dimension, implicit in

---

[66]"We will be like Che, we are internationalists."

[67]MacDonald, Theodore (1988): Making a New People. New Star Books, Vancouver.

participating in overseas service, is a natural follow-on from the oft repeated slogan of childhood. It is not entirely irrelevant perhaps that Che himself was trained as a doctor and only became an active revolutionary later.

An important feature of Cuban foreign policy since the triumph of the revolution has been the provision of "aid in kind" to other third world countries. All over the third world, for instance, one finds Cuban teachers, doctors, engineers, etc., except in those countries run by extremely reactionary regimes who do not recognise the Cuban government. It has been said, that one of Cuba's most well-known and highly valued exports has been doctors. With 19 medical schools and a domestic supply already of about 1 doctor to 310 people, Cuba has no shortage of talent to be used in this way.

In this way, Cuba likes to present itself to the third world as a country, small and poor itself, but which has succeeded in finding a social policy which allows it to solve its problems. As the reader has already seen, improvements in Cuba's domestic medical care systems soon led to the eradication of many of the health banes common to third world life elsewhere - such as diseases of malnutrition, parasitic disorders and the like. Certain medical conditions, common throughout the rest of the third world, became so rare in Cuba that medical students could receive no practical training in their cure or management. The solution arrived at was for each medical student to spend three to six months of his penultimate year of medical training as an "assistant doctor" in one of the other third world countries. Students are given some choice as to where they wish to go to and/or as to the type of medicine that they wish to practice, but medical overseas service of some kind is a requirement.

Voluntarism comes into play when the students have qualified as doctors. The government actively encourages newly qualified doctors to volunteer for overseas service for one or two years. No one is forced into it, but moral and social pressures are strong. Doctors returning from overseas service are lionised by the media and are frequently invited to talk to youth groups, etc. Moreover, such "inspirational" talks fit into the whole ethos of 'service' constantly presented to youth. The walls of public buildings in Cuba, especially where young people gather, often carry slogans - a sort of official graffiti - such as: "The true revolutionary is guided by love, said Che", "Yesterday's dream can be tomorrow's reality", "The children of the world want peace", "There is no peace without justice and no justice without dignity" - all of which are ones which I have seen in Havana. Such public expression of lofty and altruistic sentiments is further enhanced, no doubt, by the virtual absence of commercial advertising.

But what struck this author of particular interest was the unselfconscious way in which many of the medical students and doctors I spoke to defined a rationale for their action along the lines of a 'personal commitment' based on these assumptions. The arguments used invariably reflected what we would regard as unvarnished political propaganda, but in the case of all of the people to whom I spoke, they seemed totally unaware of this. They had internalised the message - including such intimate details as the names of various factions and their leaders in the countries concerned, etc. - as though by osmosis. Almost all of them claimed that they had been 'politically aware' in this way since their early teens.

This is reflected very markedly in the fulsome commentary made by Oscar Sanchez, when I asked him to discuss his medical work as a volunteer in Angola. We spent a most enjoyable afternoon over cups of Cuban coffee in the medics' common room at Pinar del Rio Maternity Hospital, as Oscar (now a trainee internist) and visiting Pinar for two months, related to me how, as a medical student, he was assigned to spend 6 months of his penultimate year in Angola (this sort of work abroad being built into the medical course) and then voluntarily went back for two further years after qualifying. His account has been pieced together from extended answers he gave to individual questions which I asked, but I record it here in continuous speech. Note how he delves into Angolan politics, as though it is the most natural thing in the world for one to be aware of those details as part of one's personal intellectual furniture.

Oscar's Account

"Well, I guess you know about the heroic people of Angola and Mozambique. I had always thought that, somehow, Portuguese colonialism was better than British. Somehow I had picked up the idea from some book I read in secondary school that Spanish and Portuguese people are not naturally racist but that English-speaking people and Afrikaners really do think they're superior to blacks. I had heard about Angola and Mozambique, but the thought had never crossed my mind to go there. When I was asked in my fourth year at medical school where I wanted to do my overseas service, I said "Ireland" just as a joke because you never get to go where you nominate anyway!"

"A couple of weeks later, the notices went up and I had been assigned to some unpronounceable town full of "c's" and "h's" in Angola! I went to the reading room to look up Angola in the encyclopaedia. Everything about the place sounded terrible, especially the medical set-up. It sounded like the white man's graveyard that they used to call West Africa last century."

"As chance would have it, an Angolan freighter came into Havana in June 1985 and my supervisor said: "There's your chance to find out more about Angola". He had to get a permit from the Superior and the Higher Education Office for me to get permission from some other guy in the Port Authority to get permission from the CDR to get permission from the district committee to get permission from ...... By now he was laughing as he waved his hands in mock exasperation.

Anyway, I got on the boat and that was where I really saw racism. All the black crew seemed to be doing the dirty work and the whites were officers - and Angola's supposed to be a Peoples' Democracy! But worse was to come. While we were eating tinned pineapple in this room where the white officers played ping pong, they kept talking about "Angolan shit". They knew I couldn't speak Portuguese, so they spoke Spanish - rather well, at that. I asked what "Angolan shit" was and they said "It's the black people. They're animals - real animals!" That visit was an education for me alright, but not quite what my supervisor had in mind when he suggested the idea!"

"Well, I was 25 then and very impressionable. It really depressed me. They asked me what I knew about Angola. So I told them all about the Independence Declaration of 1975 and the Revolution in Portugal of 1974 and they were really happy. I mean really happy. They said I knew more about it than they did."

"I guess you know what happened. I mean, they were under Portuguese exploitation for a couple of centuries and now that I know what racists those white Portuguese were I realised that it must have been hell."

At this point, as much to hear the tale from him as for any legitimate reason, I said that I wasn't too sure of the details.

"Oh, you don't know", he exclaimed so loudly that other people in the room turned and looked at us. My status as a foreigner having anti-imperialism explained to me attracted considerable interest. "I see I'll have to give you a history lesson, my companero!"

"In 1961, the Angolan nationalists started systematically revolting against the Portuguese - a bit like the Cuban revolution. Come 1974, the Portuguese military overthrew their own government back in Lisbon and established a socialist regime. Of course, you know that you can't really establish socialism by a military take-over, but that's what they called it at the time. No matter, it created so much confusion that the Angolan rebels had an easy time pushing the Portuguese authorities out."

"The only problem was that the Angolan freedom movement was divided up into this faction and that faction. There were three main ones - Movement of the People for the Liberation of Angola (MPLA), led by Agostinho Neto. He's a poet, you know, and was always being put in prison by the Portuguese for writing revolutionary verses. Then, there was the National Front for the Liberation of Angola (NFLA) led by Holden Roberto. You probably remember, he was a criminal pure and simple. Finally you have those bastards, UNITA who are causing all the trouble now. Even back then in 1985 UNITA (National Union for Total Independence) was getting its funds from the US and South Africa. Their sole duty was to betray the revolution. Well, those three groups fought against each other as much as they fought the Portuguese. When Angola's revolution succeeded, each group tried to claim it as their own. They weren't united like Cuba was."

"As you know, the MPLA were the authentic socialists and they just got busy in the areas of the country that they controlled, building schools, hospitals etc. The NFLA meanwhile gradually fizzled away and went down the drain. But UNITA kept getting funds and arms from the imperialists, especially the US and South Africa, and they spent most of their time burning down MPLA schools, etc., and murdering people. Eventually elections were held, you know, and MPLA won in every district, even in Jonas Savimba's town and he's the head of UNITA!"

As Oscar Sanchez's words rolled on, I had to keep reminding myself that he was a doctor, not a political activist or a historian. He had clearly internalised the whole situation and had made it his own - a phenomenon which I often found in interviewing professionals (mainly doctors, but not exclusively) who had done voluntary service in the third world overseas.

"When will we get to the medical bit?" I nudged him.

"Ah, but companero," he said "Surely you know that you can't practice medicine without knowing the feelings and aspirations of those people you are treating!

You must let me finish what I am saying about the political and social background. It is all relevant to health care."

"Of course, UNITA did not accept the election result and continued their diabolical activities and now appear to be winning".

"Well, anyway, you want the medical side. After I had gone back and talked about what I had learned about Angola on the freighter, my supervisor said I should definitely learn some Portuguese and two tribal African dialects. The Portuguese I did from tapes and a book. I mean, I'm no expert at it but it wasn't too difficult to get some sort of feel for it. As for the African dialects - what a laugh. They sent me once a week to this fellow in Cienfuegos who taught me some Yoruba. This went on for four weeks and then he said "Where are you going in Africa?" I told him "Angola" and he just about hit the roof. "Hey", he shouted, "Your school is one big arse-hole. No one speaks Yoruba in Angola!" I was just as glad to see the end of those lessons because I couldn't get my tongue around Yoruba. In the end, I went out there only with

Portuguese. I guess I have no ear for really exotic languages because, although I grew to love Angola - especially the area I was serving in - I have never learned any of the languages - just a few words here and there. You know, I think you learn to do better doctoring that way - you go only by what your own eyes, ears, and fingers tell you."

Oscar's First Trip

"They sent me across in September 1985. We flew to Lorenco Marcs and then I was put in a hotel for four days while waiting for a train to take me to an inland station where I was going to be working. Man, it was rough - bedbugs the size of turtles and people stealing from you. The food was like the wrath of Christ, too. But once I got to work, I never missed the good life of Cuba. Really, I felt like a missionary or something. You know, the people there had nothing - and they trusted me, especially the children. Every day I woke up and I said to myself 'Oscar, you mustn't make a mistake'. It was like Che himself was watching me and I wanted to do good. I have never felt so - how can one describe it - so revolutionary!"

"I was supposed to be assistant to a local Angolan doctor, Dr. O., who had trained in Fort Hare University in South Africa and had qualified in England somewhere. You probably know, Fort Hare is a black university. What I quickly found out was that the guy wasn't much of a doctor. Well, he might have been originally, but the whisky had got to him. He and his nurse, a local girl named Eucharistika who had trained in Zambia, ran this clinic. It was a bit like one of our polyclinicas in the countryside, but much, much bigger. I mean, the outpatients dealt with several hundred people a day and there were 40 beds as well - an amazing place in a village called Malange. Malange itself is a dump. I think the only thing you can say about it is that it is inland from Luanda, about 180 km, and the railway line ends there. It is more correct to say that the railway line did end there, having been built by the MPLA with Cuban help from about 1975 to 1981 and then work on it stopped because UNITA guerrillas kept blowing up sections of it. By 1989 the closest a train could get

215

to Malange was about 6 or 7 km down the line. After that you used the bus - but that's another story!"

"Anyway, at Malange the Portuguese had built three huge warehouse-like structures for some agricultural purpose. No one ever seemed to know what they had in mind, but I tell you, these places were huge with the ceiling being about 5 metres high and windows all around, but too high above floor level to look out of. One of these buildings had been turned into a 40 bed hospital and it also had offices in it and a classroom with desks, etc., but which I never saw in use."

"For the outpatient part they used the other two buildings. We had some expensive diagnostic equipment in there, but most of it was non-operational, with bits missing or broken and not repairable locally. Also, in one of those outpatient buildings was a pharmacy full of new equipment - but with almost none of the drugs in stock. I don't know where Dr O. got his whiskey, but he had no problem with supplies of that! He was friendly most of the time but sometimes aggressive. He pretty well had been letting Sister Eucharistika do most of the decision-making. Even on the first day she said to me - 'Never let Dr O. operate!' She had learned quite a bit of surgery on the job over the years!"

"People came to the outpatients - and even to the hospital part -from huge distances. Early in the morning, maybe 3 or even 2 in the morning you would see people gathered outside the place with their babies and children waiting for opening time, which was 8.00am. There were other nurses besides Sister Eucharistika, but she was the only properly trained one. These other people would only stay for a few months and then be replaced by others who had trained in Luanda. With these nurses (other than Eucharistika) you couldn't turn your back without them stealing bits and pieces of your equipment, which they would then sell on the black-market. Even pens and pencils and certainly thermometers and watches, would be taken. If a patient came in with any valuable possession at all, even to outpatients, he wouldn't have it any more within five minutes of being examined!"

"I'll never forget my first day. There was such a variety of complaints - from infections caused by pieces of thorn buried so deep you had to dig a hole to get them

216

out, to enteric symptoms, etc, etc. Parasitic diseases, combined with malnutrition, were what one generally found in the children. You had to work fast because by opening time the queues were immense. Here I was the qualified doctor but during that first six months, it was Eucharistika who taught me what to do. The 'clinic' where the people were treated was just a big expanse of concrete with rows of wooden benches and two examining tables. There was no privacy and while you were treating people up at the front you were aware that there were about 50 or 60 other people sitting down watching, as though it was some kind of show. I couldn't believe it when I thought of how well organised we are back in Cuba. As well, there was the noise. If there is one dominant pervasive impression I gained of Angola it was noise - all day, all night. In the night, the mosquitoes and flies. For every one biting insect we have in the worst night in Cuba you have 500 on the best night in Angola! And they buzz louder while they're at it. In the daytime the same except add to it people shouting. You could hardly hear yourself when you were talking and to be heard the patient had to shout at you!"

"The big difference between Cuba and Angola was that at Malange you could only treat 'incidents' as they called them. You couldn't check an infection out and treat it in stages by telling the person when to come back. They didn't know times and dates, I don't think, and they had sometimes been travelling 3 or 4 days through jungle to get there once. They didn't come to get cured of diseases but only if the disease's symptoms got so bad that they needed relief from the symptoms. It was very frustrating in that way for a doctor, but they were so grateful when you eased the pain for them. They often brought children and they would be willing to leave them and come back in 2 or 3 weeks if you told them that was necessary. The hospital was mostly full of children so sick that they couldn't be treated in a few minutes and then carried back through the jungles. That meant, naturally, that our death rate was very high. The thought crossed my mind than that we could do better with local education programmes so that people could look after their own better."

"You've no idea how tiring that kind of work was. By the time you had been busy two or three hours, you needed a good cup of coffee and a cigarette. Dr O.

217

belonged to some American religious sect that was against liquor, tobacco, coffee and tea. Somehow his whiskey didn't count, but when I came there he wouldn't allow his staff to drink, smoke, or have tea or coffee. He wouldn't back down on the cigarettes - which is just as good because it made me give-up, but I swore that I could not work without the coffee. He backed down on the coffee."

"By the time darkness started to fall in the evening, the people had almost all gone. There were lots of big spaces left on the benches and the floor was covered with rubbish, faeces and urine. The smell was like a wall! But you felt all clean and pure inside - that experience was all part of me becoming an internationalist and in believing that only in that way will we ever make the world a good place to live. I think many Cubans feel like that, especially medical graduates."

"My six months came to an end and I was anxious to get back to Cuba to see my family again. But I wasn't entirely glad to leave Angola. Agreed it is a terrible place if you like comfort, but you know a lot of humans live and suffer there. It also seemed to me that it could be a lot better. I mean, it seemed to me that they could organise things so that the ordinary people weren't so helpless. They could teach the local villagers what was important and what wasn't so that people didn't have to trek for days through the jungle to get someone to look at them for ten minutes! So I left thinking those thoughts."

Oscar Returns to Angola

"Back in Cuba it was a case of spending only a few days with my parents - well, my mother really - and my little sister, then I had to stick my nose in the books. Only three months to go before the Finals and then the Medical Registration Board Exams after that - plus revision classes and clinics. It was interesting talking to the other students who had done their stints in different places. One poor guy went to Upper Volta and the village he was supposed to go to didn't exist! He spent two months in the Cuban Embassy in Lagos, Nigeria, and then went to some place in the bush in Ghana. Some

218

of the guys really had funny stories to tell. One woman got to her posting and found that they had thought she was a fellow and had her in a dormitory with three men. They spent hours rigging up strings to hang sheets from all around her bed and it was all unnecessary because the guys were so afraid of offending her that they wouldn't even talk to each other unless she was asleep. She used to pretend to be asleep so as not to interfere with their social life!"

"Well, I did well on my exams[68] and I think people expected me to settle down. I mean, I had a pasantia[69] offered to me in Santiago in internal medicine. I took it, but I couldn't get Angola out of my mind. I studied everything I could find that had ever been written about the place until, you know, if there had been such a thing as a Professor of Angolan History and Culture, I could have got the job! At night I used to think of those children dying all alone away from their mothers. Women may be oppressed in most of the third world, but in terms of power over children, the village women are much more important than the village men. It may sound funny to you, but - you know -I really do love what Che stood for and I could die for internationalism if it would do any good. I thought - like Che -where is the solution? But in Angola, the solution is not military. It is to 'teach the village mothers'.

"It seemed to me that a lot of the stuff on health that we teach in Cuban primary schools would be good - things like malaria cycles, AIDS, food preservation, infection, etc. Angola also had a big tobacco problem, like Cuba did in the 70's. Most Cuban kids today know that it is no good to take up smoking - even though we are reputed to produce the finest tobacco in the world! - but in Angola, even kids smoke. Even head teachers in schools smoke. They think it means that they are important. Breast feeding was another problem I kept thinking about. A lot of Angolan villagers use powders - not even the real tinned powdered milk from South Africa, like Nestles,

---

[68]A slight understatement. He topped the National Medical Boards and won prizes in surgery, prosthetics and laryngology.

[69]Residency post at a hospital in a specialist area.

but powder that they put together. Women who suckled their babies - people clicked their teeth at them. You know, when blacks click their teeth it means "You're low class" - it's disapproval. I wanted to turn all that on its head."

"You know, in medical school in Cuba we have an expression - 'Doctor Killdeer'. He's an American TV character who runs around saving people and women faint at his glance, etc. When people say: 'Hey man, you're being Doctor Killdeer!' you know, they are saying that you are taking it too seriously and that no one is indispensable. Well, they said that to me a lot but I said to myself that I think Che is right and I wanted to go back to Angola to see if I could organise local medical care. I'm not much into politics, you know, all this shit - well, excuse, you know - about working class, etc. It's a terrible thing to say, but I get bored with the CDR people and the Young Communist meetings when they spout all that propaganda, but I like the rest of the Young Communist work - you know, doing things for the community and all that jazz. It's the talk I can't stand."

"You do quite well at it, though!" I interjected.

My irony missed its mark and he continued with barely a pause.
"So, I went to our CDR chairperson and asked her how to go about organising to do volunteer work in Angola. You know what she said? She said: 'There's lots more exciting places than Angola for a doctor to go to.' I said it had to be Angola and she said: 'I know. you've got a chiquita out there, don't you? But she got hold of me at work next day and said: 'Come this evening. There are some comrades here from ICAP[70] who want to talk to you about Angola'. I went and they asked me to give them a plan in writing of the project I had in mind. They wanted it ready in two weeks! But this was easy for me to do because I had been thinking about it so much and because I had already written down a lot. So, in two weeks he called by and asked me for my writing. I gave him 82 pages of typing. He said: 'Comrade, we asked for it in only 2 weeks so you wouldn't have time to write a whole lot for us to read. I can see that you

---

[70]ICAP - Institute Cubano por Amistad entre los Pueblos
(Cuban Institute for Friendship Among the People)

don't need to have a son or to plant a tree'.[71]

"They sent it off to the Ministry of Health in Angola and I waited and kept working. It was not until a year and a half later that my CDR got an answer. I had to go to the Ministry of Public Health in Havana and present my plan to them and to UNESCO to see if we could get funding. UNESCO said that they were afraid of offending the Americans but they could fund their own field workers who could then co-operate with me. The Angolans asked if I would be willing to spend two years, rather than one year, out there. I agreed but then they had to get permission from our own Ministry of Public Health. In Cuba they are good at organising things like that between different ministries and agencies, etc. Anything for internationalism - I know Fidel believes that, most people do. Of course, they were as mad as pissed-on cobras at the hospital because I was being trained by them. But when they saw that I was serious and that Angola was serious and the government was serious and everybody else was serious, they said 'OK - you can sit the exams when you get back from Angola'. So off I went again."

"This time, though, I worked for four months with the Rural Health Unit in Luanda, a provincial capital. It was much less primitive than Malange. There my plans for health education in the villages, especially to mothers, were discussed and I wrote a lot of material, - some of it in picture form, and I'm no Picasso! - which was translated into local dialects and distributed. I could see that they were going to use me as an ideas man and that other people would work in the field. This I did not like, but they said: 'Look you can't speak the languages. We send you out, we have to send someone out with you. What a waste.' It seemed like a good argument but, you know, I never had any trouble talking to the people of Malange -and they came to the clinic from different tribes. You know, something like medical skill - it's international, don't you believe?"

"Well, no," I countered, "diagnosis would require history-taking and the patient

---

[71]Reference to an old and widely used proverb - "A man can achieve immortality in three ways: by planting a tree, having a son or writing a book".

feeling free to talk about his/her feelings with the doctor. You can't do all that in sign language and mime!"

However, it was clear that Oscar wasn't going to buy that line.

"No, no - it's not so much <u>words</u>, it's feelings, it's non-verbal, a lot of it. If you can palpate you can find out a lot. Most GP's can't palpate for shit, you know. Anyway, eventually I did get back to Malange for a month. They said that I could re-organise the staffing and the running of the clinic and the hospital if I could do it better! Jesus - how do I know what 'better' is? - number of patients processed in a day? recovery ratio? What? But the way they were talking, I knew that Dr O. must have gone "I'll bet cirrhosis got him", I thought. So my first big surprise when I got there was that Sister Eucharistika had gone, replaced by a miserable uncommunicative girl named Sister Felicia, but Dr O. was still there! In fact, he seemed, if anything, to be more in control than he had been before. He had even cut down, as far as I could see, on the whisky."

"But how was I free to re-organise anything with him still there? So I opened up and told him what they told me in Luanda! He said - 'Fine! But what happens when you go back to Cuba?' I thought he was angry but that wasn't it. The next day he said that they used to have - just after Independence - special two week 'schools' for village midwives and tried to use them as a means of spreading a bit of health knowledge into the community. But it got too expensive so the government gradually gave it up. I suggested that we train the local nurses from the clinic and the hospital - which now had no electricity or running water - to teach their own village people by getting the nurses to tell us what they should know, rather than the other way round. You would think I was a genius the way Dr O. reacted! He shouted: 'That's it!' So we started having seminars after the clinic closed. Some of the mothers who were staying with their sick children in the hospital also wanted to come. I had to do the talking first and I couldn't use an overhead projector because there was no electricity. I tell you, I know that I couldn't do this one by sign language - ."

"Or even palpation", I suggested.

"(Laughter) Well, Dr O. translated. The more he translated, the more excited

222

he got. By the time I had finished there and gone back to Luanda, we had trained 14 village health teachers! Dr O., unknown to me, had written a letter to the Angolan Ministry of Health saying that I was Jesus Christ or something. When I got back to Luanda, they asked me to organise meetings with groups of all other Cuban medical volunteers to tell them how to organise local health management and community hygiene. I was travelling all over the place and government people couldn't believe how much I know about Angolan geography and history."

"You know, how can I tell you all I did. I wasn't only administering medical education. Everywhere I went, even in the cities, I found myself involved in basic medical work. I did surgery that they would never have let me do in Cuba because I wasn't senior enough. I did surgery that I would not have had the nerve to do in Cuba and under conditions that would never have been allowed anywhere but in Angola. I don't know but somehow when you have to do these things, you do them. You mentioned to me at lunch how scared you were when you had to take bullets out of a guy's intestines on the ground with only a flashlight on a box to guide you. Like you say, it's amazing how quickly you get used to it. Eventually you don't even log the operations. Remember the 'cut book' in Cuba - you have to record every invasive technique you do? Shit - if I'd done that in Angola, I would have been writing all day!"

"At the beginning of 1989 the Angolan Ministry of Health said to me that they wanted me to stay but that Cuba wanted me back. I went to our embassy and they said, yes, it's time I came back home. No volunteer should make a full-time career of it. We are here to help our brothers, not to take over, etc., etc. As well, you know I knew I had trained enough people to carry on and then, you know, it was starting to be a strain - not always - but sometimes I would feel the need to hear Cuban voices, to see a smiling face say something to me in Spanish. You know, you see many smiling faces in Angola and your heart fills with love to talk and then when they speak you realise you cannot reply. Like I say, it was not always, but increasingly I felt this depression of missing my country. So I was also glad to go home again."

"What", I asked Oscar, "did you find most difficulty with in readjusting to Cuban life when you got back?" I asked this because when the Americans had started having Peace Corps volunteers returning in large numbers from their first tours of duty back in the '60's, a whole lot had been written about "reverse cultural shock". I had noticed it in myself on resuming work in metropolitan countries after working extended tours in the third world and I wanted to see if Oscar had experienced the same. He paused for some moments to reflect on the matter and then said.

"This I felt. People treated you like nothing had happened to you all the time you were away. You were a junior doctor then, you are a junior doctor still. You are allowed no decisions, no initiative, no ideas of your own. Never mind you've done hundreds of hours of surgery that even your boss wouldn't dream of doing. Never mind that over there (sic. in Angola) you had authority. You were used to speaking to rooms full of significant people and saying what needed to be done. Suddenly you were nothing again. Like that story about Jesus, you know. Everybody else respected him except his own people! (He laughs loudly as I take his hands pretending to look for the stigmata).

"So that is how it is at first. You feel a bit - well, sorry for yourself. You think, if I turn around and go back, I will feel good again. But you get into the work again and the bad feelings go away. There's nothing like exams coming up to make you realise that you are still only a boy and there is a lot to be learned."

"Have you ever felt", I enquired of him, "that the time you spent in Angola had been a bit of a digression, a waste of time perhaps, in your professional development? I mean if you had not done it, you would by now be head of a department of internal medicine?"

"No. Honestly I cannot say that. Other people, who went to school with me and are already established, say this to me. But they just do not understand. You know, more than studying Marxism, Angola taught me what it means to be a human being. Che is right about that. If I get killed in the crazy traffic when we go from here today, I would know that I have already lived - the world is already a little bit better, anyway, because I lived. That to me is the most important truth. I'm not saying I want to die! But I am saying I know how to live and that life has no meaning without service. You understand?"

224

I certainly did understand, but possibly - almost certainly - at a level that Oscar did not. What I understood by his comments was that moral training can have and does have an impact, but only in a society in which public values consistently reflect such moral training. In talking about Cuba, we are talking about a country in which even labourers on a building site characteristically modify their conversation in the presence, say, of young school children because all adults in Cuba are persistently told that they are role models (not in those words!) for the country's children. Likewise, of course, children learn to honour the dignity of labour and do, on the whole, confidently look up to adults. Even in Havana, it is not uncommon for young children to be sent off on their own to various after-school educational and cultural activities in the sure knowledge that if they become lost or confused, all they need to do is ask any "uncle" or "aunt" (that is, any adult) and they will receive help. One could not imagine risking that with a child in London or New York!

Of course, Cuba is a totalitarian state and that is doubtless one advantage such a state has over more complex social forms, such as pluralistic democracies. A totalitarian state has, after all, only one morality to peddle and this makes life much more simple! But having said that, it is still clear that there are uplifting totalitarian societies and the reverse. Might it not be argued that Cuba's is of the 'uplifting' variety because socialism really does address the basic moral imperatives of peace, justice and human dignity.

Oscar has been quoted at very great length, not because his comments were extraordinary, but because they were so similar to those of dozens of other medical volunteers I spoke to. His comments faithfully reflect the values of 'socialist morality' for want of a less pretentious phrase. Like many of the other volunteers interviewed, Oscar's comments reflected impatience with rhetoric (boring political speeches were a 'pet hatred' nominated by large numbers of socially active interviewees!) while clearly manifesting the effectiveness of the message contained therein.

225

CHAPTER FOURTEEN

CUBAN MEDICINE IN THE TEETH OF THE BLOCKADE.

The Third Noose

The US Economic Embargo and Blockade of Cuba is, of course, a constant stress factor but, as already indicated, has been exacerbated three times since the mid 70's by other factors. In Cuban journalism, these three worsenings of the situation have been, rather picturesquely, described as "the three nooses". The third noose in this respect has undoubtedly been the precipitous collapse of the eastern European economies coupled with the continuing impact of the Cuban Democracy Bill. Cuba has been aware, ever since the revolution in 1959, of the need to achieve economic and technological autonomy and, although it was massively sustained by preferential trade agreements with the former USSR and the other "fraternal socialist states", it fortunately had never become a complete client state. Even ideologically, it was sharply divergent from Soviet communism in many instances, and could in no way have been regarded as a "puppet regime".

In fact, the degree of Cuban ideological and philosophical autonomy has consistently been underestimated by western media commentators, and even by many political scientists, who expected the Cuban revolution to fold within days of Gorbachev's departure from the international scene. As Adolf Hitler was quoted as saying of Britain, once France had capitulated in 1940, "England will not last long now. When we need to, we shall simply wring its neck as one does with a chicken". To which Churchill replied: "Some neck, some chicken!" Much the same spirit now pervades Cuba.

As far as health care is concerned, the Cuban Ministry of Public Health has been the first to admit that its activities are so expensive in hard currency terms that the US blockade causes it continuous problems (See Chapter Sixteen). Much of the time and energy of that ministry is directed to seeking cheaper ways of meeting the same needs. One avenue that has been looked at with increasing interest lately has been various low cost "alternative" therapies (e.g. herbal remedies, homeopathy, acupuncture, etc.)

Former Opposition to Alternative Therapies

Cuba, even prior to the revolution, regarded itself as "modern" as far as medical practice was concerned. Certainly of all the medical schools in all of Latin America, that in Havana vigorously eschewed the systematic study of "alternative" and "complementary" therapies, simply because the AMA[72] has taken such a strong line against such alternatives and complementary methods since the 1930's. By way of explanation, it needs to be pointed out that there is a subtle difference between "alternative" and "complementary" medical practices and theories.

An "alternative" modality is one which does not even recognise the epistemological basis on which "orthodox" or "allopathic" medicine (conventional medical philosophy and training such as informs most medical decisions that people take). Acupuncture is a good example, as is homeopathy, although those can - in certain circumstances - also be used as "complementary" therapies. A "complementary" medical system is one that can be used alongside orthodox medicine without conflict. For instance, people who report to their GP with low back pain may be recommended (by their GP) to also see an osteopath or a chiropractor. Osteopathy and chiropractic are common complementary therapies, although the purists in those two fields regard them as totally sufficient for all health care and would thus see them as "alternative".

---

[72] American Medical Association

228

Contending Philosophies of Medical Care

Orthodox medicine has evolved over the centuries, deriving strands along the way from various other therapies. It has always been "conservative" in the sense of trying to protect itself and its clients from questionable practices based on non-scientific foundations. Unquestionably some of the practices thus rejected by the "orthodox" establishment have subsequently been established to be valid and have had, on that account, to be reincorporated into the orthodox "canon" once an explanation for their effectiveness has been successfully expressed in terms satisfactory to orthodox medicine. For example, acupuncture was absolutely rejected by the orthodox medical establishment until the mid-sixties. At that point, a number of orthodox researchers, experimenting with acupuncture applied to pain relief, not only found that it worked, in certain cases, but elaborated a model - consistent with current physiological knowledge - of how it did so.

The fact that something "works" in curing illness is not by itself sufficient justification for regarding it as acceptable to orthodox medicine. This is because many things are done and said to help in time of illness and, if a recovery comes about, how is one really to know what has worked and what didn't? "Faith healing" works, "homeopathy" works, "drinking carrot juice" works, etc., in the sense that sometimes they are associated with cures. But this does not make them acceptable to normal medicine because none of them (as yet) can be explained in terms of standard physiology and anatomy.

Just about every nation has a medical association (like America's AMA), which determines what goes into the training of doctors and what practices can or cannot be allowed to be included in the practice of medicine in that country. But there is considerable variations in this from country to country. The American Medical Association (AMA) is extremely rigid in its stand. American doctors are absolutely forbidden by law to engage in, or recommend to patients, medical therapies alternative to orthodox medicine. In Britain, on the other hand, some alternative and complementary therapies are recognised and are even used by the Royal family. The

229

British Medical Association (BMA) is considerably less rigid about their members practising alternative therapies than is the AMA.

These factors are, and have been, reflected in the third world. For instance, in Fiji (long under British control), medical practitioners, herbalists, acupuncturists, etc., are all listed under "medical" in the Yellow Pages. Likewise, in Jamaica, orthodox doctors work alongside herbalists etc., an attitude derived from the British influence. In Cuba, on the other hand, all forms of medical treatment other than orthodox were banned, until 1960. Of course, they were still practised, especially in the rural areas, where all sorts of "healers" would operate to meet the needs of people who could gain no access to orthodox treatment and couldn't have afforded it even if it had been available!

Legalising Herbalism in Cuba?

Herbalism has, since 1990, been increasingly coming to public notice in Cuba. There is no question but that the reason for this is the Economic Blockade, rather than any recent scientific validation of its practices.

As Cino Colina, writing in Granma International of June 28th, 1992, says:

"The collapse of trade with the extinct Council for Mutual Economic Assistance (CMEA) and the subsequent lack of raw materials and products has led Cubans to put all of their ingenuity and creativity into action to sort out the difficulties. Of course, with the passage of time original ideas have arisen in order to take advantage of the available potential, and other solutions have been rescued from oblivion.

In this last case there exist various old traditions which the rhythm of modern life has discarded. Such is the case of bicycles, fruit and vegetable gardens and raising chickens and other animals in town for human consumption, as well as the use of a wide variety of plants to treat pain and diseases.

In the country today there are more than one million gardens with products for home consumption tended by families, neighbourhood groups, workers or students. Yards, gardens and empty lots have acquired new significance at home. Someone discovers the appropriate corner to place the most unimaginable container, where luxuriantly grows some plant supplying spices or a home remedy."

Note that no claim is being made that Cuba should re-embrace herbalism because it has been empirically tested and found effective, but simply because it cannot be affected by the blockade. This author perceives great dangers in this, although one can sympathise with such a strategy. Until now Cuban medicine has, against almost overwhelming odds, continued to progress and has, as indicated in previous chapters, earned itself a deserved international recognition. It would represent a disaster if, finally, all of this were lost to anti-scientific influences because of financial stringency's.

Quoting again from Cino Colino:

"Herbal medicine, as it is currently called, has gained new importance, as has grandmother's remedies, in the face of the drug shortage. Years ago most physicians would never have recommended the use of herbal teas, poultices or flower compresses. Now not only do they do so, but many have become involved in expanding their knowledge in this field.

An example of this is that, surrounding the family doctor's offices, which are increasingly more common in the country's urban and rural landscape, are gardens for growing plants with medicinal properties. The number of merchants who sell herbs and roots is also growing. Until recently their clients were primarily followers of Afro-Cuban syncretic religions, who contend that everything except Okra vines have some use.

Thus it has come into fashion to utilize plants such as the passion flower - now known as the maracuya (Passiflora quadrangularis, Lin.) - whose herbal teas together with orange, lemon and citron blossom water were used as a sedatives by our ancestors; the humble romerillo (Didens polosa, Lin.) whose leaves are a recognised cough medicine, its roots are good for combating toothache and its flowers a magnificent vocal tonic; the guajani (Pruna offidentalis, Sw.), with its peel and leaves rich in hydrocyanic acid frequently used in preparations against asthma and coughs; and the aloe vera plant (Aloe barbadensis Mill.) used for such diverse purposes as cosmetics and treatment against liver ailments."

All of this smacks very much of advocacy and, moreover, suggests "alternative" rather than "complementary" use of herbalism.

Does Herbalism have a Positive contribution to Make in Cuba?

As a medical student on a visit to one of the Caribbean islands, I was once badly stung on my face by wasps. I knew what I needed, in the way of standard pharmaceuticals, but I also knew that - remotely placed as I was - there was no way of getting them. However, the people with me - none of them with any schooling beyond two or three years of primary and certainly with no knowledge of chemistry - proceeded to collect handfuls of leaves. They carefully mixed together leaves of three different types (as determined solely by leaf shape and it didn't matter <u>which</u> three!) and, pulping them together, handed me the resulting "goo" and told me to apply it. My anger at their superstition was only superseded by the discomfort of the stings and, since the stuff was cool, I did apply it. Of course, it worked!

There is a perfectly acceptable biochemical reason as to why it would have. Some plant leaves (most) contain the right anti-inflammatory chemical, some don't. If you take three different types, the chances are pretty close to certainty that at least one of them will do the trick. Of course, I didn't understand that at the time and neither did they. All they knew was that particular insight had been handed down and it "worked". Of course, they also knew not to pick, say, poison oak as one of the leaf types!

The Possibility of Linking Herbalism to Pharmacology Research

We know that modern pharmacology owes much to old herbalism, and in that sense, Cuba might make very effective re-use of herbalism - that is, using it as a complementary therapy by fully trained personnel who are aware of what they are after pharmacologically. If this is the line taken, something very worthwhile may come out of it. The UN Food and Agriculture Organisation recognises at least 50 million "herb" species of which almost all are represented in Latin America somewhere. It is also

232

known that Cuba has the greatest plant diversity in the Caribbean, with some 6200 species.

On the other hand, as we saw in Chapter Eleven, on the basis of research prosecuted since 1981 and of its abundance of professionals and mixed-level technicians, Cuba has fantastic potential for the solution of problems relating to alternative (low tech) pharmaceutical production. As of 1992, Cuba already spends about 130 million US dollars annually on pharmaceutical preparations for medicinal use in Cuba alone. Various of these products are now being produced in Cuba by its nascent pharmaceutical industry. If a thorough study of available herbal resources can reduce this reliance on expensive high tech production methods and on factors which are threatened by the blockade, it is to be earnestly hoped that Cuba will walk that path.

Indeed, it has already made great strides. Interferons, monoclonal antibodies and antibiotics are all being investigated as possibly being derivable cheaply from primary herbal resources by intermediate level technological processes. As already indicated in Chapter Nine, drugs such as melagenina (used to combat vitiligo), the meningococcus type B vaccine and epidermal growth factor are already actually being produced in Cuba for the international market without recourse to technology outside of Cuba. Research on herbalism will doubtless suggest even more equally daring initiatives.

Some Recent Application

One possible avenue in this regard is the use of sugar-cane waste products. Already mentioned has been the use of sugar-cane stubble to produce paper, but since 1962 Cuba has run an Institute for Research on Sugar-cane By-Products (ICID-CA) and, in 1989, they succeeded in isolating important nitrofuranic pharmaceuticals through investigating the long-standing peasant habit of treating skin burns by rubbing sugar-cane juice and ash mixture on the burned areas! By continuing this line of research they have, this author was told, run across isolatable quantities of a standard pharmaceutical used in urinary tract infections. Details were sketchy and have not yet been published but, as I understand it, the compounds in question are obtained from 5 - nitrofurfuraldiacetate (5-NFDA) which, in the industrialised countries, are obtained at much greater cost, from wood pulp.

Starting early in 1992, work is being carried out on the production of sapogenin from powdered henequin plants, as well as iron dextrin (so far only for veterinary use) from supplies of 5-NFDA referred to above. The implications of such lines of research are enormous for a hungry world, for such compounds can be used to greatly increase the protein content of cattle fodder and other livestock feeds.

Other, more directly applicable, nutritional products are being extracted and re-synthesised from potato and corn yeast extracts such as hydrolysed proteins. High molecular crystalline alcohols are being distilled directly from cane froth oil. Prostaglandins - which command an extremely high price on the world market - are even being extracted from certain types of coral! That latter line of research again was suggested by long-standing folklore herbalism.

In 1990 a new medication called "biocen" was put forward for testing in geriatric medicine. It is made from horses' gastric juices mixed with cattle blood and bees' honey (another folk remedy) and is attracting interest. Again, details are lacking, but I was told that it had already passed clinical trials as a means of combating anaemia in old people.

Dangers and Challenges

It would seem, then, that the re-awakening interest in herbalism is very much a two-edged sword. Insofar as it can serve as a fertile source of suggestions for research in low or intermediate tech production of pharmaceuticals, it can lead Cuba to new levels of "health autonomy" within the confines of the Economic Blockade. But the very real danger is that the ever present stress of economic restriction may empower an anti-technology/anti-science lobby that will lead to such modalities as herbalism being accepted in toto because it is "Cuban" and "cheap". So far, it appears that such a negative scenario is only a distant possibility, although perhaps Cuban journalists themselves should take greater care as to how they report these things. The impression gained is that, in the Cuban pharmaceutical industry, scientists are daily striving to compensate for lack of access to the world's intermediate biochemical components by deriving replacements from Cuba's rich panoply of herbal remedies.

Why should a country of Cuba's medical credentials be driven to rely so heavily on outdated and questionable health care paradigms? The answer is provided, rather chillingly, in the final chapter of this book in terms of an objection analysis by American medical observers of the Cuban scene. Their unambiguous view is that the U.S. Trade Embargo has already undercut many of Cuba's hard-won health advances since 1994 and is unquestionably inflicting unnecessary suffering and death on Cuban civilians.

CHAPTER FIFTEEN

HEALTH CARE FOR THE NATION'S PEOPLE.
(Comparing and Contrasting the USA, the UK and Canada.)

Replacing Cuba's Problems in Context

While the main thrust of this book is devoted to an account of how a third world economy manages to produce first world health care statistics, it is helpful to set the whole health care issue in context. This will be attempted through a very brief overview of the history of the problem and differing approaches to it adopted in the US, the UK, and Canada. The main contribution that Canada makes to the debate is that it evolved - in many respects - in response to analyses of the differences between the British NHS and the American market economy model. As such, the Canadian approach is frequently referred to by both UK and US health care commentators.

Prior to the 20th century, health services were mediated in most countries as a commodity in exactly the same way that any other economic commodity was mediated. The sick looked for providers and the providers looked for customers who could pay. Coverage was somewhat hit and miss, prices were low, equipment meagre and results somewhat what one might expect. The rich could pay more and so tended to be healthier. Although that same connection between wealth and health persists today, even in the UK, with its National Health Service, the relationship is at least recognised as being considerably more complex than it was before. One of the assumptions behind the setting up of the NHS was that the nexus between social class and health would disappear. It did not but it became much less easily defined and the persisting relationship is not used as a criticism of the NHS by those who wish to make it more subject to "market forces".

Indeed, it was the sheer inefficiency of the old "laissez-faire" system that prompted efforts to improve it. The grossly uneven distribution of health care meant that large sectors of society remained conspicuously unhealthy and a health-threat to the rest of the community. Also the private enterprise ethic meant that providers were reluctant to modernise equipment and to contribute significantly to medical advance. Churches, and other charity institutions, found themselves called upon to provide what they could for the poor, but this was done out of a sense of moral duty, religious compassion or emotive pity, rather than as an integrated response to social health needs.

As the 20th Century unfolded, different societies responded in different ways to this unsatisfactory state of affairs. In the three societies specifically being considered in this chapter - the UK, the US and Canada - various patch-up remedies were tried to counter the inadequacies of a free-market approach to health. Especially in Britain and Canada, national health insurance laws were passed and a very large proportion of the workforce had to sign up. Attempts were made to guarantee access by the uninsured, although it is far beyond the scope of this author's remit to detail these. The basic idea was that risk pools could be defined well enough for actuarially determined rates to cover everyone's costs.

All of this is well summarised by William Glaser[73] in a recent Lancet article, in which he observes:

> "In place of the self-orientation and self-protection of the free market, social solidarity and redistributive financing became the foundations. Extra money was collected regularly from the richer and healthier persons to cover the excessive costs of the poor and unhealthy.
>
> The health sector was stabilised. If an area had fewer of poorer patients, the hospitals did not disappear through bankruptcies. Doctors did not concentrate in areas with large numbers of paying patients. Fewer resources were diverted from patient care into marketing. Money steadily flowed into health facilities for modernisation. Cut-throat economic competition was no longer necessary, but much competition of a different sort remained. Doctors competed for the respect of their peers and of the general public. Doctors also continued to compete for economic rewards, since professional reputations attracted the richer private patients and led to appointments to the

---

[73]Glaser, W (1996): The Competition Vogue and Its Outcomes.

The Lancet, Vol 341, March 27th, 1996, pg. 805 - 813.

better paid jobs. Hospitals also competed for reputations of high quality, safety, and eminence. Then they could attract the better doctors to their staffs. They could attract private and famous patients. Insurance carriers competed for the healthier and richer subscribers.

Developments in the United States tended to differ from this for a variety of reasons. Again, analysis of these reasons transcends this author's brief. Suffice to say, as a society which achieved pre-eminence in so many fields of human endeavour on the basis of free-market capitalism (or so it was widely perceived in the popular mind, but in reality there were many other factors) it was psychologically natural for a majority of Americans to eschew government control when it came to health care.

Health and Ideology

Health throughout the world has come a long way since the British National Health Service (NHS) was established in 1948. That initiative on the part of Britain's first post war government, a Labour government led by Clement Atlee, was regarded as amazingly innovatory all over the world and the public utterances of its most zealous protagonists, people like the redoubtable Emmanuel Shinwell and Aneurin Bevin, invested it with an ideological dimension that many confused with being an epistemologically necessary precursor for the existence of any kind of a national health system at all! In a sense, this gave those forces (especially in the US) who were opposed to a publicly funded health service, a convenient scape-goat on which to give street cred to their antagonism to the idea. If you want a publicly funded health service, you must want socialism!

Some of my readers will even recall an advertisement that was run by the American Medical Association in the early 50's that showed a photograph of a hand holding out a conventional collecting-can on the label of which was written "SOCIALISM". Above it was written "Would you put a nickel (5 cents) in ?" Underneath was written: "No-one wants to see socialism in America. Keep government out of your relationship with your doctor. Keep our medical care private -

239

keep it American".

In the intervening 45 years, much has changed. It is now widely recognised, in both the UK and the US, that the financing of a nation's health care is not only expensive and involved, but inexorably becomes more so as time passes. It is this pernicious growth factor, rather than the original concept, which carries serious philosophical and ideological implications.

The initial idea was that, as soon as health care became "free" at point of delivery (it is never really free, of course, but must be paid for somehow), the system would be swamped at first and even abused. However, as the health of the people improved, so went the theory, use and abuse of the system would decrease. People predicted a golden future in which the NHS would devote most of its resources to health promotion and to preventive medicine. What a pipe dream! The actual situation is that, as the health of the nation improved, so did medical knowledge. Better, more effective and more expensive medicines and interventional treatments evolved and - since now everyone had access to the system - the need for resources kept increasing exponentially.

One does not have to be an Einstein to realise that health care costs have no ceiling. In Britain, government spending on health constitutes about 6.9%[74] of the gross national product. This sounds a lot, but in the US - where the government is not even the main supplier of health care and where everyone does not have a right to public health care - the cost of government involvement alone in health comes to 14% of the gross national product. In Cuba, where the system is completely public and where there is no private health care in the domestic economy, the cost is 8% of the gross national product. And one could go on.

To reiterate, though, the pivotal point is not what the cost is now in terms of proportion of a country's GNP. It is the fact that we now all know that the original optimistic assumption was wrong. The system is never going to become less costly as people get healthier. It will only become more costly. More people will lead longer lives and require more and more capital consumption to keep themselves illness-free or to pay for increasingly involved high technology to cure themselves when they do fall ill.

Health is like no other ordinary economic commodity. Indeed, some health economists argue that it cannot be called a commodity at all. It raises enormous moral and political complications. If a government has a fixed amount of money to spend on health care, what proportion of it do they devote to routine, mass health care and what proportion to the sort of heroic heart surgery which didn't even exist in 1948 and which only a small proportion of people require anyway? So we have waiting lists in the British NHS. For instance, you're 94 and you need a cataract operation, sir. Well, I'm sorry but we have two 75 year olds who need the same surgery and even a 58 year old. Somebody has to put these people in order, because we can only do one at a time. Who makes that decision and on what basis? Who decides whether my baby dies for lack of an expensive surgical intervention in order that 9,000 other babies get routine health checks and immunisations?

No political system can claim to have resolved these problems in terms of equity. But some are clearly less just and more inefficient than others. In the UK, NHS-knocking is a popular indoor sport, but with all of its waiting lists, inefficiencies, bureaucracy, corruption's etc, it seems to compare rather favourably with, say, the US system. That is, the average Britisher seems to get more and better medical attention for his/her 7% of GNP than does the average American for his/her 14% of GNP. For his/her 8% of GNP, the Cuban in the street - any Cuban, whatever his/her status or work - gets a cradle-to-the-grave primary health care system, but when it comes to high tech medicine, choices between people again have to be made.

To complicate the moral dilemma further, it must not be imagined that "high tech" medicine somehow implies non-essential, luxury medicine. What it implies is the inexorable fruit of steady progress in medical research in often quite mundane areas. Thus, Joe Bloggs - a working man - may go for a routine medical, but because of more sophisticated equipment now in common use, a medical problem he has is revealed which ten years ago wouldn't have been revealed. Now comes the crunch. Do we say

---

[74] British Medical Association. September 14th, 1998.

to Bloggs: "Ah, I see you have such-and-such. But fixing it is damned expensive. We can do it, but only if we don't do any more FBC's for a couple of months or maybe we can leave out a dialysis or two because that patient isn't going to make it 'til Christmas anyway." As the US blockade on Cuba tightens, choices like that are going to have to be made further and further down the line in Cuba until their guaranteed primary health care becomes very primary indeed.

Thus, in making comparisons between the health systems of various countries, we are not working with moral certainties to the degree that maybe we would like to be. Party politics is great for the throwaway phrase, but is notoriously ambivalent on real answers to real questions of health resource distribution! However, having said that - and before comparing the health systems as such - the reader should realise that the present author cannot see how the issue of an adequate health system can be solved outside of some sort of socialism. This is so within any given country, and even in the context of an international administration (a world government) between nations, if resource allocation is to be rendered even remotely rational!

In briefly considering three "mainstream" (first world) national systems of health care, no claim will be made to a detailed analysis of the UK, the US and the Canadian structures. The first two have been addressed (and are still being addressed) in far greater detail than this author can hope to do in one chapter. Moreover, they have already been the subject of critical analysis - at various depths - by scholars much more knowledgeable about structure, policy and health economics than this author claims to be. The purpose of the following discussion, then, will be to set the three systems in "rough comparative context", short on detail perhaps but - it is hoped -long on general social and philosophical outlook.

The Canadian system has not as yet attracted the attention it merits, where as the systems in the UK and the US have each had a number of books written about them, rendering it unnecessary to suggest a particular one as being in any sense "Canonical"; the Canadian system has really only had a few decent publications devoted to it. For the purpose of the following description, then, I will be relying largely on a paper by Kiely and Blyton[75], which is recommended even to the general reader as a source for material on the Canadian system.

The American System

The US system of health care is in a mess. They avoided socialism and the impersonal face of state care, but they certainly did not save money! Whether it be expressed either in absolute terms (even Cuba uses the US dollar as the basic international monetary unit in discussing comparisons of costs from one country to another) or as a percentage of GNP, the US government spends much more than does the UK, Canada or Cuba, for less health care and for a lower proportion of total health care, than do any of the other three countries. Let us get this unambiguously straight!

In the US, government (Federal, State or Local) is involved in a smaller proportion of the financing of the total health bill than it is in Cuba, the UK or Canada. Most medical attention in the US, from a visit to the GP up to the most involved of high tech medical intervention, is paid for by each individual patient. Most, of course, do this through health insurance of some type or another, but very little of this is mediated in other than conventional profit-and-loss commercial terms. Yet even the small proportion that does involve government deployment of funds comes to a whacking 14% of GNP. Whatever the ideology, this has to be inefficient. An increasingly large and vocal proportion of the American electorate have known this to be so for a long time. Should the AMA run those "Would you donate a nickel to socialism?" ads again today, a surprisingly large number of Americans - more ideologically mature now, as post-Vietnam, post-recession people - might well say "Yes!"

Mary Hilary Clinton knew in 1994 that the system needed straightening out.

[75]Kiely J and Blyton P (1990) "Health Service Management - An Introductory Overview of Canada and the United Kingdom" International Journal of Health Care Quality Assurance; Vol 3, Part 3: pg.-6.

The only question is, how much ideological and financial leeway did she feel that the task required, and how much would she have been be given? Readers might remember that, immediately after her appointment, she said that she would have definitive proposals to put forward within three months. On the whole, though, Americans are generously tolerant about such miscalculations - as long as they eventually get the goods. Americans gladly gave Mrs Clinton a bit of extra time to bail them out of a system - or even to think of a way of bailing them out of a system - that is eating up 14% of GNP and is costing about $2,500 per year for each individual in health insurance. But when push comes to shove, she couldn't do it. The various 'freedom lobbies' representing the vested financial interests of wealthy medical people and insurers were called into play and the whole enterprise was allowed to fade away.

But even that 14% does not really protect the individual from anything more than treatment for acute episodes of illness. A chronic illness can send a family's insurance premiums sky high. In some cases, one's place of work pays the premium, so that one almost has an indentured labour system in which some employees cannot leave their job because, if they did so, they would lose their health cover!

In spite of this, some do decide to change their job, and join the ranks of that larger proportion of middle-class Americans who find themselves inadequately insured for health care. About 17% of the population are without any health insurance cover at all. This constitutes about 37 million people - people who are not poor enough for government assistance but whose employers do not provide a private policy.

In most states, it is obligatory by law for hospitals to treat such people, but they can then extract payment from the individuals in any way that they regard as feasible. For instance, one standard admitting office procedure is to do a "wallet biopsy" when the patient is first brought in. If his/her insurance card will not yield enough to cover costs, the debt collectors are sent around. Even if the patient does make it past the admissions office, many American state or county hospital facilities do not do routine tests unless they are specifically requested to. Never mind preventive medicine or health promotion, every medical activity is costed and one only does what the patient asks for or his/her doctor requires. That may be one reason why currently the incidence of TB is on the rise in the US and, to a lesser extent, in the UK.

Prior to Hilary Clinton's stated interest in the problem, no previous presidential incumbent had faced the problem front on. One idea, initiated in the 60's, was to give tax concessions to people who were paying health insurance premiums. But this just encouraged a spending spiral and a built up inflation. The big employers generously purchased more insurance, partly to reduce tax! This led to the hospitals charging more, the insurance companies raising their premiums and hence, the patients ultimately paying. The situation is now (1998) at the point where, if the system is not changed, the government will have to negotiate lower premiums and reduced cover.
Since 1985, there has been a marked withdrawal of government involvement in health in the US.

Medicaid and Medicare

America currently has two public health instrumentalities, Medicaid and Medicare. They only cater for less than one third of the US population. Let us briefly examine them.

Medicaid is designed to meet the health needs, or some of the health needs, of people who live below the poverty line. The private insurance companies try to avoid entanglement with Medicaid bureaucracy, so that people affected - if they do buy extra insurance cover - have to do the top-up through different private companies. When the author was in Los Angeles in 1987, one of the research staff at UCLA's Postgraduate Department of Public Health Administration told him that about 20% of total hospital floor space in American hospitals had to be set aside to accommodate the huge and complex clerical operations required to keep track of refunds and claim settlements. There are so many private health insurance companies in the US, each with slightly different claims procedures and liability clauses, that highly trained financial specialists are required to sort the claims in each hospital.

Now more and more hospitals will not accept Medicaid patients because the

245

return on the clerical work put in to secure the refund no longer covers the clerical expenses involved. Really there is only one way out of such a crazy system - provided that one is going to play by the rules - and that is the route recently taken by Oregon State. That state is going to render Medicaid more cost effective by restricting the services it will provide. If you are poor, in that context, you are only allowed to fall prey to the cheaper illnesses! This will allow Medicaid to embrace a much larger number of people, but with reduced effectiveness. Anyway, various studies have shown that the sick mathematics of the system is that the numbers of people who cannot afford private insurance always increase at a greater rate than that at which Medicaid can expand!

Medicare is the second government financed initiative. It is federally operated and is designed to serve the needs of old age pensioners. It is funded out of the social security deductions taken out of every employed American's pay cheque throughout his/her working life. Americans who are now old age pensioners, retired after good working lives, can feel quite secure with Medicare. But many middle-aged working Americans are legitimately worried. As we have already seen with respect to Cuba - and as is true almost everywhere - general improvements in medicine (and better awareness of healthy lifestyles) guarantee that the proportion of people living longer beyond retirement age is increasing exponentially. Will the Medicare funds last long enough for these people to benefit from them? Gail Wilensky, the Director of Medicare, has been quoted by American News Services[76] as saying that Medicare will be bankrupt by the turn of the century!

What strategies are open to Medicare? It has already introduced some cost-cutting strategies, such as: paying hospitals only a fixed price according to the patient's diagnosis, putting ceilings on doctor's fees to Medicare patients and even funding health education initiatives to encourage preventive medicine. It appears that Hilary Clinton was considering strategies like this in trying to impose coherence on the huge private insurance sector. No wonder she was deflected from real action!

---

[76]Kansas City Star (AP): March 24th, 1993

In order to do this, she would have had to introduce two new pieces of federal legislation. Every employer, however small the enterprise, would have been required to provide health insurance. The state of Hawaii already has such legislation. As well, though, she would have had to contrive some sort of means of control over all American private insurance companies. There are over 1,600 of them! This would have had to be done so that payments to the hospitals can be negotiated at lower levels.

Obviously even mild, patch-up legislation like this, would have had adverse effects on a free enterprise economy. Any state that follows Hawaii and introduces the first initiative will effectively discourage firms from setting up business there. Taxes of any kind scare business away! Also, both measures involve restricting profit margins for medical care. In a society which has always claimed that health is a purchasable commodity and that normal market forces should apply to its supply and demand, this is going to raise enormous psychological -and legal - problems.

These issues appear so complex only if we try to play the game by the existing rules. But surely Americans will realise that this cannot realistically be done. It is this author's assumption that somehow, somewhere - either in the near future or in the distant future - it will become accepted that the old shibolleths are too expensive. It will be seen that health, even if it is a commodity, is a different kind of commodity and that market forces don't handle it particularly efficiently.

American Solutions Vs British Solutions

The British NHS has its detractors, of course, as shall be discussed later, and it in consequence underwent a series of far-reaching "reforms" after 1988 in order to try to render it more responsive to normal market forces. What this means is that, both in the UK and the US, health care and the politics of it is a big issue. In the UK this has largely been manifested by public debate along party political lines - the Conservatives being for a market forces ideology while still being pledged to support the concept of an NHS, while some in the Labour Party (together with the Liberal Democrats) argue that the reforms were really the first steps to "privatising" the NHS!

But in the US, the debate is still about much more fundamental issues. It has been said that even President Clinton had been persuaded that socialised medicine must be avoided[77]. Henry J Aaron, a highly regarded American health economist, however, has argued that America's present system is such as to guarantee an increase in cost for a decrease in effectiveness of health care delivery[78]. In other words, he is saying that it is caught in an inescapable paradox of rising cost and falling coverage! His thesis is that health economics is such that competition among providers renders it less efficient and he argues that therefore Americans must accept the ideological nostrum of a largely government funded, government regulated health care system. This, of course, would represent a combination of the socialist and private enterprise models, but it is a model that more and more Americans are recognising is required. This is taking place in a context in which President Clinton appears to be gradually moving away from government involvement models!

Aaron proposes a 'single power' model. In it control over spending on health would be vested in the individual state legislatures, rather than federally. In that way, difficult decisions about who to accept and who to reject, which treatment to authorise and which not to, would have to be made closer to the community level in which the problems arise. The merit of Aaron's model is that it recognises the fact that there can be no realistic ceiling on health costs - either in absolute or in GNP proportion - terms - and that some people must be denied care in order that others may have it. This of course, is an unpalatable proposition for idealists.

Canada's System

Canada's system already shares some of those characteristics. In Canada the national

---

[77]ibid. 90

[78]Klein, R (1991): "The American Health Care Predicament"
British Medical Journal, Vol 303, Aug 3rd 1991, pg. 259-260

insurance system is administered by the provinces, but brings about universal coverage. Local provincial control restrains the rate of growth of spending, while a multiplicity of providers (some of them private insurance companies) provides leeway. More will be said about the Canadian system towards the end of this chapter, especially insofar as it contrasts with the UK's NHS, but what we have said so far indicates that the way in which a country elaborates a health care system is not primarily a mathematical phenomenon. It is a political phenomenon. That is, all material considerations being equal, British, Canadian, American and Cuban engineers would probably all build a bridge across a given river in roughly the same way. Politics would impinge very little. Health care, however, is not only different economically (i.e. different mathematics is required) but even the mathematics varies according to the philosophical assumptions of the people concerned!

If one knew American, British and Canadian history and politics, but nothing at all about their health systems, one might well conjecture that a Canadian health care system would share features of both - a sort of half-way house. This, in fact, is so. But surely all three systems would build bridges in the same way!

If then we agree that the problem is not solely one of justice, morality or mathematics (or even justice and morality dictating mathematics!) but is one of political feasibility, we can begin to isolate some of the variables in the mix. The problems all arise in connection with, or because of conflict between several interest groups. For instance, a health care system has to meet the conflicting needs of employers (who want to reduce cost outflow), of socialists (who want the whole population to be protected), of insurers, hospitals and the medical profession (who want to maintain their incomes) and of politicians (who don't want to increase direct taxation).

Mathematics Confronts Politics

At this point mathematics rears its ugly head and surveys the problem with cold logic. Extending coverage while also stabilising health care spending is an impossibility.

249

Either the price of individual treatments has to be reduced or the number of such treatments has to be curtailed. The question which all democratic societies must face today involves arriving at some kind of political coalition which will balance these conflicting objectives in such a way as to strike their electorate as feasible. With respect to the American and British systems, they have resolved these issues in mutually complementary ways. Britain is financially efficient overall (6.9% of GNP vs. 14% of GNP in the US), but is atrociously inefficient among individual providers at the local level. This will become more evident when we contrast the Canadian and UK systems. But basically the British system provides universal coverage cheaply and equitably while offering few direct incentives to providers. The US, on the other hand, is - on the whole - atrociously wasteful at the same time as guaranteeing efficient monetary return to providers.

The UK's NHS has traditionally given providers incentives to decrease involvement while the US system gives them incentives to increase involvement - even if this is ineffective.

At the operational level, the NHS is faced with strong pressures to either spend more or deliver less. These problems are exacerbated, not only by such factors as an ageing population and better diagnostic modalities, but by a population which now knows more about its rights and more about medicine! Private insurance companies have seen to that! The insurance companies, by advertising campaigns involving free gifts, etc., have made the average Briton more aware of health issues at the consumerist levels than did 35 years of socialised medicine. But what was the impact of this sort of thing in the US? It has led to consumer choice in health matters (a Health Charter personified!) and this has led to the sort of medical bureaucracy that uses up 25% of total health care expenditure on administrative/clerical costs[79].

This, if we are to learn anything at all from the American experience, can be expected to balance cost and effectiveness in three ways - maybe as alternatives, maybe

---

[79]Klein R (1991): "The American Health Care Predicament"
British Medical Journal Vol 303 August 3rd, 1992 pg. 259-260

all together. One can hardly do better than to quote Klein[80].

"Firstly, clinical audit has the potential to measure whether doctors can do what they claim to do: improve health, or at least decrease suffering. The potential for learning about the effectiveness of various treatments is awesome in a closed medical system such as the NHS, especially with the information technology the government has pushed and that general practitioners are adopting. The cost, however, will be great, especially in the first few years. The costs of administering audit programmes, especially in hospitals and other centres away from the general practitioner's surgery, will be great, perhaps going from an estimated 8% at present toward the United States estimate of 25% of total medical costs. Kenneth Clarke[81] believed that the costs would be offset in the long term by improved efficiency in care.

Secondly, prevention of disease is a major focus of the general practitioner's contract and the targets. However, laudable a goal that may be, the Americans have again discovered, painfully, that "prevention" often means finding disease earlier - before symptoms occur - which often increases the cost of caring for the person. In addition, some observers, such as Ivan Illich, have suggested that prevention leads to a perverse medicalisation of society, which he claims is a social problem in America.

Thirdly, any marketplace, internal or otherwise, requires that certain risks should be taken to survive. For hospitals the risks of competition will be closure."

Canada's System Compared with the UK's

While it is true that Canada's health care system might be expected to reflect both American and British psychosocial preoccupations, it obviously has to be realised within a radically different geopolitical context. Canada has a population of 26 million

---

[80]Ibid. 94.

[81]Minister of Health in the UK at the time of writing.

rattling around in an area of 3.85 million square miles. Contrast this with the UK - with a population of 57 million living in an area one fortieth the size of Canada. Of course, Canada's population is not uniformly distributed over its available area. It tends to "huddle for warmth" along the US-Canada border! But then Britain's population also is very unevenly distributed. This author has hiked for days in northern England, and in parts of Scotland, through desolate countryside, without catching sight of human habitation. To make up for its refusal to live horizontally throughout much of their real estate, the British - in large numbers - live vertically in square mile after square mile of urban high rise in areas such as London.

Canadians tend to enter hospital with greater frequency than do their British counterparts. But this is because - probably as a consequence of the distances between settlements - entering a hospital is the only way many Canadians can get medical care. Altogether the Canadian system is much more hospital-oriented than is the UK system. The break-up of costs, between the private and public sector in Canada, is organised around this phenomenon. Private insurance cannot be allowed for services covered by public health insurance (such as hospital beds) but is allowed for drugs and dentistry. All of this means that, per patient, Canada has a larger number of beds and a greater variety of hospital facilities than does Britain. In the NHS in Britain, 95% of care is provided outside hospitals, while in Canada only about 71% of care is so provided[82].

As has already been observed, Canada has ten health care systems -one for each province. Of course, there are many similarities from one provincial system to another, but the electorate within each province have a direct political say in how their health system is to be run and this can, and does, reflect regional cultural differences. That cannot be said of the UK. At the fiscal level, these cultural factors also have expression. For instance, many hospitals in Canada are built as religious or community endeavours, reflecting local value judgements.

Like its UK counterpart, though, the Canadian health care system also finds

---

[82]Keily J and Blyton P A (1990) "Health Service Management: An Introductory Overview of Canada and the UK" International Journal of health Care Quality Assurance, Vol 3, Part 3, pg. 4-6.

itself the subject of heated public debate. The difference is that the Canadian system is far less subject to change introduced as an expression of national party politics than is the case in the UK. How can it be when there is only one federal government but ten autonomous provincial health systems?

But the provinces, although they each run their own health care systems, cannot play political dice with the funding of it because the money does not go into the federal treasury to be allocated according to competing demands made on the treasury by other public services. This does happen in the UK.

In fact, provincial politics is much less subject to radical change in the way it handles the health care systems than is any federal system. Various polls have shown that, while Canadians may criticise various aspects of their system, they do not like sudden changes to it. They can energetically kick out a party and its leader at federal level, but remain confident that their provincial health care system will change only in response to local pressures.

Because the system is not federally run in Canada, it is more expensive - about 8.1% of GNP and therefore similar in proportional cost to the Cuban system. This makes it more expensive than the British NHS but not nearly as expensive as the American system.

At the operational level, what do Canadians and British get out of their respective systems? Life expectancy and infant mortality are two of the customary health indices cited, although no one would claim that these two statistics in any exact sense reflect the efficiency of a society's health care system. Life expectancy (as of 1991) was higher in Canada (76.5 years) than in Britain (74.7). Britain also lags behind in infant mortality (9.4) compared with Canada's (7.9). Both of these should be contrasted with the American figure of 10.6.

In a survey quoted by Maureen Dixon[83] (1990) an attempt was made to gain some sense of relative consumer satisfaction among Britons and Canadians for their

---

[83] Dixon M (1990) "Health Care: A Critical Comparison of Canada and the UK" International Journal of Health Care Quality Assurance, Vol 3 Part 3, pg. 8-15.

respective systems. When asked if they thought their system required fundamental change; 42% of Canadians responded affirmatively, while 69% of the British did. 73% of the Canadian sample claimed to be "very satisfied" with their last contact with a physician, whereas only 63% of the British sample so claimed. With respect to their last stay in hospital, 71% of the Canadian sample was positive about the experience, but only 57% of the British sample were.

When asked whether they had ever been refused medical care for financial reasons, only 0.17% of the British sample answered affirmatively while 0.6% of the Canadian sample did. Compare these with 7.5% for an American sample.

In summary, it can be said that both the Canadian and the UK systems are more responsive to the needs of a wider range of the population than is true of the US system. They both make strenuous efforts to adjust on the basis of geographical equity and are relatively comprehensive in the range of services they provide. At the financial level, the Canadian system is more wasteful because GP's in Canada are not "gatekeepers" to the specialist services in the way that they are in the UK. This means, in effect, that anyone in Canada can, say, make an appointment to see an eye specialist without any medical advice that this is necessary. In the UK, whatever the health problem is or appears to be, one's first port of call is always the GP. He/she makes the decision as to what, if anything, to do next.

Perhaps it is routine for authors to allude to the forbearance of their families in the authorship of a book, but in this case the sentiments are all too genuine. Who but saints could put up with a paterfamilias coming home every night after work to a small flat and saying "Please don't talk to me to even to each other. I have to finish this chapter!"? Therefore, to my wife, Chris, and son, Matthew, I accord the most heartfelt thanks. Both share with me - and exemplify it with more purity than I - a commitment to social justice worldwide and a profound respect for the people of Cuba.

CHAPTER SIXTEEN

THE MEDICAL VIEW OF CUBA FROM AMERICA

America - More than its Government

The intransigence of successive US governments in maintaining the blockade against Cuba has had a number of psychosocial effects on the way people outside of Cuba see the situation - independently of what is really happening. For instance, in the US itself a widespread view among ordinary people is that Cuba must be extraordinarily dangerous (remember, President Reagan in 1986 likened it to a virus!) and/or uniquely evil. There are lots of countries the US government does not like, but only three which are actually "blockaded" in any way - Cuba, Iraq and Libya - with Cuba sustaining the most thorough-goingly complete blockade and over the longest period of time. But there is also a long tradition of fair play in American daily life and one runs across all sorts of minority groups vociferously arguing that the blockade of Cuba is morally wrong and/or politically unwise. These people and groups are always coming up with various devious means of breaching the blockade, especially to get educational and medical supplies through.

One even runs across a strong sentiment in favour of lifting the blockade among some American middle level and small businessmen. They see Cuba as a great potential trading partner. Its people are highly educated and technologically minded and appear to be versatile and adaptable at the entrepreneurial level.

Major opposition to Cuba comes from the Cuban American National Foundation, a Miami-based group of anti-Castro political exiles. CANF was indeed founded by leading figures in the Batista regime who fled Cuba with the dictator and they were very well endowed financially. Many of its leading figures today are prominent business people and, for such a small group, they are extraordinarily powerful. They would be just one of several US-based groups of anti-Castro Cubans, but for one major difference. Florida is a pivotal state in US politics and because

CANF has such immense political power in Florida, its member are able to influence American government (whether Democrat or Republican) policy on Cuba to a degree out of all proportion to their small numbers.

Thus, even if one runs across a broadly less extreme view about quarantining Cuba among many sectors of American public opinion, US Government invariably seem to stand by CANF values in their reaction to and policy towards Cuba.

American Doctors Speak

But Cuba's remarkable achievements in primary health care have not gone unnoticed by American medical opinion. Those American medical people who have enquired into the health situation in Cuba, have generally commented in praiseworthy terms about it. but such commentary does not often reach the popular media. It has tended to be buried away in the more esoterically academic journals and, for that reason, often constitutes preaching to the converted. However, in 1997 the American Association for World Health (AAWH) made a report on the impact of the American blockade on Cuban health called - rather appropriately - Denial of Food and Medicine. This report was, moreover, widely circulated to American medical organisations and the press. It appeared on the Net in early 1998. One can hardly do better, in a book dedicated to a fair analysis of Cuba's health care system, than to end the book with a summary of the AAWH report.

The AAWH, although founded in 1953 as a private educational organisation, now serves as the US Committee for the World Health Organisation (WHO) and the Pan American Health Organisation (PAHO). Its remit is to educate the American people about any health problems that are likely to affect people either in the US or overseas. It is dedicated to the promotion of co-operative solutions, but especially those that are grass-roots based.

How the AAWH Views the Blockade Generally

In their report they observe that the U.S. embargo against Cuba has
the early 1960s. It is one of the few embargoes of recent years that
foods and medicines in its virtual ban on bilateral commercial ties. Prompted by their
40-year commitment to international health, especially in the developing world, and by
tightening of the embargo since 1992, the American Association for World Health
launched a study of the impact of U.S. policy in the health of the Cuban population.

Over a twelve-month period between 1995 and 1996, a multi-disciplinary
research team traced the implications of embargo restrictions on health care delivery
and food security in Cuba. The team reviewed key U.S. regulations and their
implementation, conducted a survey of 12 American medical and pharmaceutical
companies and documented the experience of Cuban import firms with the embargo.
The team assessed the impact of the U.S. sanctions on health in Cuba through on-site
visits to 46 treatment centres and related facilities; it conducted 160 interviews with
medical professionals and other specialists, government officials, representative of non-
government organisations, churches and international aid agencies. In October 1996,
the AAWH sent a delegation of distinguished medical experts to Cuba to validate the
findings of the draft report through first-hand observation.

The full report of more than 300 pages is the first comprehensive study of its
kind. It is intended to provide a factual basis for informed decision-making on Cuba,
and indeed on the wisdom of including food and medicine in any embargo as a means
to achieve foreign policy objectives.

Summary of Findings

After a year-long investigation, the American Association for World Health has
determined that the U.S. embargo of Cuba has dramatically harmed the health and
nutrition of large numbers of ordinary Cuban citizens. As documented by the summary

257

of the report given here, it is their expert medical opinion that the U.S. embargo has caused a significant rise in suffering - and even deaths - in Cuba. For several decades the U.S. embargo has imposed significant financial burdens on the Cuban health system. But since 1992 the number of unmet medical needs - patients going without essential drugs or doctors performing medical procedures without adequate equipment - has sharply accelerated. This trend is directly linked to the fact that in 1992 the U.S. trade embargo - one of the most stringent embargoes of its kind, prohibiting the sale of food and sharply restricting the sale of medicines and medical equipment - was further tightened by the 1992 Cuban Democracy Act, referred to in the Foreword to this book.

A humanitarian catastrophe has been averted only because the Cuban government has maintained a high level of budgetary support for a health care system designed to deliver primary and preventive health care to all of its citizens. Cuba still has an infant mortality rate half that of the city of Washington D.C.. Even so, the U.S. embargo of food and the de facto embargo on medical supplies has wreaked havoc with the island's model primary health care system. The crisis has been compounded by the country's generally weak economic resources and by the loss of trade with the Soviet bloc.

Recently four factors have dangerously exacerbated the human effects of this 37-year-old- trade embargo. All four factors stem from little-understood provisions of the U.S. Congress' 1992 Cuban Democracy Act (CDA):

1   **A Ban on Subsidiary Trade** Beginning in 1992, the Cuban Democracy Act imposed a ban on subsidiary trade with Cuba. This ban has severely constrained Cuba's ability to import medicines and medical supplies from third country sources. Moreover, recent corporate buy-outs and mergers between major U.S. and European pharmaceutical companies have further reduced the number of companies permitted to do business with Cuba.

2.   **Licensing** Under the Cuban Democracy Act, the U.S. Treasury and Commerce Departments are allowed in principle to licence individual sales of medicines

258

and medical supplies, ostensibly for humanitarian reasons to mitigate the embargo's impact on health care delivery. In practice, according to U.S. corporate executives, the licensing provisions are so arduous as to have had the opposite effect. As implemented, the licensing provisions actively discourage any medical commerce. The number of such licenses for medical equipment and medicines have been denied on the ground that these exports "would be detrimental to U.S. foreign policy interests."

3.   **Shipping** Since 1992, the embargo has prohibited ships from loading or unloading cargo in U.S. ports for 180 days after delivering cargo to Cuba. This provision has strongly discouraged shippers from delivering medical equipment to Cuba. Consequently shipping costs have risen dramatically and further constricted the flow of food, medicines, medical supplies and even gasoline for ambulances. From 1993 to 1996, Cuban companies spent an additional $8.7 million on shipping medical imports from Asia, Europe and South America rather than from the neighbouring United States.

4.   **Humanitarian Aid** Charity is an inadequate alternative to free trade in medicines, medical supplies and food. Donations from U.S. non-governmental organisations and international agencies do not begin to compensate for the hardships inflicted by the embargo on the Cuban public health system. In any case, delays in licensing and other restrictions have severely discouraged charitable contributions from the U.S.

Taken together, these four factors have placed severe strains on the Cuban health system. The declining availability of foodstuffs, medicines and such basic medical supplies as replacement parts for thirty-year-old X-ray machines is taking a tragic human toll. The embargo has closed so many windows that in some instances Cuban physicians have found it impossible to obtain life-saving medicines from any source, under any circumstances. Patients have died. In general, a relatively sophisticated and

259

comprehensive public health system is being systematically stripped of essential resources. High-technology hospital wards devoted to cardiology and nephrology are particularly under siege. But so too are such basic aspects of the health system as water quality and food security.

Specifically, the AAWH's team of nine medical experts identified the following health problems affected by the embargo:

1. **Malnutrition** The outright ban on the sale of American foodstuffs has contributed to serious nutritional deficits, particularly among pregnant women, leading to an increase in low birth-weight babies. In addition, food shortages were linked to a devastating outbreak of neuropathy numbering in the tens of thousands. By one estimate, daily caloric intake dropped 33 percent between 1989 and 1993.

2. **Water Quality** The embargo is severely restricting Cuba's access to water treatment chemicals and spare-parts for the island's water supply system. This has led to serious cutbacks in supplies of safe drinking water, which in turn has become a factor in the rising incidence of morbidity and mortality rates from water-borne diseases.

3. **Medicines & Equipment** Of the 1,297 medications available in Cuba in 1991, physicians now have access to only 889 of these same medicines - and many of these are available only intermittently. Because most major new drugs are developed by U.S. pharmaceuticals, Cuban physicians have access to less than 50 percent of the new medicines available on the world market. Due to the direct or indirect effects of the embargo, the most routine medical supplies are in short supply or entirely absent from some Cuban clinics.

4. **Medical Information** Though information materials have been exempt
   from the U.S. trade embargo sine 1988, the AAWH study concludes that in
   practice very little such information goes into Cuba or comes out of the
   island due to travel restrictions, currency regulations and shipping
   difficulties. Scientists and citizens of both countries suffer as a result.
   Paradoxically, the embargo harms some U.S. citizens by denying them
   access to the latest advances in Cuban medical research, including such
   products as Meningitis B vaccine, cheaply produced interferon and
   streptokinase, and as AIDS vaccine currently under-going clinical trials with
   human volunteers.

Finally, the AAWH stresses the stringent nature of the U.S. trade embargo against
Cuba. Few other embargoes in recent history - including those targeting Iran, Libya,
South Rhodesia, Chile or Iraq - have included an outright ban on the sale of food. Few
other embargoes have so restricted medical commerce as to deny the availability of life-
saving medicines to ordinary citizens. Such an embargo appears to violate the most
basic international charters and conventions governing human rights, including the
United Nations charter, the charter of the Organisation of American States, and the
articles of the Geneva Convention governing the treatment of civilians during wartime.

Cost in Lives of the U.S. Blockade

The cost of the embargo in human terms can be calculated both statistically and
anecdotally. Here are some highlights from the report:

- Surgeries dropped from 885,790 in 1990 to 536,547 in 1995, a glaring
  indicator of the decline in hospital resources. Surgical services face shortages
  of most modern anaesthetics and related equipment, specialist catheters, third
  generation antibiotics and other key drugs, sutures, instruments, fabric for
  surgical greens, air conditioning equipment and disposable supplies.

261

- The deterioration of Cuba's water supply has led to a rising incidence of water-borne diseases-such as typhoid fever, dysentery's and viral hepatitis. Mortality rates from Acute Diarrheal Disease (ADD), for instance, increased from 2.7 per 100,000 inhabitants in 1989 to 6.7 per 100,000 inhabitants in 1994. Amebic and bacillary dysentery morbidity rates showed marked increased during the same period.

- The U.S. embargo is limiting the access of Cuban AIDS patients to a variety of medicines. The AAWH found that the embargo was directly responsible for up to six month delays in AZT treatment for a total of 176 HIV patients in Cuba at a time when AZT was the only approved medication heralded for slowing the progress of the virus. As one AIDS professional told the AAWH, "The problem is that our patients don't have the time to wait."

- AAWH visited a paediatric ward then on its 22nd day without metoclopramide HCI, a drug used in combination with others such as betamethasone for paediatric chemotherapy. Without this drug's nausea-preventing effects, the 35 children in the ward were vomiting an average of 28-to-30 times a day.

- Heart disease is the number one case of death in Cuba. Mortality rates for men and women have increased since 1989: with 189.3 deaths per 100,000 in 1989 and 199.8 deaths per 100,000 in 1995. In one instance Cuban cardiologists diagnosed a heart attack patient with a ventricular arrhythmia. He required an implantable defibrillator to survive. Though the U.S. firm CPI, which then held a virtual monopoly on the device expressed a willingness to make the sale, the U.S. government denied license for it. Two months later the patient died.

- In 1993 the U.S. Treasury Department denied a license, ostensibly for reasons of foreign policy, to the German subsidiary of Pfizer to sell Cuba one pound of the active ingredient methotrexate for trials of an anti-cancer drug.

- Some 48 percent of the 215 new U.S. medications in phase 1-111 FDA trials in 1995 are specifically for breast cancer. None will be fully accessible to Cuban women as long as the embargo remains in place.

- Cuban children with leukaemia are denied access to new, life-prolonging drugs. For example, the FDA has already approved Oncaspar (pegaspargase), patented by the U.S. company Enzon for patients allergic to L-Spar (l-asparaginase). Both drugs produce longer remission when included in treatment for lymphoblastic leukaemia (ALL). However, L-Spar has an allergy rate of 40 percent for first-time use and 70 percent for relapsed ALL patients. Further, Oncaspar is less traumatic to a child suffering from ALL, since it requires only one-sixth the number of injections of L-Spar. But the embargo deprives Cuban children of this innovation. Left untreated, this type of leukaemia is fatal in two to three months.

- In general, the embargo effectively bans Cuba from purchasing nearly one half of the new world class drugs on the market.

Embargo Restrictions Today

The bulk of U.S. prohibitions against trade with Cuba are set forth in regulations enforced by the Treasury Department's Office of Foreign Assets Control and the Commerce Department's Bureau of Export Affairs. These include a ban on U.S. exports to Cuba, Cuban imports into the U.S. and even third-country U.S. subsidiary transactions with Cuba. Also banned are family remittances, credits, the transfer of money or property by U.S. nationals to Cuban nationals. Several provisions of the U.S. embargo constitute major obstacles to any kind of medical commerce for humanitarian purposes:

263

Direct flights between the two countries are banned.

Entry is denied to U.S. ports by any ship which has docked in Cuba during the prior 180 days. U.S. ports are also closed to third-country vessels carrying "goods in which Cuba or Cuban nationals have an interest whatever the cargo's origin or destination. This prohibition applies to a third-country vessel carrying third-country goods which incorporate even trace amounts of Cuban-origin products or produce."

Re-exports to Cuba of U.S.-origin goods and technical data are banned.

Exports are banned to Cuba by third-country companies of goods containing 20% or more U.S. origin components; individual licenses are required for those goods containing over

10% U.S.-origin components.

On paper a procedure exists under which application can be made to the U.S. Departments of Treasury and Commerce for licenses to sell (or even donate) medicines and medical equipment to Cuba. In reality, these licensing procedures are a charade. Ostensibly, licensing should have opened a window in the embargo for medical commerce. As implemented however, by the Treasury and Commerce Departments, licensing has closed this window. The complexity of these procedures and their arbitrary interpretation have created inordinate delays and costs which pose an insurmountable obstacle to commercial interests. For all practical purposes an absolute ban exists on sale of medicines and medical equipment to Cuba by U.S. companies and their foreign subsidiaries. Licenses are also required for humanitarian donations that can only go to non-governmental organisations, of which there are very few in Cuba. Under no circumstances is the sale of food authorised.

Cuba's Health Under the Blockade

Such a stringent embargo, if applied to most other countries in the development world, would have had catastrophic effects on the public health system. Cuba's health care system, however, is uniformly considered the pre-eminent model in the Third World.

The Cuban constitution makes health care a right of every citizen and the responsibility of the government. The system is based on universal coverage and comprehensive care, essentially free of charge to the population. Over the year the cental government has placed a top priority on public health expenditures, the national budget and allocated considerable human resources to public health strategies that have earned praise from the World Health Organisation, the Pan American Health Organisation, UNICEF and other international bodies and individual health care authorities. See the WHO comment as reported in the Forward.

Consequently, in the 1990's Cuba's health statistics more closely approximated those of the nations of Europe and North America than of developing countries with 195 inhabitants per physician, and 95 percent of the population attended by family doctors living in the communities they serve. The infant mortality rate in Cuba is roughly half that in Washington, D.C. Primary care is bolstered with 400 polyclinics; and secondary and tertiary facilities include 284 hospitals and 11 national institutes with impatient and research capacities. See table 16.1

Table 16.1 : Selected Health Indicators[84]

	Cuba	Latin America*
Life Expectancy (1994)	75 years	68 years
Infant Mortality (1994)	9.4/1,000 live births	38
Under Five Mortality (1994)	12/1,000 live births	47
Maternal Mortality (1980-92)	39/100,000 live births	178
Access to health services	98% of population	73%

* 22 countries of the region

While the U.S. embargo has always exerted a negative effect on the Cuban economy, its impact particularly on the health care system, was significantly ameliorated by

---

[84] UNICEF (1996): State of the World's Children. Paris

Cuba's relationship with the Soviet bloc until the 1980's. Besides the obvious advantages of subsidised trade and aid, the relationship also kept 85 percent of Cuban trade outside the reach of the embargo. Havana's inability to obtain U.S. medical supplies was largely offset by imports from the socialist bloc countries and western Europe. (Nevertheless a handful of U.S.-produced drugs still could not be obtained from any other source.) In the 1990's, this situation was dramatically reversed : as the socialist bloc crumbled, the embargo suddenly became extremely effective. After 1989, Cuba lost an annual $4-6 billion in subsidised and bartered trade. Overnight, all imports required hard currency. In a two-year span, the economy contracted by 60 percent, evaporating an annual average growth of 4.3 percent in the previous decade.

Suddenly, Cuba's health system no longer had access to East bloc raw material for its pharmaceutical industry, and at the same time shortages of hard currency made it increasingly difficult to purchase drugs and medical equipment in Western Europe and elsewhere.

The Cuban Democracy Act (CDA) of 1992, severely aggravated the situation, prohibiting foreign subsidiaries of U.S. companies any trade with Cuba. Ninety percent was in food and medicines. Business with U.S. subsidiaries had continued to grow well after the Soviet collapse, reaching $718 million in 1991, the last full year before the CDA cut off.

To compound matters, the CDA prohibitions were enacted during a period when U.S. firms are particularly active in buy-outs and take overs of third-country medical companies. Many of these companies were prime suppliers to the Cuban health care system. While in some instances Cuba managed to continue such purchases through intermediaries at greatly inflated prices, as a rule Cuban hospitals and physicians had to cope with abrupt cut-off of key medicines, medical equipment, medical texts, imputs for diagnostics, vaccinations, and pharmaceutical and biotechnology research and development. In 1995, for instance, Upjohn, a major U.S. pharmaceutical company, merged with a Swedish concern, Pharmacia, which since 1970 has logged multi-million dollar sales to Cuba of protein purifying equipment (HPLCs), reagents for clinical laboratories and production plants, chemotherapy drugs, and growth hormones. Though technically Upjohn could have applied for a U.S. export licence to continue supplying Cuba with some of these items, the company opted instead to terminate pharmacies sales and close down its Havana office within three months of the merger. Cuba suddenly lost another supplier of plates for HIV-tests and other diagnostic kits to screen for hepatitis B and C, when Sybron International of Wisconsin bought out Nunc of Germany. Cuba lost two main sources for pace-makers under similar circumstances.

The human consequences of these decisions are all too evident in the wards of Cuban hospitals. When the AAWH delegation visited the cancer ward at the Julio Manuel Marquez Paediatric Hospital in Havana, their doctors found the oncologists do not have access to U.S.-manufactured cell-site-ports for chemotherapy. (The U.S. is the leading producer of this item.) As a result, nurses and physicians must repeatedly puncture and search for new veins in young children, causing them added pain and suffering. In order to treat one five-year-old girl suffering with sarcoma, doctors were compelled to use the girl's jugular vein because all other veins had already collapsed. As a result, she developed a heamatoma that almost killed her. The child was in excruciating pain. The availability of the cell-site-port implantofix would have prevented the child's suffering. This product however, is manufactured by Braun Medical, Inc, of Bethlehem, Pennsylvania. Although Braun is associated with a German company and has an affiliate in France, the cell-site-port is produced in the United States and is thus subject to the embargo. The other obvious supplier - indeed, the world market leader in cell-site-ports is the previously mentioned Swedish-American firm, Pharmacia, which is also covered by the embargo.

Even when Cuba is able to find a third-country supplier of medical equipment, penalties under the embargo have proved to be a serious impediment. The CDA extraterritorial provision barring entrance to U.S. ports of any ship docking in Cuba during the preceding 180 days has not only impeded normal commercial shipping to the island, but cost Cuban importers up to 30 percent more in shipping charges over the world scale rate. Within months of the CDA's passage, shipping problems caused major delays in deliveries in soap, fuel, powdered milk, cooking oil, wheat, beans, rice

267

and medical supplies. Steeper rates require Cuba to spend more of a limited budget on shipping and less on purchases of food and medicines critical to the welfare of the Cuban population.

The 1996 Helms-Burton law seeks to discourage foreign investment in Cuba by threatening third-country investors with suits in U.S. courts and by applying sanctions against their executives. The law has had a chilling effect, further discouraging American suppliers in the health care industry from even contemplating trade with Cuba.

The Cuban government has responded to the challenges posed by the stiffened embargo by boosting its health care spending. During the years from 1989 to 1996 - a period of general economic trauma - the national budget remained static but public heath outlays nevertheless increased by 30.4 percent, reaching $1.1 billion pesos. This added investment in public health came at the expense of other sectors, such as public administration, defence, culture and the arts. While priority was also afforded to health in hard currency spending, the devaluation of the Cuban peso and general hard currency shortfall reduced dollars for the health sector by 30 percent from 1989 to 1993, the year after the Cuban Democracy Act went into effect. The slow climb to $104.2 million in hard currency expenditure in 1995 remained less than half the 1989 spending levels.

Both the embargo and the hard currency shortfalls have resulted in an acute shortage of medical products. Of the 1,297 medicines in the country in 1991, only 889 can be obtained today, many of them only intermittently. Lack of spare parts has slowed equipment repair and replacements are virtually unobtainable. The Ministry of Health reports, for example, that 13 per cents of Cuba's X-ray machines are out of commission, as are 21 percent of their cobalt therapy units.

In addition, the nation's health care infrastructure has suffered from diminished access to electricity, oil, diesel and gasoline. Many ambulances and mobile mammography vehicles stand idle for lack of gasoline. Pharmaceutical plants are operating at one third their 1980's levels, and power outages risk spoilage of medications and vaccines in refrigerated warehouses and threaten the lives of patients in

268

the midst of surgery.

Lack of spare parts for U.S.-outfitted water treatment plants, and shortages of chlorine, detergents and disinfectants have led to an increase in water-borne disease, with higher mortality rates among the elderly; outbreaks of scabies and other dermatological disorders are on the rise, as are incidents of hospital infections and sepsis.

Sharp declines in food imports and inputs for agriculture have resulted in significant signs of nutritional deficits, most notably in the 1993 neuropathy epidemic that temporarily blinded over 50,000 Cubans. Workplace and school dining halls serve fewer calories and less protein, while the daily litre of milk once assured to all children up to age 13 is now limited to children through age six. The population over 65 no longer receives special dietary supplements.

Quite clearly, Cuba's health care delivery system has been severely weakened, particularly at the secondary and tertiary levels of care. Only the pre-existing excellence of the system and the extraordinary dedication of the Cuban medical community have prevented infinitely greater loss of life and suffering.

Details of the AAWH Study

This study was conducted over a year-long period of time by an inter-disciplinary team of researchers. Visits were made to 28 patient-care facilities and 15 non-governmental and international organisations. More than 160 professionals were interviewed, as well as innumerable patients and families. Data was obtained from the Cuban Ministry of Health, international agencies and U.S. government sources. Several lawyers in the United States contributed to the section of the report dealing with the history and legal aspects of the embargo. The impact on the pharmaceutical industry and the human rights implications of including food and medicine in the embargo.

The study examined Cuba's public health system sector by sector, including such critical area as: food security and nutrition, water resources, women's health, children's health, family relations, national health emergencies, hospital care,

269

humanitarian donations and international co-operation, oncology, cardiology, the HIV/AIDS programme, nephrology, endocrinology, ophthalmology, diagnostic and protection of the blood supply, scientific information and medical education.

While signs of deterioration abound, a herculean effort is underway to try to maintain the previous high standard of health care. The public health system has adapted its resources to address specific problems: community clinics, for instance, have expanded their facilities to include emergency services. The study includes, however, that the embargo is driving the system towards crisis and causing significant suffering and death. The AAWH finds that while present law, as set forth in the Cuban Democracy Act, has been construed as a loosening of the embargo on medicine, in practice, new and almost insurmountable obstacles to free trade have been created. The embargo has been extended to include U.S. subsidiaries and any product from the third-country companies which contain U.S. components. The result has been to tighten - not loosen - the embargo on medicines and medical supplies. The Cuban Democracy Act of 1992 (CDA) permits U.S. firms and their subsidiaries to apply for licenses to sell medicines or medical equipment to the island, provided they meet a number or pre-requisites. These include the following: that there is no reasonable likelihood the item will be used for torture or human rights abuses; that it will not re-exported; that it will not be used to treat any of the several thousand foreign patients who come to Cuba each year and pay for medical care; and that it not be used in the production of any biotechnology product. The law also requires end-use certification, which in practice means companies must supply detailed information on distribution in Cuba, and the Cuban's must be willing to accept the possibility of independent on-site verification to prove the end is what is claimed. The U.S. government further constricts the trade by interpreting "medical exports" to mean only finished products, thereby denying any license for inputs or equipment for Cuba's pharmaceutical industry, which are banned from sale. Embargo regulations prohibits third-country company sales to Cuba of any medical products containing over 20 percent U.S. components and require individual licenses for goods containing over 10 percent U.S. components.

Obtaining licenses from the departments of Commerce and Treasury to sell medical goods to Cuba on a contract-by-contract basis is a laborious process. The severe restrictions imposed such a disincentive that only our foreign subsidiaries of U.S. companies sought and obtained such licenses from October 1992 through May 1995. There is no record of government licenses approved for direct sales to Cuba from parent companies in the United States. AAWH surveyed 12 top U.S. pharmaceutical medical supply companies: Baxter Health Care Corporation, Bristol-Myers Squibb Eli Lilly and Company, Johnson and Johnson, Merck and Co., Ohmeda Pharmaceutical Products, Schering-Plough Corperation, Searle, Siemens U.S.A., SmithKline Beecham Pharmaceuticals, TPLC Pacemakers and WyethAyerst Laboratories. Ten companies stated that the embargo prevented or discouraged them from selling products to Cuba, citing licensing red tape, additional financial burdens and shipping difficulties created by CDA. The executive of one pharmaceutical company told AAWH that so few apply primarily because they are discouraged by the CDA provision requiring certification of end use. Some feared U.S. government appraisals against them in other areas if they traded with Cuba.

Six of the 12 mistakenly believed that the embargo completely banned sales to Cuba. Two to the companies cited political reasons for not selling to Cuba. And the four that had made verbal enquires regarding export found government licensing officials dampened such initiative with inaccurate, confusing and misleading information on the law itself.

In the rare instances where licenses have been granted, the process itself creates delays of weeks to month or even years. For example, from initial enquiry, to purchase, documentation, licensing and final delivering, the sale spare parts for over 300 Siemens-Elema (of Sweden) Servo-900-C respirators took over two years and involved seven agencies in four countries. Since 1992 the U.S. government has required Johnson and Johnson's Belgium subsidiary to apply for a separate license for each sale of the anaesthesia Thalamonal. An average period of six months elapses between each contract closure and delivery.

271

Examples of the Embargo's Impact

1. **New Drugs Inaccessible:** Due to U.S. embargo law, Cuban patients are deprived of any drug internationally patented by a U.S. manufacturer since 1980. Since the United States boasts the world's leading pharmaceutical research and production capability, the embargo effectively bans Cuba from purchasing nearly one half of new world class drugs on the market. Of 265 "major global drugs" developed between 1972 and 1992, nearly 50 percent were of U.S. origin.

2. **Medical Equipment Blocked:** The embargo virtually proscribes Cuban purchase of U.S. medical equipment, parts and accessories. U.S. firms, such as the hospital supplier Thomas Compressors, commonly refused even price information to Cuban importers, citing the U.S. embargo. Foreign companies have refused sale of X-ray equipment, operating tables, respirators, and other medical supplies containing over 20 percent U.S. components, since such sales are prohibited under the embargo.

   For example, in December, 1994, the commerce department denied license for a CAN $705.30 contract for 110 X-ray parts to the Canadian subsidiary of the Cleveland-based Picker International. The parts contained 27 percent U.S. components, valued at CAN $193. Though Picker had received a previous license in August 1992 authorising replacement parts for the same equipment, in July, 1994 Dr Eugene W. Lewis, Chief of Capital Goods and Production Material Branch of the Department of Commerce Office of Export Licensing, wrote Picker with the new exports would be "detrimental to United States foreign policy" and that "it is the policy of the United States not to approved (SIC) license applications to Cuba, except for shipments to meet basic human needs". The parts were designated 20-year-old X-ray machines in maternity, paediatric, and rural hospitals.

   In another instance, a programme of the National Oncology institute that evaluates 360 patients per month for blood and coagulation information uses an Italian platelet aggregometer know as the Omniscribe Series D-500. But the metallic tape used to inscribe the test results is produced in Texas. Cuba has been unable to purchase the tape. Without it, the Omniscribe can read only one half of the information from each patients test's.

Equipment donated on a humanitarian basis faces the same repair problem: Cuba has been unable to purchase parts or accessories for equipment ranging from 30 Cobe Dialysis Units to Preemicare Respirators for new-borns.

3. **Pharmaceutical and Biotechnology Input Banned:** The U.S. government refuses to license export of raw materials for Cuba's pharmaceutical industry. That industry has the capability of producing some 464 drugs at approximately one third of the price of importing comparable medications. As a direct result, Cuba is now producing only 119 drugs for its domestic market. The Cuban Democracy Act also explicitly bans exports for Cuba's biotechnology research and production. Cuban biotech research has not only added several vaccines to the national immunisations programme but is also responsible for drugs such as recombinant streptokinase, the "clot-buster" for heart attack victims produced at a fraction of the price of imports and thus stocked in all Cuban hospitals.

4. **Financial Constraints:** Effectively barred from the U.S. medical market, Cuba now pays higher prices for comparable European and Asian goods. Purchasing refurbished dialysis units directly from the United States, for instance, would save Cuba as much as 75 percent, multiplying by three or even four the number of units procured. The embargo also prohibits Cuba from using the U.S. dollar for international transactions. Thus, even when Cuba buys medical supplies from wholly-owned foreign companies, converting currencies increases costs.

5. **Delivery Delays:** The Cuban Democracy Act discourages even foreign companies from allowing their vessels to dock in Cuba. For example, just after the law took effect in October 1992, delivery to Cuba of 1500 metric tons of tallow for hospital soap was delayed by several months because the Argentine supplier refused to send its ships to Cuban ports. During an epidemic in 1981 of hemorrhagic dengue the

inability to acquire U.S. fumigation equipment on a timely basis resulted in a long delay in controlling the mosquito vector and a significant increase in the number of cases and unnecessary deaths.

The AAWH finds that the U.S. embargo directly threatens the food security of the Cuban population. U.S. sanctions reduce the island's import capacity for basic foodstuffs, agriculture and the food industry. Moreover, shipping regulations and the ban on direct and subsidiary trade in food close Cuba from an otherwise natural market.

Subsidiary Trade-Ban

With the post-1989 decline in east-bloc trade, Cuba's purchases from U.S. subsidiaries abroad increased, with grain, wheat and other consumables reaching 71 percent (or $500 million) of Cuba's total imports from the United States by 1990. There was no prohibition on such sales prior to the passage of CDA in 1992.

By 1992 (the last year before the CDA eliminated subsidiary trade) soybean products, wheat, sunflower oil, corn, rice and palm oil constituted 89% of total Cuban imports from U.S. foreign subsidiaries, such as Cargi Central Soya, Continental Grain, Del Monte, Dow Chemical, HB.J. Heniz, Hoechst Celanese, and International Multifoods. The AAWH found that, after the CDA took effect, suppliers were forced to cancel contracts with Cuba, including purchased of baby food from H.J. Heinz of Canada and of $100 million in wheat, soy, beans, peas and lentils from the Argentine subsidiary of Continental Grain (New York) and Cargill (Minneapolis).

Shipping Costs

The embargo's prohibition on vessels docking in U.S. ports if they have been in Cuba during the previous six months has deterred shippers, causing long delays in the importation of basic foodstuffs and dramatic increases in cost. The AAWH found that

274

by 1993 Cuba was paying as much as 43 percent over pre-CDA shipping rates. Indeed, high fuel costs were partially responsible for many shut-downs in the food industry during the worst years of the crisis. A New Zealand milk producer cancelled a long-standing contract to sell Cuba 1500 metric tons of powdered milk when its regular shipper refused to carry cargo bound for Cuba. Several months later Cuba found a new, more expensive source of powdered milk in Europe. Cuba was similarly forced to pay a high-cost shipper to bring in 9,000 metric tons of soy cooking oil from an Italian supplier unable to find a tanker willing to take the risk of docking in Cuba. Likewise, the CDA'a shipping ban forced Cuba to send one of its freighters to China to pick up 20,000 metric tons of beans held up for seven months. If goods could be sent to Cuba from the United States, Cuba would save $215,800 for each ship replacing a European freighter and $516,700 for each replacing as Asian freighter.

Food Imports

Cuban domestic agriculture - meats, grains, fruits, vegetables, rice, tubers - supplied, in 1985, 22.7 percent of the calorie intake per capita and 53.1 percent of the protein. But the economic crisis of the 1990's has taken its toll on harvests and on meat and dairy yields, obliging Cuba to continuing relying on imports. The embargo explicitly bans the sale of food either directly by U.S. companies or by their subsidiaries abroad. There is licensing provision even though such an absolute ban directly violates international human rights conventions. The ban includes the sale of fertilisers, pesticides, animal feed, and fuel for domestic food production. In the absence of the embargo Cuba could buy grain from U.S. suppliers and ship it from a U.S. port at approximately $13 per ton. The embargo obliges Cuba to buy wheat from Europe at $25-28 per ton, including freight, a difference in 1994 of $9,441,000. In 1994 alone, Cuba paid an additional $35,881,896 to non-U.S. suppliers and shippers for deliveries of wheat flour, wheat, soy flour, corn, soy beans, chicken and milk. The same year, an extra $8.3 million was paid for agricultural chemical imports, bringing embargo-related costs to a total of $204.6 million through 1994, or 47 percent of the previous year's entire food import budget.

Baking and distribution of bread, a ration card staple, illustrates the toll the embargo has taken on basic foodstuffs in Cuba. Up until October 1992, Cuba bought wheat and other grains from U.S. subsidiaries. Since then, we estimate Cuba has paid about $7.8 million more each year for wheat flour alone.

Agriculture

The study found that the U.S. embargo's ban on exports of fertilisers, pesticides, animal feed and fuel has seriously damaged product and crop yields.

For example, in September, 1992, Bayer AG of Germany halted sales of the pesticide "Sencor" because the company transferred production of the pesticides' active ingredient to a plant in Kansas City. Bayer sought, but was flatly denied, a U.S. license for continued export. Eventually, Cuba replaced "Sencor" with more expensive potato pesticide. The switch cost money and delayed planting of the staple crop. Major fertiliser shipments have been cancelled or delayed for similar reasons.

Nutritional Deficit

Such embargo-imposed expenses have compounded food shortages and contributed to the deterioration of he Cuban population's nutritional intake. Between 1985 and 1989, calorie intake in Cuba exceeded 2800 per day, with protein level at 76 grams per day. By 1993, daily caloric intake had dropped by 33 percent to 1863 and protein level had dropped by 39 percent to 46 grams per day. By 1993, nutrition deficiencies began to emerge in the general population: the median weight of males and females in 1993 dropped, with adolescents registering weight loss of at least two kilograms compared to 1982 figures; children born in 1993 or after were notably smaller than those of the same age in 1982; and men and women age 20 to 60 registered a marked weight loss. Cuba also began to register deficient nutritional status in women at the beginning of their pregnancies, as well as an increase in the incidence of low-birth-weight babies.

Neuropathy Epidemic

In 1992 and 1993, over 50,000 Cuban men and women between 25 and 64 years of age were afflicted with a widespread outbreak of neuropathy. After exhaustive research, Cuban and international specialists concluded that the nation's food shortages were a central cause of the epidemic, most likely complicated by the presence of an environmental toxin and heavy tobacco usage. They determined that the sudden decline in nutrition had left the Cubans particularly vulnerable to toxic factors.

Cuban researchers as well as those from the U.S. Centres for Disease Control and Prevention and the Pan American Health Organisation also concluded that women, children and the elderly had been less affected by the epidemic because they received extra nutrients under the government's foreign distribution system. Investigators concluded that the U.S. embargo had significantly contributed to the appearance of this nutrition-related condition by leading to further cuts in foodstuffs and other key imports.

The U.S. embargo has always posed serious obstacles to expanding water supplies and treatment in Cuba. The more stringent embargo restrictions of the 1990's deny Cuba competitively-priced water treatment chemicals and prevent ready purchase of spare parts and equipment for aqueducts, piping meters, and other equipment upon which Cuba's clean water supply depends. The AAWH finds that the embargo contributes to serious cutbacks in supplies of safe drinking water and is a factor in the rising incidence in morbidity and mortality rates from water-borne disease.

Water Services and U.S. Parts

Water services were progressively extended among both urban and rural settlements after 1959. In 1960, 65 percent of the urban population had ready access to water,

277

while running water in rural areas was virtually unknown. By 1994, the figures reached 94.2 percent and 83 percent respectively. By 1993, budget cuts and embargo-related importation obstacles resulted in deficient services for nearly one third of the population.

Cuba's water supply and sewerage systems generally mirror the U.S. construction model, which separates drainage from sewers, as distinct from the European model. Until 1959, all but two water pumping stations in Cuba were manufactured in the United States. Gradually, Cuba diversified its suppliers, and today the island relies on Russia, Chinese, Spanish and French suppliers. Nevertheless, the water supply program still requires the U.S. parts, such as meters and couplings, and still uses the National Pipe Thread (N.P.T.) system, with all compatible fittings patented in the United States. All these items are fully embargoed.

The water treatment plants that use chlorine gas - treating 72 percent of Cuba's drinking water - are built with components from the U.S. firm Wallace and Tiernan and their subsidiaries. Since 1992 when the Cuban Democracy Act banned subsidiary sales to Cuba, Cuba can no longer purchase parts for the Wallace chlorination systems. That single embargo-related prohibition jeopardises safe drinking water for every city in Cuba with over 100,000 inhabitants - a total of four million people. all reserve equipment has been exhausted, and in 1994, Havana (the semi-rural province outside the capital) shut down all 12 of its chlorination plants. Pinar del Rio province closed all 18 of its factories.

By 1993, 40 percent of chlorination installations were shut down due to lack of parts and equipment breakdown, while 46 percent were shutdown because of chemical shortages. In 1994, for example, a shipment of Canadian chlorine was delayed by two months, leaving Havana at one point with only a one month margin of supplies to keep the capital's water safe.

Disease

The deterioration of Cuba's water supply has led to a rising incidence of water-borne disease such as typhoid fever, dysentery's and viral hepatitis. Measured by the number of physician visits, the incidence of Acute Diarrheal Disease (ADD) in 1989 was 888,318. By 1993, the figure jumped to 1,115,616. Curbed slightly by 1995, the incidence of ADD was particularly higher in adults over the age of 65. Mortality rates from ADD increased from two point seven per 100,000 inhabitants in 1989 to six point seven per 100,000 inhabitants in 1994. Amebic and bacillary dysentery morbidity rates show marked increases during the same period.

Such diseases as scabiosis and pediculosis - both related to inadequate water supply - are running to epidemic proportions in Cuba's boarding schools. Dirty water is also related to hospital infections which in 1995 alone accounted for 51 outbreaks involving 349 patients and 60 deaths.

The AAWH found a strict correlation between cutbacks in water chlorination services and the outbreak of disease. Havana Province, the semi-urban and rural province just outside the capital city, is a case in point. In 1989, three-fourths of the 120.9 million cubic metres of water supplied was treated and safe to drink. By 1993, only 34,6% of Havana Province's 107.1 million cubic meters of water was safe to drink. The decline caused serious outbreaks of Hepatitis A, with 3,813 reported cases, or 22.1% of the national total. In 1994-95, the province showed viral hepatitis reacts well above the national average.

The AAWH finds that the U.S. embargo limits access to life-prolonging drugs for Cuban HIV and AIDS patients, and otherwise impairs prevention diagnosis, treatment and research in this field. The families of AIDS patients have also been negatively affected by limitations on travel between the United States and Cuba.

From 1986, when the first HIV-positive cases were identified in Cuba, until January of 1996, the cumulative number of Cubans testing seropositive was 1200, including 440 AIDS patients, 292 of whom have died. The incubation time from HIV infection to full-blown AIDS is 11 years, and the average survival time from the onset of AIDS is 18 months. In 1987, Cuba introduced a broad screening program using domestically produced diagnostic kits. Until 1993, when an outpatient program was developed, all patients testing seropositive were hospitalised in 13 sanatoriums.

The U.S. embargo has jeopardised AIDS testing, diagnosis and protection of the blood supply. Mergers of European suppliers with U.S. companies have suddenly cut off parts and equipment, supplies of reagents and plastic modules for lab work, increasing long-term costs. For example, the Pharnacia Upjohn merger eliminated supplies of reagents for bloodwork to follow the progress of patients, making it impossible to carry out Cd4, Cd22, Cd38 and Cd25 tests for specific T-lymphocytes until substitutes could be found.

Limiting the access of Cuban AIDS patients to medicines is the most damaging result of the U.S. embargo that the AAWH team observed. Cuba does not have ready access to FDA-approved medications manufactured by U.S. firms to have been internationally patented in the last 17 years. As one AIDS professional told the AAWH, "The problem is that our patients don't have time to wait." Cuba make illegal purchases of some of these drugs through third parties, although at steeper rates, which in turn limits quantities procured.

U.S. manufacturers are an important source of AIDS medications for Cuba. A recent study reveals that for 22 years (between 1970 and May of 1992) the United States was the world's number one source for new immunological drugs. By 1995, the number of U.S.-developed and FDA-approved medications for AIDS and AIDS-related conditions had reached 30.

The case of AZT is illustrative: Approved by the FDA in early 1987, it took several months for Cuban importers to locate suppliers willing to sell them even small amounts at virtually prohibitive cost. The AAWH found that the embargo was directly responsible for up to six month delays in AZT treatment for a total of 176 HIV patients in Cuba.

The outlook is even more bleak for U.S. medications still under development, to which Cuban patients will not have ready access for 17 years following international patent. The 1995 survey on AIDS medication in the pipeline, published by the

Pharmaceutical Research and Manufacturing of America, indicates that 110 medicines have begun the FDA approval process-only three of them by manufacturers outside the United States. Cuban specialists are particularly interested in the protease inhibitors, a new class of AIDS drugs, which are being developed by at least four U.S. pharmaceutical corporations.

Approximately 70% of all Cuban AIDS patients receive interferon as part of their treatment. This drug is produced relatively cheaply in Cuba, but enjoys only limited use in the U.S. because of the prohibitive cost in this country. Studies carried out in Cuba indicate the beneficial effects of interferon: Approximately half the HIV patients treated with interferon showed a greater delay in the onset of AIDS, adding five point five to six years to the incubation period, and interferon also prolonged survival time. At the same time, the embargo's biotech ban has hampered research on a promising Cuban AID vaccine, one of 18 worldwide, 14 of which are being developed in the United States. Ironically, should the Cuban vaccine prove successful, the embargo's ban on imports from Cuba would deny U.S. citizens access to it.

The AAWH concludes that the U.S. embargo directly contributes to lapsed prevention, diagnosis, therapeutic and surgical treatments of breast cancer; diminished alternatives for contraception; gaps in availability of in-vitro genetic testing resources; reduced access to medications associated with pregnancy, labour and delivery, and deficient nutrition during pregnancy.

Breast Cancer

Breast cancer, a primary cause of death for women worldwide, is often preventable with early detection and treatment. Until 1990 all Cuban women over 35 received mammograms on a regular basis at no cost. Today mammograms are no longer employed as a routine preventative procedure and are used only for women considered to be at high risk.

Cuba has two mammogram units based at medical institutions in Havana and 15 mobile units. When functioning, each unit can carry out some 400 mammograms

281

per week. Shut-downs in the entire screening program occurred in 1994 and 1995 for lack of x-ray film. The embargo prevents the Eastman Kodak company or any subsidiary from selling the U.S. product Kodak Mini-R film - a product specifically recommended by the World Health Organisation because it exposes women to less radiation. Cuba has attempted to buy the film from third-party trading companies, but their mark-ups prices the film out of Cuba's reach. Moreover, intermediaries were reluctant to purchase sufficient quantities that might have called U.S. attention to the illegal sale.

Treatment for breast cancer has also been severely compromised. During the 1980's an average of 15 surgical interventions were performed daily. Now due to lack of surgical supplies that number has dropped to two or three with up to 100 women on a two-month waiting list. Cuban oncologists normally apply a chemotherapy protocol that includes cyclophosphamides and 5-fluorouracil, combined with either methotrexate or adriamycin. These drugs are not always in sufficient stock, and supplies often arrive at erratic intervals. Further, the U.S. dominance of the cancer drug market, combined with the 17-year patent for drug manufacturers, make breast cancer therapies developed as far back as 1980 inaccessible to Cuban women. Some 48 percent of the 215 new medications in phase 1-111 FDA trials in 1995 are specifically for breast cancer. None will be fully accessible to Cuban women as long as the embargo remains in place.

To compound this tragedy, the embargo directly interferes with Cuba's own ability to produce some anti-cancer drugs. For example, in 1993 the U.S. Treasury Department denied a license to the German subsidiary of Pfizer to sell Cuba one pound of the active ingredient methotrexate for trials of the anti-cancer drug by the same name. The embargo also bars purchase of U.S.-origin equipment necessary for domestic manufacture of chemotherapy drugs. For example, Cuba's Centre for Medical Research and Development (CIDEM) has been unable even to obtain a quotation for a freeze dryer for dehydration of injectable chemotherapy compounds. The unit is sold by the British firm Edwards, but produced in the United States.

282

Access to contraception alternatives

Until 1990 most Cuban women remained on birth control pills for contraception. Cuba's domestic pharmaceutical industry produced pills for most of the country's consumers. However, when in 1995 Swedish Pharmacia merger with Upjohn, Cuba was suddenly denied access to repair parts for lab equipment essential for quality control, delaying the release of millions of pills. The cut-off forced Cuban women to rely on donated pills that can change month-to-month - with uncomfortable fluctuations in hormone levels.

Genetic Testing

In 1985 Cuba initiated a comprehensive testing program detecting congenital malformations, with alpha fetoprotein (AFP) and corollary analysis, covering 95 percent of pregnant women. The tests determine the presence of congenital hypothyroidism, infant allergy predisposition, HIV 1 and 2 viruses, and hepatitis B and C. The programme uses reagents and kits produced by the National Immunoassay Centre, which is responsible for some eight million laboratory diagnostic tests every year, and for supplying reagents, technology and equipment for over 100 Cuban laboratories.

When Pharmacia merged with Upjohn, and Nunc (Germany) with Sybron International of Milwaukee, Wisconsin, they were forced under CDA to cancel their contracts with Cuba. This eliminated two key suppliers of components necessary for quality control in genetic testing laboratories. These mergers forced Cuba to find substitutes for these products at substantially higher costs. Delays of as much as six months have undermined Cuba's diagnostic testing regime, by decreasing the use of amniocentesis (by 80 percent between 1989 and 1995), thereby limiting the diagnosis of congenital malformations, and other conditions.

Basic indicators for new-borns, infants and children underscore their priority

283

status in Cuban health care. For example, infant mortality has declined from 60-65 per 1,000 live births in 1960 to 9.4 per 1,000 live births in 1995, the lowest in Latin America. The AAWH finds, however, that the economic crisis, aggravated by embargo restrictions, is exacting a toll on children's health, particularly in neo-natology, immunisations, paediatric hospital care, access to medicines, and treatment of acute illness.

Neonatology

Since 1992, the CDA food embargo has caused an increase in maternal malnutrition leading to a significant rise in low-birth-weight babies and premature births. This occurred despite Havana's efforts to provide supplemental feeding for pregnant women. The AAWH found underequipped and under-stocked neo-natology services, with neonatal deaths becoming the third leading cause of infant mortality by 1995. Lack of hard currency and embargo restrictions impair purchases of essential equipment. For example, Cuba received 25 Preemicare Model 105-4 Neonatal Respirators as a donation, but the embargo prohibits sale of spare parts, accessories and provisions of services to train specialists in their use.

Immunisations

Cuba's immunisation program covers 11 infectious diseases: polio, diphtheria, tetanus, whooping cough, measles, rubella, mumps, meningococal meningitis, hepatitis B, Typhoid Fever and tuberculosis. Fuel shortages, power outages, refrigeration cuts, and transportation lags impede delivery of vaccines. Though Cuba produces all its own vaccines except polio, domestic production remains vulnerable to embargo-related shifts in suppliers. Sine 1992, mergers of U.S. companies with third-country companies have resulted in sudden cancellation of contracts for vaccine production inputs.

284

Paediatric Hospital Care: Equipment

Cuba's National Medical Supply company (EMSUME) prioritises purchases for paediatric hospitals. Still, hard currency shortfalls oblige Cuba to depend upon donations of equipment that frequently require U.S. parts and accessories procured through intermediaries. But third-parties cannot always substitute for direct trade with the United States. For example, the AAWH found donated refurbished Eli Lilly-IVAC 560 infusion pumps out of commission in hospitals in both Pinar del Rio and Havana. Infusion pumps are critical for administration o anaesthesia and for intensive care units. We also found Bird, Babylock, Siemens USA and Preemicare respirators in Cuban hospitals that are in and out of commission for want of spare parts. X-rays in Pinar del Rio's Pepe Portillo Paediatric hospital are down 70-80 percent because the United States denied licenses for the sale of Picker X-Ray unit parts described above.

Medicines

In the nine paediatric hospitals and neo-natology units we visited we found the following drugs in critical short supply:

Fluconazole, or "Difulcan," an important systemic anti-mycotic, produced by Pfizer and patented in 1983. It is used in ICU's for pseudomonas; post-surgically, in immunidepressed patients (cytoto) chemotherapy and radiation patients, bone marrow transplant patients particularly susceptible to candidiasis.

Vancomycin, an important antibiotic without substitute, for patient with antibiotic resistance, gramm positive supra-infections.

Third generation antibiotics, in general; cephalosporins: Often more effective drugs are not readily available in Cuba because they are still under U.S. patent.

Ceftriaxone (Rocephin): life-saving paediatric medication especially meningitis in infants.

Bronchodilators: asthma medication (Note that paediatric deaths from asthma have risen.)

Anti-convulsants: for epilepsies and other neuropaediatric disorders.

Cancer medications. These critical medicines are always in short supply, particular the combinations needed for typical protocols.

Dobutamine and dopamine: lifesaving in shock and heart failure, particularly in ICUs.

Growth hormone (soatropin) for dwarfism.

Oral analgesics and anti-pyretics (the team found no acetaminophen or ibuprofen anywhere): In Pinar del Rio they found acupuncturists on 24 hour duty in emergency rooms to help compensate the nearly complete absence of these medications. High fevers in children were generally brought down by injection, when available.

Steroid medications.

Anaesthetics: especially scarce in 1993-94 and cause for numerous surgery cancellations.

Erythropoietin and other medications needed by renal patients.

Heart medications, including Prostin V-R, and I.V.-administered substance produced by Upjohn and patented in 1981 to maintain patency of the ductus arteriosus in new-borns [blue babies] who have cyanotic congenital heart disease.

Other medications denied to Cubans of all ages because of the embargo include third generation antibiotics, various cardiac and hypertensive drug chemotherapy agents, antimycotics, analgesics, anti-inflammatory and psychoactive drugs, and steroids. Cuban physicians specifically cite shortage or absence of the following:

Aprotinin (Trasylol), Miles Laboratories. Antifibrinolytic used to reduce preoperative blood loss and for transfusion in select corona patients.

Captopril, Bristol Myers Squibb. Treatment of left ventricular dysfunction following myocardial infarction.

Enalapril Maleate, Merck. Treatment of asymptomatic left ventricular dysfunction.

Doputrex (Dobutamina 259). Treatment of coronaries.

Megestrol Acetate (Megace), Bristol Myers Squibb. Progesterone derivative for treatment of anorexia or unexplained weight loss in patients with AIDS.

Our researchers encountered numerous cases where individual children were suffering needlessly with terrible pain merely because some drugs are unavailable due to the embargo.

Rosabel Cano Guerra, a 35-day-old baby girl, was hospitalised in the Pinar del Rio with a serious fungal infection. Care providers searched for the U.S. patented anti-mycotc, Fluconazole, which would allow the baby to recover for pending surgery. Though they obtained a small amount from donations, it was not enough for a full course of treatment. The operation had to be postponed, endangering the life of the baby. Eventually, the operation took place and the baby survived.

Cuban children with leukaemia are denied access to new, life-prolonging drugs. For example, the FDA has already approved Oncaspar (pegaspargase), patented by the U.S. company Enzon for patients allergic to L-Spar (l-asparaginase). Both drugs produce longer remission when included in treatment for lymphoblastic leukaemia (ALL). However, L-Spar has an allergy rate of 40 percent for first time users and 70 percent for relapsed ALL patients. Further, Oncaspar is less traumatic to a child suffering from ALL since it requires only one-sixth the number of injections of L-Spar. But the embargo deprives Cuban children of this innovation. Left untreated, this type of leukaemia is fatal in two to three months.

Cuba has 278 hospitals that provide general, paediatric, maternity and neo-natology, ob-gyn, clinical, surgical and other specialised care. The AAWH study of 20 hospitals in the city of Havana and in the Province of Pinar del Rio suggests that the economic crisis and the U.S. embargo have seriously eroded surgery, radiology, clinical services and access to medication, hospital nutrition and hygiene.

Surgery

The drop in surgeries from 885,790 in 1990 down to 536,547 in 1995 is a glaring indicator of the decline in hospital resources. Surgical services face shortages of most modern anaesthetics and related equipment, specialised catheters, third generation antibiotics and other key drugs, sutures, instruments, fabric for surgical greens, air conditioning equipment, and disposable supplies. The United States is a leading producer of state-of-the-art anaesthesia and related equipment. In one of the rare instances in which the U.S. government has issued a license, Cuba has been able to import the anaesthesia Thalmonal, produced by a Johnson and Johnson subsidiary. Even so, each shipment has taken six to nine months for delivery because Washington bureaucrats have quibbled over the specifics of the eventual use certification. When Thalamonal runs out, other anaesthetics can be substituted, but are subject to considerably greater side effects.

Radiology

Over the last 20 years, the Cuban health system has made major investment to outfit the country's hospitals and specialised institutes with x-ray units, CAT scans, ultrasounds, image enhancers and even MRIs. Since 1992, maintenance costs associated with this equipment have risen dramatically due to the embargo. For example, by the end of 1995, out of a total of ten hospitals with CAT scans, five reported their units out of order for lack of tubes or other components. European prices for parts tend to be higher than those produced in the United States. A tube produced by Siemens in Germany costs $40,000, while Varian X-Ray Tube products of Salt Lake City, Utah, lists prices at $16,000-$33,000.

On the basis of visits to diagnostic and treatment facilities, adult and paediatric wards, and interviews with specialists, the AAWH concluded that the U.S. embargo has significant direct and indirect impact on the quality of patient care and even on the chances for survival of Cuba's cancer victims. The U.S. embargo bars Cuban access to state-of-the-art cancer treatment under U.S. patent, subjecting all diagnosis and treatment-related imports to delays due to the shipping bans and hinders domestic research, development and production due to the embargo's ban on biotechnology-related exports.

Prevention and Diagnosis

Since 1960 Cuba has developed nationwide programs for prevention and early detection of paediatric cancers and cancer of the lung, cervix, breast and mouth. The embargo constantly frustrates the ability of Cuban doctors to provide the quality of diagnosis and follow-up of cancer patients they would wish. For instance, their ability to treat patients with intra-ocular tumours was frustrated by the inability to purchase

289

parts for the Oncology Institute's opthamological ultrasound equipment. In 1985, the Institute purchased 10 Cooper-Vision Model System IV ultrasound units through Mexico from a U.S. company located in Redding, California. The embargo has since prevented the acquisition of spare parts for the equipment even from third parties.

Radiation Therapy

Cuban oncologists regard U.S. cobalt radiation therapy equipment and accelerators as among the best on the market. Cut off from that market, Cuba pays higher prices for inferior quality from non-U.S. sources. As a result, there is one cobalt therapy unit working at the National Oncology Institute. The unit is in use from 6:00 am to 1:00 am the next day, with technicians rotating on round-the-clock duty. Such schedules cause untold hardship on sick patients and greater stress for medical staff. The equipment also suffers: In the last four years the unit has used up eight years of its normal 12-year lifespan.

Chemotherapy

We have already seen in the section on Breast Cancer that Cuban cancer patients have limited if any access to U.S. medicines under patent. They miss out not only on leading U.S. state-of-the-art cancer therapies but also on medications that ameliorate side effects. Gaps in availability of these medications, such as hormones, antiemetics, analgesies or antibiotics, increase patient suffering and prolong hospital stays and can be life-threatening. For example, the AAWH visited a paediatric ward then in its 22nd day without metoclopramide HCl, a drug used in combination with others such as betamethasone for paediatric chemotherapy. Without these drugs' nausea-preventing effects, the 35 children in the ward were vomiting an average of 28-to-30 times a day.

Based on hospital visits and extensive interviews with cardiologists, the AAWH concluded that the U.S. embargo constitutes a direct threat to patient care, by denying

Cuban heart patients access to lifesaving medications and equipment available only in the United States.

Heart disease is the number one cause of death in Cuba. Mortality rates for men and women have increased since 1989: with 189.3 deaths per 100,000 in 1989 and 199.8 deaths per 100,000 in 1995. One hospital, the Cardiology Institute in Havana, implants nearly two-thirds of all pacemakers nationwide. The Institute performed an average of 400 major operations per year through 1990 but by 1995 carried out only 174 surgeries. As of early 1996, nearly 300 patients were on a waiting list for surgery, increasing the risk of death by 10 percent.

Pacemakers and Implantable Defibrillators

Lack of access to this specialised equipment poses a particular problem. In one instance Cuban cardiologists diagnosed a heart attack patient with a ventricular arrythmia. He required an implantable defibrillator to survive. Though the U.S. firm CPI, which held a virtual monopoly on the device, expressed a willingness to make the sale, the U.S. government denied a license for it. two months later the patient died.

Cuba was able to purchase pacemakers from Siemens-Elema of Sweden and Telectronics Pacing Systems of Australia until 1993 when both parent companies transferred production and ownership to the United States and were required to cut off sales to Cuba. Replacing the long-time suppliers involved purchasing new lines of accessory equipment and re-training personnel to program the pacemakers. While no fatalities resulted from the change in supplier, the case illustrates the vulnerability of life-saving procedures to the unpredictable and sudden consequences of the U.S. embargo. In addition, Telectronics' moves to South Florida left 19 patients with defibrillators that expired in 1996, some requiring hospitalisation until replacements could be procured.

In this highly specialised field of medicine, devices are often needed for a handful of patients, or even just one. The U.S. embargo is particularly costly when Cuba must find reasonably priced quality equipment for immediate delivery. The

291

purchase of an internal pacemaker for a baby boy in 1992 is a case in point. While hooked up to an external pacemaker, five months passed before Cuba could find and buy the U.S.-manufactured Medtronic device in Peru at an inflated price through intermediaries. Such delays and heroics cost time and money, when without the embargo finding the item would have required little more than a phone call and a trip to the airport.

Medicines

U.S.-manufactured medications under patent remain for the most part inaccessible to Cuban physicians and their patients. Among these are Dobutrex, produced by Eli Lilly for shock; Capoten, produced by Squibb left ventricular dysfunction and hypertension; Vasotec, produced by Merck for asymptomatic left ventricle dysfunction and hypertension; and Inocor, produced by Winthrop for shock.

Paediatric Cardiology

Infants with cyanotic heart disease, including tetralogy of fallout and pulmonary atresia, need drugs such as Upjohn's Prostin V-R, patented in 1981. These babies frequently die before surgery because the Prostin is not administered in time: There is no substitute. Cuba purchased the drug through third-country trading companies until 1995. But at the end of that year, the Havana Cardiocentre faced a sudden cutoff when Upjohn declared the medication "for hospital use only," requiring the name of the hospital for which it was destined. Disclosing that the product was for a hospital in Cuba prevented intermediaries from making any further purchases. On January 18, 1996, the Cardiocentre used its last vial of Prostin V-R for a 14-day-old baby. Unless more Prostin V-R was rapidly acquired the next child with a similar condition would die.

Nor do Cuban children have access to U.S. cardiac equipment. The stent

292

produced by Cordiss Corporation for Johnson and Johnson is a tubular device that props open damaged blood vessels, preventing deterioration that might otherwise require a heart transplant. Cuban cardiologists have never had access to the stent, nor to U.S.-produced specialised catheters and umbrella devices used for angioplasty.

On the basis of on-site visits to nephrology services and institutes and interviews with nephrologists, the AAWH finds that the U.S. embargo limits the change for survival of Cuban patients with chronic renal failure; increasing their suffering; and adds significant expense to already costly care. Renal failure occurs when the kidneys cannot maintain normal biochemical balance. In the chronic form, the nephrons are progressively destroyed. If reversed, this leads to end-stage renal disease (ESRD) and death. Thus, early recognition and management are critical. Kidney failure affects the whole body, and patients often suffer from anaemia, hypertension, central nervous system disturbances, skeletal affectations, biochemical and mineral imbalances, and increased susceptibility to infection. All require higher calorie and protein intake, and children need growth hormones to tackle retardation of bone development.

The incidence of renal failure in Cuba (including acute, chronic and end-stage) is 355 per one million. Each year, approximately 80 per million (or 840) are added to the group with end-stage renal disease: These patients require dialysis to survive while they await transplant. Between 160 and 250 transplants per year are conducted in Cuba, with a survival rate of 55 percent.

Dialysis

By the end of 1995, 1,094 patients with end-stage renal disease were eligible for regular dialysis. However, only 712 were enrolled, and due entirely to the shortage of hemodialysis units in the country, not all of them were receiving the necessary number of dialysis sessions. In fact, the AAWH found that the shortage of equipment has led to a situation in which each new patient added to the program reduces the hours of dialysis available to all.

The embargo closes off the nearest, most technologically developed and often most competitively priced market for dialysis equipment, accessories and maintenance. Baxter HealthCare, a leader in dialysis sales to Latin America, refuses to sell equipment to any country embargoed by the United states. Drake Whillock is another U.S. firm that, for the same reason, does not send equipment to Cuba because of the embargo. Vitalmex Interamericana, S.A., a Mexican distributor for the U.S. dialysis manufacturer Cobe, also cited the embargo when it refused to quote prices to Cuban medical importers for 20 dialysis units in July 1995. That fall, even the Pan American Health Organisation (PAHO) had trouble obtaining bids from some U.S. firms on 18 dialysis units requester by Cuba, until PAHO assured them it would handle all negotiations with the U.S. licensing bureaucracy and arrange for shipping.

Like used equipment for other tertiary care, refurbished dialysis units are readily available from the United States, but inaccessible to Cuba. Prices of this equipment run one-third to one-fourth of new machines. Cuban importers who resorted to purchasing in Europe could have 54 U.S.-made refurbished units for the price of the 18 new ones they ended up buying. As a result, another 180 Cuban patients are not receiving the dialysis prescribed by their doctors.

There are currently 21 youngsters under 18 suffering from end-stage renal disease. They are receiving dialysis as they await possible transplant. The primary difficulty in treating these patients is the absence in Cuba of modern peritoneal dialysis methods, critical to survival for smaller patients. Some of these children may be as old as five years of age, and yet they weigh less than 30 pounds because of disease-induced growth retardation. They cannot undergo standard hemodialysis; and yet, the embargo has made the alternative treatment - continuous cycling peritoneal dialysis (CCPD) - extremely expensive. Because Cuban hospitals are barred from the more competitively-priced U.S. equipment in this field, there is little hope for these low-weight children; most will quickly progress to end-stage renal disease and die.

294

Kidney Transplants

As in other nephrology technology, a U.S. company, One-Lambda, produces what Cuban physicians consider the most useful protocol for HLA (histocompatibility lymphocyte antigen) blood analysis, essential matching kidney transplant patients with potential donors. Cuba cannot purchase these kits, which test for 70 specificity's and require only 2-3 ml of blood from the patient. The European alternative purchased by Cuba tests only 20-30 specificity's, making matches less secure, and requires drawing 50 ml of blood from already weak and anaemic patients. In another case, when Cuba's main supplier of reagents and other chemicals, Pharmacia of Sweden merged with Upjohn, Cuban specialists faced a gap of weeks to months in supplies of Ficoll-400 and Ficoll Paque, the key reagents to organ matching.

Cyclosporins, the first drugs known to inhibit organ rejection, are costly for Cuba to import, and therefore only guaranteed to paediatric patients and adults who have shown highly reactive immunologic responses. The Cuban biotechnology industry could provide an alternative to this dilemma, with domestically produced monoclonal antibody known as "ior t-3." The antibody has shown promising results in inhibiting organ rejection and has been used so far in Cuba, Uruguay, Chile, Argentina, Russia and India. However, production of ior t-3 depends on the Biopilot unit at the Centre for Molecular Immunology, sold to Cuba by Pharmacia of Sweden before its 1995 merger with Upjohn after which the sale of necessary components were banned.

The United States generates more medical and scientific information than any country in the world. Access to its vast body of hard-copy and on-line information, ranging from findings in professional journals to indices and other bibliographic information, is fundamental to continuing education in any country. But despite recent openings in the exchange of information between the two countries, the AAWH finds that the U.S. embargo remains a formidable barrier to the free flow of ideas and scientific information between Cuban medical researchers and their colleagues in the United States.

In 1988, an amendment to the Foreign Trade Act introduced by Congressman

Howard Berman (D-CA) legalised trade with Cuba in U.S. books, journal and other informational materials. Though the 1988 law did not include electronic materials such as news wire feeds or computer information, by 1994 the U.S. Congress adopted the Free Trade in Ideas which stipulated that the President can no longer regulate or prohibit the import or export of "any information, including but not limited to publications, films, posters, phonograph records, photographs, microfilms, microfiches, tapes, compact discs, CD ROMs, art works and news wire feeds."

Cuba's 28 medical schools, four dental schools and numerous facilities for health technicians currently face severe shortages in textbooks and other teaching tools. The embargo's ban on subsidiary trade with Cuba is partly to blame. For example, in 1990 the Spanish firm Editorial Interamericana became a subsidiary of McGraw Hill. The U.S. firm advised Intermericana that the latter's personal could neither attend an upcoming book fair in Havana nor conduct future sales to the island. McGraw Hill's decision reflects the embargo's "chill factor," wherein companies are discouraged from trading with Cuba despite U.S. laws - in this case the 1988 Berman Amendment - that legalise sales of Intermericana's medical textbooks. By 1992, of 73 titles Cuba wished to purchase in the field of oncology, only 12 were available.

The dearth of medical literature on computer disk or CD-ROM would serve to offer inexpensive alternatives to importing bulk texts and periodicals. Yet U.S. companies remain under the impression that the embargo excludes their sale. For example, the Sciences Citation Index, a standard CD-ROM resource published by the Institute for Scientific Information (ISI) in Pennsylvania, lists abstracts and bibliographic references. ISI was under the mistaken impression that selling the $17,000 CD-ROM to Cuba would violate embargo laws and thus refused the sale. Likewise, despite the 1994 Free Trade in Ideas Act's expanded definition of "informational materials," DH refuses to ship to Cuba packages containing floppy disks.

Embargo regulations continue to limit the free flow of information. For example, the ban on bilateral banking activities prohibits direct subscription to and payment for U.S. journals or other informational materials; the virtual ban on export to

Cuba of computer hardware limits options to support software programs, Internet connections and on-line services.

While the donation of professional services is legal. The related licensing process can act as a red flag. This occurred when the U.S. denied travel licenses to a group of opthalmological surgeons to operate on dozens of Cuban patients in a professional exchange between Project Orbis and Cuban teams at the Pando Ferrer Opthalmological Hospital in Havana. After significant lobbying, licenses were eventually granted. But the dispute delayed operations on nearly 50 patients.

The AAWH finds that donations from U.S. NGO's, international agencies and third countries do not compensate to any major degree for the hardship inflicted by the embargo on the health care system and the health of the Cuban people. Restrictions placed on charitable donations from the U.S. which are similar to those imposed on commercial trade have the same discouraging impact, severely limiting what might otherwise be contributed. In addition, contributions rarely match needs in terms of specific drugs, equipment or related parts. Delays in licensing, shipping and end-use certification requirements make charity an unacceptable alternative to free trade.

The U.S. embargo regulated various categories of humanitarian donations of U.S. nationals to Cuba; export and shipping licenses are required in the carriage of medicines, medical supplies and equipment, while food only requires a shipping license. Since March 1996, humanitarian goods require only shipping licenses as long as the donor is experienced in verifying that the donations reach their intended recipients. The American public has been generous in providing humanitarian donations, with Catholic Relief Services being in the forefront.

According to Treasury Department figures, between October 1992 and March 1995, 82 licenses for sales and donations valued at almost $63 million were granted, while two licenses valued at just over $23 million were denied. But in 1990 alone, prior to the enactment of CDA, Cuba imported from U.S. subsidiaries $500 million in food and medicines. (The Treasury Department combines figures for sales and donations which obscures the minimal number of sales they have permitted.) thus, licensed sales and donations during the 31 months after the October 1992 implementation of the Cuban Democracy Act reached just 12 percent of U.S. food and medical sales to Cuba in the months before the law took effect.

Family visits have over the years become an exceptionally important source for medicines and medical equipment, such as wheelchairs. From the late 1970's until August 1994, the United States permitted persons visiting close relatives to travel to Cuba under a general license. In August, 1994, new presidential restrictions revoked this general license. Thereafter, the Treasury Department announced that "travel-related transactions by persons demonstrating a compelling need to travel to Cuba for humanitarian reasons involving extreme hardship...will be considered for a specific license on a case-to-case-basis." The case-to-case stipulation gave the Treasury Department's Office of Foreign Assts Control the juristriction to define "compelling need," "extreme hardship," or "extreme humanitarian need." It also created a backlog in license requests that reached into the thousands at one point in 1995.

Until 1994, the law permitted a U.S. resident to send a monthly $200 gift parcel to individual Cubans or Cuban educational, charitable or religious organisations. But the August 1994 Presidential ruling limited gift parcels to food, vitamins, seeds, medicines in dosage form, medical supplies and devices, hospital supplies and equipment, equipment for the handicapped clothing, personal hygiene items, veterinary medicines and supplies, fishing equipment and supplies, soap-making equipment, radio equipment capable only of receiving and batteries for the same. New U.S. Commerce Department regulations issued in March 1996 permit unlimited gift parcels of food. But sending gift parcel to Cuba became significantly more expensive with the end of direct charter flights between Miami and Havana in late February 1996.

The licensing process also kept Cuban families apart. For example, on May 7, 1995, the Treasury Department denied a travel license to Isabel and Amando G. Munoz to visit their ill mother in Cuba. The Munozes presented documents showing their mother had cancer, but OFAC found that her illness did not constitute "extreme humanitarian need." When the Treasury Department granted a license on appeal two months later, it acknowledged "that the applicant's relative is in a final state of cancer." But the license arrived just days before the Munozes mother died, too late to make the trip.

On October 6, 1995, President Clinton announced changes governing Cuban-American travel to the island. The new regulations new permit travel once a year under a general licence for "extreme humanitarian need."

Air Travel

Despite loosened regulations governing donations, U.S. NGO's must still procure licenses for donations of medicines and medical supplies. In addition, travel licenses are required from the Treasury Department, which can take anywhere from three weeks to six months. The Cuban Council of Churches, for instance, has experienced up to three-month delays in U.S. donations re-routed through Canada. The AAWH found that the Catholic Church's CARITAS-Cuba spent an additional $30,000 to re-route through Canada. U.S. donations of $2.5 million in cephalosporins [broad-spectrum antibiotics] for Cuban intensive care units. The additional shipping costs could have been spent for more medicine. (During the autumn of 1996, the Clinton administration did waive the travel restrictions to allow hurricane relief supplies to be flown directly to Cuba.)

Third-Countries and International Agencies

Third countries donate a substantial portion of the $20 million each year that Cuba receives in health care-related assistance. The extraterritorial reach of the embargo affects those donations in at least two ways. First, the Cuban Democracy Act's effective blacklisting on ships that have docked in Cuba, preventing them from stopping within 180 days in U.S. ports, applies to purchases and donations. Second, like their U.S. counterparts, international donors must apply for licenses from U.S. government agencies if the material they will send to Cuba contains over 10 percent U.S.-origin components.

Delays and increased costs, according to one international NGO, the Spanish

Medicos Sin Fronteras (Doctors Without Borders), reduce "the effectiveness of every dollar spent" to assist Cuba. Medicos could have purchased far more water supply and purification equipment with its $1.8 million budget if it could buy calcium hypochlorite in Georgia, rather than in the United Kingdom.

In November, 1994, Tropical Storm Gordon displaced 2,570 families in the Eastern Cuban provinces, leaving some 11,967 refugees in its wake. The European Union contributed nearly $500,000 in disaster relief assistance, the International Federation of the Red Cross Societies in Central America purchase materials ranging from fumigation equipment, insecticides, electrical wiring, and housing repair supplies. Currency and shipping restrictions imposed by the embargo, however, delayed delivery of the storm relief assistance by a total of six months.

The inclusion of food and medicine in an international trade embargo is a violation of international human rights conventions which uphold the principle of a free flow of food and medicines, even in wartime, to serve the basic needs of civilian populations.

The U.S. embargo's ban on food and de facto ban on medical exports to Cuba violates international and inter-American resolutions, charter and conventions governing human rights, among them the United Nations Charter, the charter of the Organisation of American States, the American Declaration and American Convention, and Geneva Convention articles regarding the treatment of civilians during wartime. Moreover, the embargo's prohibition on food and its virtual prohibition on medicines is extremely rare among trade embargoes of the post-World War II era.

The United Nations

In four consecutive sessions the United Nations General Assembly has passed resolutions condemning the U.S. embargo against Cuba and calling on the nation to rescind those aspects of the statutes that violate principle international law and the United Nations Charter. In November 1995, for instance, the U.N. General Assembly registered its concern with the embargo's extraterritorial reach and the manner in which measures related to the Cuban Democracy Act extended "the economic, commercial and financial embargo against Cuba...and the adverse effects of such measures on the Cuban people and on Cuban nationals living in other countries." In 1994, the United Nations Commission on Human Rights characterised unilateral coercive measures such as trade embargoes as a "clear contradiction of international law," and noted that "such unilateral coercive economic measures create obstacles to trade relations among states, adversely affecting the socio-humanitarian activities of developing countries, and hinder the full realisation of human rights by the people subject to those measures."

The Organisation of American States

In 1975, the OAS resolved to permit each member state to decide independently whether to trade with Cuba. One month later, the United States lifted its own ban on subsidiary trade with Cuba. But the embargo-tightening measures of 1992 describes in this report violate not only the intent of the 1975 OAS ruling but also U.S. obligations under the OAS charter, the American Declaration of the Rights and Duties of Man the American Convention on Human Rights. Together with the OAS change the Declaration is among the "sources of international obligation" binding member states, the United States included.

Article 31 of the OAS charter, for example, notes that "...member states agree to dedicate every effort to....protection of man's potential through the extension and the application of modern medical science....[and] proper nutrition, especially through the acceleration of national efforts to increase the production and availability of food." As documented herein, U.S. restrictions on the sales of medicines and food to Cuba directly impair the ability of the Cuban population and their government to preserve health and welfare through adequate and proper medical care. As such, the punitive extraterritorial reach of U.S. embargo laws are in violation of the regional system of inter-American rights set forth by the Organisation of American States.

301

The Geneva Convention

The Geneva Conventions, to which some 165 countries included the United States are
party, require free passage of all medical supplies and food intended for civilian use
during war time. The United States and Cuba are not at war. Indeed, the two
countries maintain Interest Sections in one another capitals. Nevertheless, the AAWH
findings suggest that the embargo's restrictions amount to the purposeful impeding of
foods and medicines-in peacetime.

Twentieth Century Trade Embargoes and Humanitarian Exemptions

International practice in applying trade sanctions for political ends has come to include
an exception for medicines, medical supplies and certain basic foodstuffs in order to
prevent unnecessary suffering amongst civilian populations. The multilateral
embargoes imposed against Southern Rhodesia, North Korea, Vietnam, South Africa,
Chile, El Salvador, the Soviet Union and Haiti featured humanitarian exceptions
permitting the free flow of medicines and food. In recent United Nations-supported
embargoes against Iraq and the territories of the former Yugoslavia, the United Nations
upheld the principle that food and medicines must be allowed to enter these areas in
order to serve the basic needs of the civilian populations. In the case of Iraq, a special
Sanctions Committee was established within the United Nations in order to ensure free
passage.

The United States government itself has acknowledged that embargoes of food
and medicines violate international humanitarian law. To note, during the 1992 siege of
Sarajevo, the United States joined numerous other countries in proposing a resolution
before the U.N. Security Council which:

> "Condemns all violations of international humanitarian law,
> including....deliberate impeding of the delivery of food and medical
> supplies to the civilian population of Bosnia and Herzegovina, and

reaffirms that those who commit or order the commission of such acts
will be held individually responsible in respects of such acs."
[November 13, 1992]

It seems only reasonable that if international law requires a humanitarian exception to a
blockade for food and medicines even in the midst of armed conflict, then it requires
such an exception to the embargo against Cuba.

APPENDIX

DEMOGRAPHIC DATA

1990

Issued by the Ministry of Public Health in Havana 1990 and as
published by WHO 1990

305

)f Population On 30 June Each Year By Sex
1965-1988

Year	Both Sexes	Male	Female
1965	7 808 291	4 006 646	3 801 645
1966	7 955 352	4 081 375	3 873 977
1967	8 105 208	4 157 516	3 947 692
1968	8 257 942	4 235 112	4 022 830
1969	8 413 635	4 314 202	4 099 433
1970	8 572 376	4 394 826	4 177 550
1971	8 669 625	4 441 466	4 228 159
1972	8 831 830	4 521 402	4 310 428
1973	9 002 338	4 605 263	4 397 075
1974	9 154 366	4 679 666	4 474 700
1975	9 292 104	4 746 658	4 545 446
1976	9 470 968	4 839 665	4 631 303
1977	9 592 974	4 893 420	4 699 554
1978	9 693 736	4 942 875	4 750 861
1979	9 774 616	4 984 116	4 790 500
1980	9 779 795	4 986 762	4 793 033
1981	9 756 714	4 972 906	4 783 808
1982	9 814 114	5 000 658	4 813 456
1983	9 879 495	5 032 288	4 847 207
1984	9 952 699	5 067 765	4 884 934
1985	10 058 400	5 075 600	4 982 800
1986	10 191 748	5 134 848	5 056 900
1987	10 288 350	5 182 390	5 105 960
1988	10 404 900	5 233 400	5 171 500

Source: State Committee for Statistics

Selected Indicators

Indicators	1960	1970	1980	1988**
Percentage of deaths (50 years of age and over)	60,8	65,9	76,7	79,9
Percentage of population (65 years of age and over)	4,8	5,9	7,3	8,5
Annual rate of population increase per 1000 population	18,7	12,5	6,1*	10,7***
Sex ratio (males per 100 females)	105	105	102	101

*   Figure for 1981
**   Provisional
***   Figure for 1987

Nationality, Selected Indicators
1963-1988

Year	Estimate of live births	Birth rate per 1000 population	Live birth occurred in health facilities	
			Number	%
1963	260 244	35,1	164 396	63,2
1964	266 554	35,0	177 153	66,5
1965	267 611	34,3	194 172	72,6
1966	264 022	33,5	204 260	77,4
1967	257 942	31,7	202 021	78,3
1968	251 857	30,4	213 342	84,7
1969	246 005	29,2	219 722	89,3
1970	237 019	27,7	216 926	91,5
1971	256 014	29,5	245 188	95,8
1972	247 997	28,1	242 078	97,6
1973	226 005	25,1	221 522	98,0
1974	203 066	22,2	198 256	97,6
1975	192 941	20,8	190 356	98,7
1976	187 555	19,9	183 932	98,1
1977	168 960	17,7	163 916	97,0
1978	148 249	15,4	145 559	98,2
1979	143 551	14,8	141 103	98,3
1980	136 900	14,1	134 830	98,5
1981	136 211	14,0	134 709	98,9
1982	159 759	16,3	158 087	98,9
1983	165 284	16,7	162 633	98,4
1984	166 281	16,7	164 077	98,7
1985	182 067	18,1	179 907	98,8
1986	166 049	16,3	164 873	99,3
1987	179 477	17,4	178 449	99,4
1988*	187 911	18,1	187 529	99,8

* Provisional

Births Occurred At Health Facilities By Month
1984-1988

Month	1984	1985	1986	1987	1988
January	14 508	14 642	15 439	13 828	16 545
February	13 069	12 980	12 735	12 750	14 900
March	12 140	14 070	12 301	13 087	14 252
April	10 795	13 027	11 796	12 216	12 258
May	11 156	12 998	12 232	12 608	12 145
June	11 566	12 866	11 801	12 990	12 349
July	13 011	15 303	13 583	14 763	14 485
August	14 964	16 863	15 229	16 047	17 135
September	15 213	17 310	16 340	17 326	18 667
October	16 463	17 542	15 757	18 085	18 785
November	15 582	16 187	13 942	17 708	18 174
December	15 610	16 119	13 718	17 041	17 834
TOTAL	164 077	179 907	164 873	178 449	187 529

Fertility Rate By Mother's Age
1975, 1980, 1985, 1986, 1988

Age of mother	1975	1980	1985	1986	1988*
15-19	127,3	86,3	92,9	80,9	82,2
20-24	179,6	116,8	126,8	110,0	124,0
25-29	118,3	70,9	95,7	85,8	88,3
30-34	68,8	37,4	46,5	45,1	53,5
35-39	37,4	16,2	18,5	17,8	18,7
40-44	13,5	4,6	3,9	3,2	3,3
45-49	2,3	1,8	1,2	1,6	1,1
TOTAL	90,9	56,3	66,1	59,0	64,1

Rate per 1,000 women in every age group.

Source: 1975-1986 State Committee for Statistics
1988 Estimate made by the Ministry of Public Health.

*   Provisional.

Life Expectancy At Birth By Sex And Five-Year Periods 1950-2000

Period	Men	Women	Both Sexes
1950-1955	56,69	61,01	58,79
1955-1960	59,81	63,88	61,79
1960-1965	63,26	67,05	65,10
1965-1970	66,80	70,30	68,50
1970-1975	69,33	72,63	70,93
1975-1980	71,15	74,45	72,75
1980-1985	71,38	75,21	73,59
1985-1990	72,21	75,83	73,97
1990-1995	72,52	76,33	74,37
1995-2000	72,72	76,72	74,66

Source: State Committee for Statistics

Life Expectancy At Birth By Province
1977-78, 1982-83

Province	1977 - 1978	1982 - 1983
Pinar del Rio	72,87	74,91
La Habana	74,27	75,25
Ciudad de la Habana	72,01	73,42
Matanzas	73,53	74,75
Villa Clara	73,87	75,66
Cienfuegos	74,30	75,16
Sancti Spiritus	73,83	75,29
Ciego de Avila	72,87	74,96
Camaguey	72,09	74,49
Las Tunas	73,21	75,31
Holguin	72,83	75,36
Granma	72,70	74,97
Santiago de Cuba	72,34	74,17
Guantanamo	72,15	74,97
Isla de la Juventud	73,01	74,77
CUBA	72,72	74,22

Source: State Committee for Statistics

311

Deaths Per 1000 Population By Age Group
1969-1988

Year	Under 1 year*	1-4	5-14	15-49	50-64	65 and over	Total
1969	46,7	1,8	0,5	1,8	9,2	54,4	6,6
1970	38,7	1,3	0,5	1,0	9,3	52,9	6,3
1971	36,1	1,0	0,4	1,6	8,9	50,5	6,0
1972	28,7	1,0	0,4	1,6	8,7	47,7	5,6
1973	29,6	1,2	0,4	1,6	8,9	48,7	5,7
1974	29,3	1,2	0,4	1,6	9,2	49,9	5,8
1975	27,5	1,1	0,4	1,6	8,7	47,2	5,5
1976	23,3	1,0	0,4	1,6	9,4	48,4	5,6
1977	24,9	1,2	0,5	1,7	9,3	49,8	5,9
1978	22,4	1,1	0,4	1,7	9,1	48,8	5,7
1979	19,4	1,0	0,5	1,7	9,1	46,9	5,6
1980	19,6	1,0	0,5	1,7	8,8	47,3	5,7
1981	18,5	1,0	0,5	1,7	9,2	47,0	6,0
1982	17,3	0,9	0,5	1,7	8,7	46,3	5,7
1983	16,8	0,8	0,4	1,6	8,8	48,2	5,9
1984	15,0	0,8	0,4	1,7	9,2	48,3	6,0
1985	16,5	1,0	0,5	1,7	9,4	49,4	6,4
1986	13,6	0,8	0,5	1,7	9,0	47,8	6,2
1987	13,3	0,8	0,4	1,7	9,2	49,1	6,3
1988**	11,9	0,8	0,4	1,7	9,2	49,3	6,6

*   Per 1000 live births
**   Provisional

Main Causes Of Death (All Ages)
1970, 1980, 1987, 1988

Causes	1970	1980	1987	1988*
	Rate per 100,000 population			
Heart disease	148,6	166,7	185,5	191,4
Malignant neoplasm	98,9	106,6	119,7	123,9
Cerebrovascular disease	60,3	55,3	64,7	62,1
Accidents	36,1	38,0	43,6	48,5
Influenza and pneumonia	42,1	38,6	39,3	34,3
Suicide and self-inflicted injury	11,8	21,4	22,4	21,3
Diabetes mellitus	9,9	11,1	17,0	20,5
Bronchitis, emphysema and asthma	12,5	7,0	7,7	10,1
Certain perinatal conditions	41,7	13,2	10,8	9,5
Congenital anomalies	14,1	8,1	8,3	8,7

*   Provisional

Main Causes Of Death (Under 1 year of age)
1980, 1986-1988

Causes	1980	1986	1987	1988*
	Rate per 1,000 live births			
Certain perinatal conditions	9,4	5,9	6,2	5,2
Congenital anomalies	3,9	3,3	3,0	3,0
Influenza and Pneumonia	1,6	1,1	1,1	0,9
Enteritis and other diarrheal diseases	1,1	0,6	0,7	0,4
Accidents	0,6	0,4	0,4	0,3

*   Provisional

Main Causes Of Death (1 to 4 years of age)
1980, 1986-1988

Causes	1980	1986	1987	1988*
	Rate per 10,000 population			
Accidents	2,2	2,1	2,1	2,3
Congenital anomalies	0,9	1,1	1,3	1,1
Malignant neoplasm	0,9	0,6	0,8	0,7
Meningococcal infections	0,5	0,7	0,6	0,7
Influenza and Pneumonia	1,2	0,7	0,5	0,5

)
*   Provisional

Main Causes Of Death (5 to 14 years of age)
1980, 1986-1988

Causes	1980	1986	1987	1988*
	Rate per 100,000 population			
Accidents	18,2	18,3	18,3	20,4
Malignant neoplasm	5,8	5,9	5,3	5,0
Congenital anomalies	2,8	3,3	3,3	3,5
Meningococcal infections	1,5	2,6	1,7	1,6
Heart disease	1,5	1,7	0,8	1,0

*   Provisional

Main Causes Of Death (15 to 49 years of age) 1980, 1986-1988

Causes	1980	1986	1987	1988*
	Rate per 100,000 population			
Accidents	36,6	38,8	38,8	42,7
Malignant neoplasm	25,1	24,5	24,0	25,4
Suicide and self-inflicted injury	28,0	26,3	26,6	23,5
Heart disease	22,7	23,3	22,1	21,1
Cerebrovascular disease	9,5	9,7	9,8	9,3

* Provisional

Main Causes Of Death (50 to 64 years of age) 1980, 1986-1988

Causes	1980	1986	1987	1988*
	Rate per 100,000 population			
Heart disease	274,1	267,7	270,8	268,1
Malignant neoplasms	246,7	252,3	255,8	252,6
Cerebrovascular disease	99,8	99,0	109,5	97,2
Accidents	39,6	42,0	42,8	48,3
Diabetes Mellitus	22,1	34,7	34,8	40,7

* Provisional

Main Causes Of Death (65 years of age and over) 1980, 1986-1988

Causes	1980	1986	1987	1988*
	Rate per 100,000 population			
Heart disease	1719,0	1718,0	1747,4	1753,5
Malignant neoplasms	903,4	923,0	939,0	939,5
Cerebrovascular disease	545,0	570,6	575,1	540,0
Influenza and Pneumonia	414,6	392,4	401,7	334,5
Diseases of arteries, arterioles and capillaries	300,5	257,0	272,0	306,6

* Provisional

Mortality From Heart Disease 1980, 1986-1988

Causes	1980	1986	1987	1988*
	Rate per 100,000 population			
Chronic rheumatic heart disease	2,3	2,4	1,9	2,0
Hypertensive disease	7,3	7,9	7,9	7,6
Ischaemic heart disease	136,5	148,6	151,9	161,7
Other forms of heart disease	20,6	24,9	23,8	20,1

* Provisional

Accidents (Selected Causes)
1980, 1986-1988

Causes	1980	1986	1987	1988*
	Rate per 100,000 population			
Motor vehicle accidents	15,5	19,3	19,7	23,8
Other transport accidents	1,8	2,1	2,4	2,1
Accidental poisoning	0,4	0,5	0,6	0,6
Accidental falls	6,8	7,7	8,9	9,8
Accidents caused by fire and flames	2,8	1,9	1,7	1,6
Accidental drowning and submersion	4,0	3,8	3,5	3,5
Occupational accidents	3,2	3,3	3,3	3,5

*   Provisional

Mortality From Selected Malignant Neoplasms
1980, 1986-1988

Malignant Neoplasm	1980	1986	1987	1988*
	Rate per 100,000 population			
Lip, oral cavity and pharynx	3,8	4,0	3,7	3,7
Esophagus	2,9	2,9	3,3	2,7
Stomach	6,5	6,0	6,0	7,1
Intestine, except rectum	7,6	8,8	9,1	10,1
Rectum, rectosigmoid junction and anus	2,2	2,4	2,2	2,5
Larynx	3,1	3,1	3,6	3,7
Trachea, bronchus and lung	24,6	28,7	28,8	30,0
Bone and connective tissue	1,0	1,0	1,1	1,2
Skin	1,1	1,5	1,5	1,2
Female breast **	13,3	14,8	16,0	15,9
Cervix uteri **	3,7	6,4	6,2	6,8
Uterus, other and unspecified	8,6	7,5	6,9	7,3
Prostrate ***	16,4	20,6	21,3	23,7
Leukaemia	4,5	4,6	4,6	5,4
Other neoplasms of lymphatic and hemopoietic tissue	5,0	5,8	5,5	4,1

*   Provisional
**   Female Population
***   Male Population

Mortality From Infectious And Parasitic Diseases
1962-1988

Year	Number of deaths	Rate per 100,000 pop.	% of total
1962	6 847	94,4	13,3
1963	5 526	74,5	11,1
1964	4 721	62,0	9,8
1965	4 150	53,1	8,3
1966	3 792	48,1	7,5
1967	3 771	46,3	7,4
1968	4 218	50,9	7,8
1969	5 281	62,7	9,5
1970	3 886	45,4	7,2
1971	3 640	41,9	7,0
1972	2 401	27,1	4,9
1973	2 413	26,7	4,7
1974	1 964	21,4	3,7
1975	1 575	16,9	3,1
1976	1 462	15,4	2,8
1977	1 633	17,0	2,9
1978	1 320	13,6	2,4
1979	1 138	11,6	2,1
1980	986	10,1	1,8
1981	1 249	12,8	2,2
1982	1 105	11,3	2,0
1983	1 148	11,6	2,0
1984	942	9,5	1,6
1985	1 168	11,6	1,8
1986	930	9,1	1,5
1987	929	9,0	1,4
1988*	968	9,3	1,4

*   Provisional

Mortality From Acute Diarrheal Diseases
1962, 1967-1988

Year	Number of deaths	Rate per 100,000 population	% of total	% of total infectious and parasitic diseases
1962	4 157	57,3	8,2	60,7
1967	1 694	20,8	3,3	44,9
1968	1 481	17,9	2,7	34,5
1969	1 896	22,5	3,4	36,0
1970	1 510	17,7	2,8	38,9
1971	1 533	17,6	2,9	42,1
1972	848	9,6	1,7	35,3
1973	875	9,7	1,7	36,3
1974	754	8,2	1,4	38,4
1975	637	6,8	1,3	40,4
1976	519	5,5	1,0	35,5
1977	634	6,6	1,1	37,5
1978	448	4,6	0,8	34,0
1979	361	3,7	0,7	31,7
1980	307	3,1	0,6	31,1
1981	343	3,5	0,6	27,5
1982	400	4,1	0,7	36,2
1983	385	3,9	0,7	33,5
1984	287	2,9	0,5	29,8
1985	437	4,3	0,7	37,4
1986	295	2,9	0,5	31,7
1987	346	3,4	0,5	35,6
1988*	321	3,0	0,5	33,2

*   Provisional

Mortality By Selected Reportable Diseases
1970, 1980, 1987-1988

Causes	1970	1980	1987	1988*
	Rate per 100,000 population			
Typhoid fever	0,0	0,0	0,0	-
Tuberculosis	7,3	1,4	0,6	0,0
Diphtheria	0,0	-	-	-
Tetanus	0,9	0,1	0,0	0,0
Poliomyelitis	-	-	-	-
Measles	0,5	0,0	-	-
Malaria	-	0,0	0,0	0,0
Syphilis	0,3	0,0	0,0	0,0
Whooping cough	0,3	0,0	-	-

*   Provisional

Incidence Of Selected Reportable Diseases
1970, 1980, 1987-1988

Disease	1970	1980	1987	1988*
	Rate per 100,000 population			
Typhoid fever	4,9	1,0	0,7	0,9
Tuberculosis	30,5	11,6	6,1	5,9
Tuberculosis of meninges	0,0	-	0,0	-
Leprosy	4,0	3,1	3,4	2,8
Diphtheria	0,1	-	-	-
Whopping cough	13,9	1,3	1,0	0,3
Tetanus	2,6	0,3	0,1	0,0
Infant tetanus	0,0	-	-	-
Measles	104,2	38,9	8,3	1,2
Rabies	0,0	-	-	-
Meningococcal meningitis	0,5	4,4	5,5	5,1
Acute gonococcal infection, genitourinary tract	2,8	168,4	353,2	371,7
Syphilis	7,2	44,7	84,3	82,4
Polomyelitis	0,0	-	-	-

*   Provisional

Incidence Of Selected Reportable Diseases By Age
1987

Disease	under 1 year	1-14	15 and over
	Rate per 100,000 population		
Typhoid fever	0,6	1,6	0,4
Meningococcal meningitis	77,5	10,1	2,4
Meningococcemia	20,8	7,9	1,1
Measles	157,3	20,6	1,0
Rubella	128,3	25,4	5,2
Chickenpox	469,6	1203,4	117,8
Viral hepatitis	93,9	585,9	135,0
Parotiditis	50,8	177,0	12,5
Infectious Mononucleosis	9,3	13,5	2,3
Whooping cough	35,5	1,5	0,0
Tetanus	-	0,1	0,0
Tuberculosis	-	0,3	8,1

Incidence Of Tuberculosis By Age Group And Site
1975, 1980, 1988

Age	Site	1975 Num.	1975 Rate*	1980 Num.	1980 Rate*	1988*** Num.	1988*** Rate*
Under	Total	37	2,4	29	2,1	3	0,1
15	Pulmonary	25	1,6	22	1,6	-	-
	Extrapulmonary	12	0,8	7	0,5	3	0,1
15-44	Total	617	15,8	464	10,3	234	4,4
	Pulmonary	555	14,2	399	8,9	193	3,6
	Extrapulmonary	62	1,6	65	1,4	41	0,8
45-64	Total	395	28,6	357	24,0	195	11,2
	Pulmonary	367	26,6	324	21,8	173	9,9
	Extrapulmonary	28	2,0	33	2,2	22	1,3
65 and	Total	271	44,6	273	38,5	184	20,9
over	Pulmonary	257	42,3	252	35,6	174	19,8
	Extrapulmonary	14	2,3	21	3,0	10	1,1
**Total	Total	1326	14,2	1130	11,6	616	5,9
	Pulmonary	1210	13,0	1004	10,3	540	5,2
	Extrapulmonary	116	1,2	126	1,3	76	0,7

*	Per 100,000 population
**	Includes cases of unknown age
***	Provisional

Incidence Of Leprosy By Age Group And Clinical Type
1975, 1980, 1988

Age	Clinical Type	1975 Num.	1975 Rate*	1980 Num.	1980 Rate*	1988** Num.	1988** Rate*
	Total	14	0,1	11	0,4	5	0,2
Under	Indeterminate	9	0,1	2	0,1	1	0,0
15	Dimorphous	1	0,0	2	0,1	1	0,0
	Tuberculoid	1	0,0	-	-	1	0,0
	Lepromatous	3	0,0	7	0,2	2	0,1
	Total	325	5,5	295	4,4	282	3,6
15 and	Indeterminate	82	1,4	96	1,4	69	0,9
over	Dimorphous	16	0,3	50	0,7	43	0,5
	Tuberculoid	91	1,5	49	0,7	48	0,6
	Lepromatous	136	2,3	100	1,5	122	1,5
	Total	339	3,6	306	3,1	287	2,8
	Indeterminate	91	1,0	98	1,0	70	0,7
TOTAL	Dimorphous	17	0,2	52	0,5	44	0,4
	Tuberculoid	92	1,0	49	0,5	49	0,5
	Lepromatous	139	1,5	107	1,1	124	1,2

*   Per 100,000 population
**   Provisional

Prevalence Rates Of Ambulatory Hypertensive Patients Under Follow-Up In General Population And In The Population Served By Family Physicians
1987

Province	Prevalence rates	
	General Population	Population served by Family physicians
Pinar del Rio	27,7	61,5
La Habana	34,5	70,0
Ciudad de la Habana	50,8	74,9
Matanzas	68,7	66,6
Villa Clara	23,0	46,3
Cienfuegos	28,9	28,5
Sancti Spiritus	19,9	38,6
Ciego de Avila	19,0	79,1
Camaguey	14,7	61,8
Las Tunas	7,2	51,0
Holguin	28,2	56,9
Granma	9,5	28,7
Santiago de Cuba	19,8	51,4
Guantanamo	25,2	51,3
Isla de la Juventud	9,1	-
TOTAL	32,7	60,9

Rate per 1000 population

Prevalence Rates Of Ambulatory Diabetic Patients Under Follow-Up In General Population And In The Population Served By Family Physicians
1987

Province	Prevalence rates	
	General population	Population served by Family physicians
Pinar del Rio	12,2	20,9
La Habana	17,1	25,5
Ciudad de la Habana	19,4	22,3
Matanzas	13,4	14,8
Villa Clara	13,5	13,8
Cienfuegos	10,4	7,5
Sancti Spiritus	10,3	9,5
Ciego de Avila	9,4	22,7
Camaguey	6,1	17,5
Las Tunas	8,0	9,0
Holguin	8,4	8,8
Granma	4,5	5,8
Santiago de Cuba	11,8	13,5
Guantanamo	8,7	9,8
Isla de la Juventud	4,0	0,0
TOTAL	13,2	16,9

Rate per 1000 population

327

Prevalence Rates Of Ambulatory Asthmatic Patients Under Follow-Up In General Population And In The Population Served By Family Physicians
1987

| Province | Prevalence rates | |
	General population	Population served by Family physicians
Pinar del Rio	16,6	37,1
La Habana	17,6	44,1
Ciudad de la Habana	24,8	44,3
Matanzas	15,0	39,5
Villa Clara	8,0	16,4
Ciefuegos	9,5	27,4
Sancti Spiritus	6,3	2,0
Ciego de Avila	8,1	59,9
Camaguey	7,4	50,2
Las Tunas	16,0	45,7
Holguin	6,3	23,1
Granma	7,5	20,2
Santiago de Cuba	6,3	40,5
Guantanamo	3,7	42,7
Isla de la Juventud	18,3	-
TOTAL	14,6	36,7

Rate per 1000 population

328

Prevalence Rates Of Ambulatory Patients Under Follow-Up In The Population Served By Family Physicians 1987

Age	Diabetes Mellitus	Asthma	Hypertension Arterial
Under 1 year	0,1	17,2	0,0
1-11 years	0,7	56,0	0,3
12 - 17 years	1,9	48,1	2,4
18 - 44 years	6,4	31,6	34,8
45 - 59 years	34,0	29,0	140,7
60 and over	74,5	31,3	203,2
Total	16,9	36,7	60,9

Rate per 1000 population

Number Of Women Screened By The Program For Early Detection Of Cervical Cancer 1970-1988

Year	Women Screened	Rate	Year	Women Screened	Rate
1970	176 307	78,5	1980	426 186	156,4
1971	284 382	124,4	1981	428 001	151,7
1972	362 802	155,2	1982	482 445	170,9
1973	391 418	164,2	1983	523 457	174,0
1974	435 080	177,9	1984	533 806	173,1
1975	432 093	172,8	1985	550 951	176,2
1976	412 225	162,2	1986	637 867	197,9
1977	404 585	156,8	1987	710 255	218,3
1978	395 889	150,4	1988*	788 170	232,0
1979	395 066	147,1			

*   Provisional

Rate per 1000 women

329

Number Of Women Screened By Age
1985, 1988

Age	1985		1988*	
	Number	Rate	Number	Rate
20-24	132 288	233,3	180 916	315,7
25-29	86 555	238,4	137 744	290,5
30-34	79 310	227,7	106 030	307,9
35-39	70 266	206,0	97 031	269,8
40-44	58 011	192,9	82 763	254,4
45-49	45 834	180,1	67 014	237,5
50 and over	78 680	82,7	116 648	112,3
TOTAL**	550 951	176,2	788 170	232,0

*   Provisional
**   Includes cases of unknown age
Rates per 1000 women in each age group

Number Of Patients Screened By The Program For Early Detection Of Cancer Of The Oral Cavity By Age And Sex
1986, 1988

Age	Sex	1986 Patients Screened	Rate*	1988 Patients Screened	Rate*
Under 15	Female	131 660	106,0	96 615	80,3
	Male	109 515	84,6	88 488	70,2
15-34	Female	626 551	326,5	686 581	349,7
	Male	436 936	223,6	482 858	241,4
35-49	Female	207 923	226,4	220 850	228,4
	Male	163 775	180,1	174 544	184,2
50-59	Female	61 729	153,1	65 608	153,9
	Male	56 449	141,2	61 182	144,5
60-69	Female	31 069	103,2	36 755	123,1
	Male	32 027	106,5	35 717	119,5
70 and over	Female	12 507	45,4	17 820	56,8
	Male	15 643	57,3	20 320	67,0
	Female	1 071 439	211,9	1 124 229	217,4
Total	Male	814 345	158,6	863 109	164,9
	Total	1 885 784	185,0	1 987 338	191,0

*   Per 1000 population in each age group

Medical And Dental Ambulatory Visits Per Inhabitant
1963, 1968-1988

| Year | MEDICAL | | | DENTAL | Total |
	Ambulatory	Emergency	Sub-Total		
1963	1,4	0,5	1,9	0,1	2,0
1968	2,3	0,9	3,3	0,4	3,7
1969	2,6	1,0	3,6	0,4	4,0
1970	2,5	0,9	3,4	0,4	3,9
1971	2,5	1,0	3,6	0,4	4,0
1972	2,7	1,1	3,7	0,5	4,2
1973	2,7	1,2	3,9	0,6	4,5
1974	2,7	1,3	4,0	0,7	4,7
1975	2,7	1,3	4,1	0,7	4,8
1976	2,7	1,3	4,0	0,8	4,8
1977	2,8	1,4	4,2	0,8	5,0
1978	3,0	1,5	4,5	0,9	5,3
1979	2,9	1,5	4,5	0,9	5,4
1980	3,1	1,6	4,6	1,0	5,6
1981	3,2	1,8	5,0	1,1	6,1
1982	3,3	1,8	5,0	1,1	6,2
1983	3,4	1,8	5,2	1,1	6,4
1984	3,6	1,9	5,6	1,2	6,8
1985	3,9	2,0	5,9	1,4	7,3
1986	4,2	2,1	6,3	1,5	7,8
1987	4,4	2,0	6,4	1,5	8,0
1988*	4,4	2,0	6,5	1,5	8,0

*   Provisional

Percentage Distribution Of Ambulatory Visits By Type
Of Medical Facility
1970, 1980, 1988

Facility	1970	1980	1988*
AMBULATORY			
		NUMBER	
Hospital**	5 292 181	6 518 669	9 377 737
Polyclinic	14 973 670	21 962 705	34 404 516
Other	1 238 761	1 518 791	2 465 409
TOTAL	21 504 612	30 000 165	46 247 662
		PERCENTAGE DISTRIBUTION	
Hospital**	24,6	21,7	20,3
Polyclinic	69,6	73,2	74,4
Other	5,8	5,1	5,3
TOTAL	100,0	100,0	100,0
EMERGENCY WARD			
		NUMBER	
Hospital**	6 255 291	12 160 548	16 604 514
Polyclinic	1 474 201	2 870 210	4 360 902
Other	65 949	134 700	287 636
TOTAL	7 795 441	15 165 458	21 253 052
		PERCENTAGE DISTRIBUTION	
Hospital**	80,2	80,2	78,1
Polyclinic	18,9	18,9	20,5
Other	0,9	0,9	1,4
TOTAL	100,0	100,0	100,0

*   Provisional
**   Includes facilities directly under supervision of the Ministry of Public
      Health

Ambulatory Visits Per 100 Population By Specialty
1970, 1980, 1988

Speciality	1970	1980	1988*
Medicine (subtotal)	118,8	147,5	240,7
General Medicine	94,7	107,4	151,3
Internal Medicine	5,0	3,7	7,0
Phthisiology	2,9	0,2	0,7
Dermatology	6,0	6,1	9,5
Psychiatry	3,6	4,8	6,7
Cardiology	1,5	1,2	2,0
Gastroenterology	1,2	1,0	1,9
Endocrinology	0,6	1,0	1,6
Pre-employment physical exam (1)	0,3	6,2	8,9
Other	3,1	18,9	55,0
Surgery (subtotal)	40,0	41,2	54,6
General Surgery	4,9	4,9	6,5
Angiology	3,7	2,0	2,7
Ophthalmology	9,0	10,8	14,5
Othorhinolaringology	5,7	5,6	6,9
Orthopaedics and Traumatology	11,6	7,9	15,7
Urology	3,3	2,9	3,6
Other	1,8	7,2	4,7
General Paediatrics (2)	145,4	213,9	306,1
Puericulture (3)	60,3	208,3	369,8
Obstetrics (4)	7,0	11,4	14,6
Ginecology (5)	40,9	58,2	60,8
TOTAL	251,5	308,3	444,5

(1)   Working age population
(2)   Population under 15 years of age
(3)   Population 0-4 years
(4)   Per delivery
(5)   Female population 15 years and over

Number Of Paediatric Visits* By Age Group
1977-1988

Year	Under 1 year Visits	Under 1 year P/Inh	1 - 4 Visits	1 - 4 P/Inh	5 - 14 Visits	5 - 14 P/Inh	TOTAL** Visits	TOTAL** P/Inh
1977	1 783 652	9,7	2 353 574	2,7	3 080 667	1,3	7 842 068	2,2
1978	1 658 499	10,0	2 382 876	3,0	3 410 927	1,4	8 227 982	2,4
1979	1 582 768	10,8	2 297 578	3,1	3 457 438	1,4	8 048 478	2,4
1980	1 692 535	13,3	2 322 265	3,4	3 369 458	1,5	8 153 030	2,7
1981	1 965 051	14,7	2 413 970	4,2	3 996 984	1,8	8 385 031	2,9
1982	2 136 457	13,3	2 309 322	3,9	3 707 336	1,7	8 153 661	2,8
1983	2 447 807	14,8	2 503 518	3,9	3 496 478	1,7	8 447 803	3,0
1984	2 520 206	14,7	2 649 499	4,4	3 454 494	1,7	8 624 199	3,1
1985	2 841 905	17,3	2 997 286	5,1	3 841 446	2,1	9 680 637	3,7
1986	3 057 124	16,9	3 365 331	5,3	3 971 553	2,3	10 394 008	4,1
1987	3 152 697	17,2	3 624 422	5,7	3 779 642	2,2	10 556 761	4,1
1988***	3 555 005	19,7	3 530 156	5,3	3 602 851	2,2	10 668 012	4,3

*   Includes Puericulture
**   Includes visits of patients of unknown age
***   Provisional

Number Of Puericulture Visits By Age Group
1970-1988

Year	Under 1 year		1 and over		TOTAL*	
	Visits	P/Inh	Visits	P/Inh	Visits	P/Inh
1970	647 445	3,0	65 050	0,1	712 495	0,6
1971	845 404	3,6	76 217	0,1	921 621	0,8
1972	1 072 939	4,6	93 806	0,1	1 166 947	1,0
1973	1 121 885	4,8	102 924	0,1	1 225 510	1,1
1974	1 138 043	5,0	121 447	0,1	1 263 196	1,0
1975	1 188 944	6,1	204 995	0,2	1 443 206	1,3
1976	1 223 493	6,8	204 250	0,2	1 429 741	1,3
1977	1 067 457	5,8	274 598	0,3	1 445 817	1,4
1978	997 878	6,0	355 964	0,4	1 478 178	1,5
1979	984 914	6,7	431 885	0,6	1 497 866	1,7
1980	1 055 029	8,3	498 623	0,7	1 630 595	2,0
1981	1 133 445	8,5	490 575	0,9	1 624 048	2,3
1982	1 248 025	7,7	577 587	1,0	1 825 612	2,4
1983	1 434 172	8,7	718 189	1,2	2 152 361	2,9
1984	1 487 806	8,7	881 423	1,5	2 369 229	3,1
1985	1 607 689	9,8	975 028	1,7	2 582 717	3,4
1986	1 735 917	9,6	1 124 485	1,8	2 860 402	3,5
1987	1 775 962	9,7	1 185 024	1,9	2 960 986	3,6
1988**	1 994 582	11,1	1 155 943	1,4	3 150 525	3,7

*   Includes visits of unknown age
**   Provisional
1977 - 1979 includes visits to primary health care facilities only

Number Of Dental Visits By Selected Specialties
1980, 1985, 1988

Specialty	1980		1985		1988***	
	Visits	P/100 Pop.	Visits	P/100 Pop.	Visits	P/100 Pop.
Endodontics	259 159	2,7	350 280	3,5	433 823	4,2
Periodontics	347 450	3,6	568 603	5,6	635 560	6,1
Oral Surgery	88 679	0,9	83 093	0,8	118 303	1,1
Prosthesis*	977 455	14,6	1 329 793	17,8	1 286 820	16,2
Orthodontics**	573 496	26,4	929 692	53,9	977 525	67,1

*   Population over 15 years of age
**   Population 6 to 14 years
***   Provisional

Hospital Admissions
1965-1988

Year	Number of Admissions	Admissions per 100 population
1965	815 998	10,6
1966	844 065	10,7
1967	923 608	11,5
1968	963 507	11,7
1969	1 033 631	12,4
1970	1 073 439	12,6
1971	1 123 119	12,9
1972	1 160 420	13,1
1973	1 292 775	13,2
1974	1 213 467	13,2
1975	1 249 798	13,4
1976	1 214 424	12,7
1977	1 199 648	12,5
1978	1 224 975	12,6
1979	1 202 581	12,3
1980	1 263 593	13,0
1981	1 358 547	13,9
1982	1 404 687	14,3
1983	1 443 801	14,6
1984	1 500 139	15,1
1985	1 608 551	16,0
1986	1 611 401	15,8
1987	1 598 693	15,5
1988*	1 610 592	15,5

*   Provisional

Indicators Of Bed Utilisation By Selected Types Of Hospitals
1980, 1985, 1988

Type of Hospital**	Average length of stay			Occupancy Index		
	1980	1985	1988*	1980	1985	1988*
General	7,0	7,2	7,3	80,7	87,1	82,2
Clinical and Surgical	12,4	11,9	12,5	86,5	89,7	87,5
Gynaecological and Obstetric	5,0	5,9	5,8	80,7	84,1	81,0
Maternal and Child	5,2	5,5	6,0	72,4	84,2	75,2
Paediatric	6,3	5,9	6,4	75,3	81,6	71,9
Rural	6,8	6,1	6,7	80,7	78,1	67,4
	Rotation Index			Substitution Interval		
General	42,4	44,3	41,0	1,7	1,1	1,6
Clinical and Surgical	25,5	27,6	25,6	1,9	1,4	1,8
Gynaecological and Obstetric	58,6	51,7	51,4	1,2	1,1	1,4
Maternal and Child	50,6	56,0	46,2	2,0	1,0	2,0
Paediatric	43,5	50,1	41,3	2,1	1,3	2,5
Rural	43,3	46,8	36,7	1,6	1,7	2,3
	Admissions per 100 population			Patient-Days per 100 population		
General	(1) 4,0	5,1	5,2	27,8	36,8	38,0
Clinical and Surgical	(1) 2,4	3,0	3,2	29,5	36,0	39,4
Gynaecological and Obstetric	(2) 6,1	5,2	5,4	30,6	31,1	31,2
Maternal and Child	(3) 1,7	1,7	1,0	8,9	9,5	6,1
Paediatric	(4) 7,1	12,6	11,2	44,7	74,9	71,0
Rural	(5) 1,0	2,1	2,2	5,0	12,6	15,0

*   Provisional
**   Does not include specialised hospitals
(1)   Total population
(2)   Female population
(3)   Female population 15 and over and live births estimate
(4)   Population under 15 years
(5)   Rural population

339

Blood Donations Per 100 Population And Per 100 Hospital Admissions 1973-1988

| Year | Total | DONATIONS | | |
| | | Suitable | | |
		Number	Per 100 Population	Per 100 Admissions
1973	335 932	319 077	3,5	27,5
1974	319 557	303 116	3,3	25,6
1975	330 128	312 352	3,3	25,6
1976	331 059	311 291	3,3	26,2
1977	314 858	294 101	3,1	25,0
1978	334 678	315 063	3,2	26,2
1979	379 745	354 734	3,6	29,5
1980	437 248	409 040	4,2	32,4
1981	419 191	387 114	4,0	28,5
1982	493 718	457 060	4,7	32,5
1983	497 894	461 939	4,7	32,0
1984	513 727	472 363	4,8	32,4
1985	548 259	498 746	5,0	31,0
1986	564 830	518 440	5,1	32,2
1987	603 101	553 972	5,4	34,7
1988*	654 364	605 057	5,8	37,6

*   Provisional

340

Low Birth Weight Rate
1974-1988

Year	Low Birth Weight	%
1974	23 170	11,7
1975	21 795	11,4
1976	19 878	10,8
1977	17 295	10,6
1978	15 115	10,4
1979	14 407	10,2
1980	13 178	9,7
1981	12 820	9,5
1982	13 819	8,7
1983	13 794	8,5
1984	12 961	7,9
1985	13 693	8,2
1986	13 244	8,0
1987	14 141	8,0
1988*	14 031	7,5

*   Provisional

Immunised Population By Type Of Vaccine
1974-1988

Year	BCG	Triple	Duplex	Tetanus
1974	297 174	467 843	357 944	2 009 679
1975	250 653	450 524	333 852	2 287 818
1976	305 006	395 201	295 591	1 907 447
1977	326 287	352 565	253 326	1 435 724
1978	285 089	384 902	267 375	1 528 967
1979	328 253	369 188	266 694	1 453 038
1980	372 689	298 751	305 573	1 583 275
1981	340 430	247 810	283 761	1 501 977
1982	371 912	241 527	259 417	1 402 766
1983	387 769	278 681	230 294	1 547 396
1984	382 350	305 784	196 529	1 760 182
1985	409 192	341 265	156 943	1 715 599
1986	318 226	350 139	115 522	1 269 471
1987	380 601	333 338	154 934	1 278 942
1988*	336 451	341 985	155 743	1 129 262
Year	Typhoid	Measles	Polio	
1974	1 003 315	314 562	1 140 519	
1975	1 188 824	123 983	1 120 530	
1976	177 905	143 883	1 077 025	
1977	529 525	147 521	980 034	
1978	729 534	224 139	928 608	
1979	492 401	307 965	939 584	
1980	762 546	167 176	852 129	
1981	708 334	197 965	861 264	
1982	726 159	303 463	787 522	
1983	842 690	241 952	781 119	
1984	971 511	229 163	777 462	
1985	825 364	335 377	801 145	
1986	529 546	175 617	842 963	
1987	920 050	923 135	824 209	
1988*	691 725	185 834	827 983	

*   Provisional

342

Medical Care And Social Service Beds
1958, 1975-1988

	MEDICAL CARE	Beds/1000	SOCIAL SERVICE	Beds/1000	TOTAL	Beds/1000
Year	Beds	Population	Beds	Population	Beds	Population
1958	28 536	4,2	3 965	0,6	32 501	4,8
1975	43 299	4,6	7 945	0,9	51 244	5,5
1976	43 234	4,6	8 279	0,9	51 513	5,4
1977	42 815	4,5	8 377	0,9	51 192	5,3
1978	43 103	4,4	8 492	0,9	51 595	5,3
1979	43 998	4,5	8 678	0,9	52 676	5,4
1980	44 339	4,5	9 078	0,9	53 417	5,5
1981	46 244	4,7	10 248	1,1	56 492	5,8
1982	47 416	4,8	10 855	1,1	58 271	5,9
1983	49 042	5,0	10 995	1,1	60 037	6,1
1984	51 872	5,2	11 143	1,1	63 015	6,3
1985	52 267	5,1	11 517	1,1	63 784	6,3
1986	54 172	5,3	11 806	1,2	65 978	6,5
1987	57 424	5,6	12 411	1,2	69 835	6,8
1988*	59 720	5,7	13 172	1,3	72 892	7,0
1988 BY PROVINCE						
Pinar del Rio	3 568	5,2	346	0,5	3 914	5,7
La Habana	1 323	2,1	761	1,2	2 084	3,3
Ciudad Habana**	21 325	10,3	4 633	2,2	25 958	12,6
Matanzas	2 662	4,4	860	1,4	3 522	5,9
Villa Clara	3 283	4,1	836	1,0	4 119	5,2
Cienfuegos	1 474	4,1	356	1,0	1 830	5,1
Sancti Spiritus	2 144	5,1	531	1,3	2 675	6,3
Ciego de Avila	1 039	2,9	467	1,3	1 506	4,2
Camaguey	4 627	6,4	1 204	1,7	5 831	8,0
Las Tunas	2 234	4,6	540	1,1	2 774	5,8
Holguin	3 865	4,0	725	0,7	4 590	4,7
Granma	3 408	4,4	437	0,6	3 845	4,9
Santiago de Cuba	5 959	6,1	885	0,9	6 844	7,0
Guantanamo	2 250	4,6	566	1,2	2 816	5,8
Isla de la Juv.	559	7,8	25	0,4	584	8,2

*   Provisional
** Includes beds from facilities directly under the supervision of the Ministry of
     Public Health

Medical Care And Social Service Facilities By Type And Province
31 December 1988

Type of Facility	Cuba	Pinar del Rio	La Habana	Ciudad de la Habana	Matan-zas	Villa Clara	Cien-fuegos	Sancti Spiri-tus
MEDICAL CARE								
Hospitals:								
General	75	6	5	2	4	4	1	6
Clinical and Surgical	30	3	-	13	2	2	1	2
Paediatrics	28	1	-	10	1	1	1	1
Ginegological and Obstetric	21	2	2	5	1	2	1	1
Maternal and Child	15	4	-	1	-	-	-	1
Rural	66	2	-	-	1	6	2	9
Oncological	2	-	-	-	-	-	-	-
Orthopaedic	2	-	-	2	-	-	-	-
Psychiatric	18	-	1	8	1	2	-	1
Ophtalmological	1	-	-	1	-	-	-	-
Antituberculosis	1	-	-	1	-	-	-	-
Leprosarium	1	-	-	1	-	-	-	-
Rehabilitation	1	-	-	1	-	-	-	-
Other Hospitals	3	-	-	2	-	-	-	-
Total Hospitals	264	18	8	47	10	17	6	21
Research Institutes	11	-	-	11	-	-	-	-
Polyclinics	421	22	41	79	38	36	19	21
Dental Clinics	161	9	19	37	12	14	7	8
Medical Post	254	28	40	1	13	8	18	21
Spas	3	1	-	1	-	-	1	-
Maternal Homes	139	15	17	-	9	1	4	8
Blood Banks	23	1	2	7	1	1	1	1
SOCIAL SERVICE								
Homes for the Aged	133	6	19	15	12	9	4	8
of these: Day Homes	30	4	10	2	4	1	2	-
Homes for the Handicapped	21	-	2	9	2	1	1	-

Medical Care And Social Service Facilities By Type And Province
31 December 1988

Type of Facility	Ciego de Avila	Cama-guey	Las Tunas	Hol-guin	Granma	Santia-go de Cuba	Guanta-namo	Isla de la Juv.
MEDICAL CARE								
Hospitals:								
General	4	6	6	17	9	1	2	2
Clinical and Surgical	-	3	-	-	1	3	-	-
Paediatrics	1	2	2	1	3	3	1	-
Ginegological and Obstetric	-	1	-	1	1	4	-	-
Maternal and Child	2	2	-	-	-	2	3	-
Rural	3	7	4	4	8	11	9	-
Incological	-	1	-	-	-	1	-	-
Orthopaedic	-	-	-	-	-	-	-	-
Psychiatric	-	1	-	1	1	1	1	-
Ophtalmological	-	-	-	-	-	-	-	-
Antituberculosis	-	-	-	-	-	-	-	-
Leprosarium	-	-	-	-	-	-	-	-
Rehabilitation	-	-	-	-	-	-	-	-
Other Hospitals	-	-	-	-	-	1	-	-
Total Hospitals	10	23	12	24	23	27	16	2
Research Institutes	-	-	-	-	-	-	-	-
Polyclinics	17	24	16	33	24	33	15	3
Dental Clinics	4	14	2	12	5	12	4	2
Medical Post	13	17	12	19	25	11	26	2
Spas	-	-	-	-	-	-	-	-
Maternal Homes	3	10	10	20	15	15	11	1
Blood Banks	-	1	-	3	2	2	1	-
SOCIAL SERVICE								
Homes for the Aged	8	11	7	9	8	9	7	1
of these: Day Homes	1	-	-	3	1	2	-	-
Homes for the Handicapped	-	1	1	1	-	2	1	-

Physicians And Dental Surgeons
1965, 1970, 1975, 1980-1988

Year	PHYSICIANS			DENTAL SURGEONS		
	Total	Per 10,000 Population	Pop. per physician	Total	Per 10,000 Population	Pop/dental surgeons
1965	6 238	8,0	1 252	1 200	1,5	6 507
1970	6 152	7,2	1 393	1 366	1,6	6 276
1975	9 328	10,0	996	2 319	2,5	4 007
1980	15 247	15,6	641	3 646	3,7	2 682
1981	16 210	16,6	602	4 188	4,3	2 330
1982	16 836	17,2	583	3 986	4,1	2 462
1983	18 828	19,1	525	4 380	4,4	2 256
1984	20 490	20,6	486	4 711	4,7	2 113
1985	22 910	22,8	439	5 335	5,3	1 885
1986	25 567	25,1	399	5 752	5,6	1 772
1987	28 060	27,3	367	5 923	5,8	1 737
1988*	31 229	30,0	333	6 134	5,9	1 696
1988 BY PROVINCE						
P. del Rio	1 445	21,2	472	325	4,8	2 097
La Habana	1 326	21,0	477	456	7,2	1 386
C. Habana	13 160	63,7	157	1 960	9,5	1 055
Matanzas	1 624	27,1	369	358	6,0	1 672
Villa Clara	2 113	26,4	378	364	4,6	2 195
Cienfuegos	808	22,7	440	199	5,6	1 786
S. Spiritus	811	19,2	521	200	4,7	2 111
C. de Avila	633	17,8	562	179	5,0	1 988
Camaguey	1 624	22,4	447	352	4,8	2 064
Las Tunas	772	16,0	625	182	3,8	2 649
Holguin	1 642	16,8	594	382	3,9	2 552
Granma	1 211	15,6	642	301	3,9	2 584
Stgo. Cuba	2 845	29,2	342	576	5,9	1 691
Guantanamo	973	20,0	501	244	5,0	1 996
I. Juventud	242	33,9	295	56	7,9	1 273

*   Provisional

Dental Chairs By Province
1988

Province	Number of chairs	Population per chair	Dental surgeons per chair
Pinar del Rio	306	2 227	1,1
La Habana	379	1 668	1,2
Ciudad de la Habana*	1 196	1 728	1,6
Matanzas	270	2 217	1,3
Villa Clara	300	2 663	1,2
Cienfuegos	192	1 851	1,0
Sancti Spiritus	219	1 928	0,9
Ciego de Avila	143	2 489	1,3
Camaguey	287	2 531	1,2
Las Tunas	156	3 091	1,2
Holguin	320	3 047	1,2
Granma	261	2 980	1,2
Santiago de Cuba	406	2 399	1,4
Guantanamo	163	2 988	1,5
Isla de la Juventud	48	1 485	1,2
Total	4 646	2 240	1,3

*   Includes facilities directly under the supervision of the Ministry of Public
Health

Middle Level Medical Training Graduates From Basic Courses By Specialty
1959-1988

Courses	1959-80	1981-85	1986	1987	1988**
General Nursing	11585	21445	5317	5202	2134
Paediatric Nursing	2707	5758	1587	1332	509
Obstetric Nursing	1154	1083	421	463	-
Auxiliary Nursing	29337	1837	-	-	-
SUB-TOTAL	44999*	30123	7325	6997	2643
Dentistry	1428	379	-	-	531
Pharmacy	5639	1853	409	235	93
Gastroenterology	225	2	-	-	-
Ophthalmology	406	286	71	32	-
Psychometry	378	414	66	23	-
Hygiene and Epidemiology	2398	1780	256	13	43
Social Work	431	749	97	97	105
Pathological Anatomy	468	178	114	39	-
Blood Bank	828	373	254	98	-
Clinical Laboratory	6048	2765	500	295	237
Microbiology	829	497	362	142	-
X Rays	2059	1875	265	109	-
Physiotherapy	537	950	108	111	-
Logopedics and Phoniatrics	29	114	37	15	-
Dental Prosthesis	373	909	111	107	2
Occupational Therapy	84	131	15	-	-
Library Science	242	171	32	52	-
Dietetics	487	378	71	65	-
Statistics	1486	893	157	83	-
Cytology	307	45	56	15	-
Psychiatric Ergotherapy	91	207	77	34	-
Other Courses	2266	115	76	174	-
Dental Assistance	5767	3078	428	-	-
Electromechanics	325	104	-	-	-
SUB-TOTAL	33131	18246	3562	1739	1011
TOTAL	78130	48369	10887	8736	3654

*   Includes other specialties
**   Provisional

Enrolment In Basic Courses Of Middle Level Medical Training By Specialty And Academic Year 1988-1989

| Specialty | Total | ACADEMIC YEAR | | |
		First	Second	Third
General Nursing	17997	5575	6976	5446
Paediatric Nursing	18	-	14	4
SUB-TOTAL	18015	5575	6990	5450
Dentistry	1775	494	845	436
Pathological Anatomy	119	65	31	23
Blood Bank	61	21	19	21
Orthopaedics	31	5	6	20
Library Science	93	34	36	23
Cytology	23	4	11	8
Dietetics	68	24	44	-
Psychiatric Ergotherapy	69	23	28	18
Public Health Statistics	241	83	108	50
Dispensary Pharmacy	1058	440	415	203
Industrial Pharmacy	41	14	16	11
Physiotherapy	254	69	120	65
Hygiene and Epidemiology	420	188	189	43
Clinical Laboratory	644	241	256	147
Logopedics and Phoniatrics	18	5	4	9
Microbiology	55	7	6	42
Dental Prosthesis	297	135	89	73
Orthopaedic Prosthesis	9	-	2	7
Psychometry	114	28	55	31
Medical Radiophysics	21	4	5	12
X Rays	159	56	66	37
Social Work	214	86	97	31
Podiatry	177	33	60	84
Ophthalmology	137	26	49	62
SUB-TOTAL	6098	2085	2557	1456
TOTAL	24113	7660	9547	6906

Provisional

349

Middle Level Medical Training Graduates From
Advanced Courses By Specialty
1961-1988

Year	Nursing	Other Technicians	Total
1961	129	27	156
1962	123	-	123
1963	156	25	181
1964	236	6	242
1965	215	57	272
1966	255	-	255
1967	100	-	100
1968	114	20	134
1969	48	-	48
1970	113	-	113
1971	46	-	46
1972	73	-	73
1973	75	-	75
1974	236	19	255
1975	178	-	178
1976	434	-	434
1977	358	102	460
1978	416	146	562
1979	385	136	521
1980	416	235	651
1981	463	215	678
1982	617	191	808
1983	688	354	1 042
1984	1 207	506	1 713
1985	1 417	547	1 964
1986	1 575	360	1 935
1987	1 411	466	1 877
1988	1 094	535	1 629

Medical And Dental Schools By Province
1988

Province	Medical	Dental	Total
Pinar del Rio	1	-	1
La Habana	-	-	-
Ciudad de la Habana	8*	1	9*
Matanzas	1	-	1
Villa Clara	1	1	2
Cienfuegos	1	-	1
Sancti Spiritus	1	-	1
Ciego de Avila	1	-	1
Camaguey	1	1	2
Las Tunas	1	-	1
Holguin	1	-	1
Granma	1	-	1
Santiago de Cuba	2	1	3
Guantanamo	1	-	1
Isla de la Juventud	-	-	-
Total	21	4	25

* Includes "Victoria de Giron" School of Basic Sciences

Graduates From Higher Education By Specialty
1959-1988

Year	Medicine	Dentistry	B.S. Degree in Nursing	Total
1959	728*	61	-	789
1960	-	56	-	56
1961	335	42	-	377
1962	434	20	-	454
1963	334	48	-	382
1964	312	29	-	341
1965	395	115	-	510
1966	380	-	-	380
1967	433	141	-	574
1968	616	20	-	636
1969	940	145	-	1085
1970	700	101	-	801
1971	432	173	-	605
1972	853	333	-	1186
1973	951	260	-	1211
1974	1269	300	-	1569
1975	1361	294	-	1655
1976	1477	142	-	1619
1977	1105	241	-	1346
1978	579	250	-	829
1979	683	193	-	876
1980	764	218	10	992
1981	1012	441	32	1485
1982	1087	3**	48	1138
1983	2114	433	45	2592
1984	1945	571	41	2557
1985	2551	545	163	3259
1986	3041	478	159	3678
1987	2841	290	513	3644
1988***	3401	323	604	4328
TOTAL	33073	6266	1615	40954

*   Includes two graduating classes
**   Course duration extended from 4 to 5 years
**   Provisional

Enrolment In Higher Education By Specialty And Academic Year 1988-1989

Academic Year	Medicine	Dentistry	B.S. Degree in Nursing	Total
1	5 637	634	1 925	8 196
2	5 104	627	1 724	7 455
3	4 786	650	1 307	6 743
4	4 284	557	858	5 699
5	4 274	378	-	4 652
6	3 776	-	-	3 776
Total	27 861	2 846	5 814	36 521

Provisional

Physicians And Dental Surgeons Graduated As Specialists 1962-1988

Specialty	1962-80	1981-86	1987	1988
Comprehensive General Medicine*	-	28	21	144
Internal Medicine	442	418	138	238
Paediatrics	539	338	136	157
General Surgery	445	201	89	58
Ginecology and Obstetrics	484	274	147	159
Other surgical specialties	1278	699	215	365
Other clinical specialties	921	665	199	248
Diagnostic specialties	586	283	86	97
Organisation and Public Health Administration	249	442	183	178
Dentistry	481	438	70	107
Basic Sciences**	-	62	66	80
Total	5425	3848	1350	1831

*   The specialty of Comprehensive General Medicine includes family
        physicians practising in schools, workplaces and other institutions

**   Not reported in previous years

Source: National Bureau for Postgraduate Training

Bibliography

British Medical Association. *September 14th*, 1998.

British Medical Journal *Vol 303* August 3rd, pg. 259-260, 1992.

Cannon, James: *Revolutionary Cuba*, Casa de las Americas Publishing, Havana, 1984.

Cannon, Terence: *"Revolutionary Cuba"*. José Marté Publishing House, Havana (Foreign Language Section), 1983.

Chadwick, Lee. *"Cuba Today"* Lawrence Hill & Co, 1975.

Constitucion de la Federacion de las Mujeres Cubanas, Department of Social Welfare, Havana, 1962.

Desarrollo Economico y Social Durante el Periodo 1958-1980, Comite Estatal de Estadisticas, Diciembre, 1981.

Dixon M *"Health Care: A Critical Comparison of Canada and the UK" International Journal of Health Care Quality Assurance,* Vol 3 Part 3, pg. 8-15, 1990.

Dr Joaquin Percy Labrador, Vice - Director of Medical Social Assistance for province of Pinar del Rio, in an interview granted April 4, 1993.

Franklin, J., *'The Cuban Revolution and the United States: A Chronological History'* Centre for Cuban Studies, Berkeley, 1992.

Franqui, Carlos *"Cuba: Le Livre des Douge"* Gallimaid, Paris, 1959.

Gerassi, J. Venceremos - *The Speeches and Writings of Che Guevara.* Pp 112-119 New York. Simon Schustes., 1961.

Glaser, W *The Competition Vogue and Its Outcome,* 1996.

Harnecker, Marta: *Cuba, Dictatorship or Democracy*, Lawrence Hill & Co, 1975.

Health Provision in the Caribbean, WHO, Geneva, 1975

Huberman, L & Sweeney, P. *"Socialism in Cuba"*, Monthly Review Press, New York, 1969.

Huberman, L. `Cuba: Anatomy of A Revolution'*, Monthly Review Press, New York, 1962.

Hugh Thomas' balanced account "*The Cuban Revolution*", pp. 120,121 Wiedenfield and Nicolson, London, 1986 .

Inter-American Development Bank, *Economic and Social Progress in Latin America.* Washington D.C, 1984.

Kansas City Star (AP): March 24th, 1993.

Keily J and Blyton P A *"Health Service Management: An Introductory Overview of Canada and the UK"*, Vol 3, Part 3, pg. 4-6. International Journal of Health Care Quality Assurance, 1990.

Klein R *"The American Health Care Predicament"*, 1991.

Lalonde M, *A New Perspective on the Health of Canadians*: Ottawa: Information Canada, 1975.

Life Magazine: 28 August 1964.

Lomax, P: *Child Health in the Caribbean 1948-1958. Forum -J of the American Paediatric Council.* Vol 3 No 1. January 1960 University of Chicago Press, 1960.

M. Harnecker, "*Cuba: Dictatorship or Democracy*", Lawrence Hill & Co. Westport, Conn, 1974.

MacDonald, T. *"Perspectives On Illiteracy"*. Newcastle University Press, Newcastle, Australia, 1968.

MacDonald, T. *Schooling The Revolution*: An analysis of development in Cuban education since 1959. London, Praxis Press, 1996.

MacDonald, T. "*The Two Illiteracies*". University of Newcastle Press Monograph in Education, 1984.

MacDonald, T. *Making A New People.* Vancouver, New Star Books, 1986.

MacDonald, T.H. "*Making a New People: Education in Revolutionary Cuba*" New Star, Vancouver, 1985.

MacDonald, Theodore, *Making a New People.* New Star Books, Vancouver, 1988.

Miller, W : *The Last Plantation*, Secker & Warburg, London,

Minh, Ho Chi, *Step-by Step to an Independent Vietnam*. Foreign Language Press, Hanoi, 1968.

356

MINSAP (together with UNICEF, UNFDA, OPS and OMS), *Cuba's Family Doctor Programme* (English translation by Cynthis Slade) ISBN 92/806/0999/8, 1992.

Murray, Mary, *Cruel and Unusual Punishment - The US Blockage Against Cuba.* Ocean Press, Melbourne, 1992.

Personal conversation with Dr. Augusto Hernandez Batista, Director of Health Administration For Havana province. 1993.

Personal correspondence with Dr Jorge S Pino Perez, Editor of the journal "Gencias Medicas", published by ECIMED in Havana January 1972.

Private Correspondence : *Infectious Diseases Centre*, UWI Hospital, Mona, 1998.

Rimmer, Percival. *"Can Caring Be Taught As A Medical Skill?"* Journal of the World Educational Fellowship, Oregon. Aug. 1982.

Santamaría, Heydée*: Moncada - Memories of the Attack that launched the Cuban Revolution.* Lyle Stuart, Inc, New Jersey 1980.

Sinclair, Andrew, *"Guevara"* p.16, Fontana/Collins, London, 1970.

Sklar, H, `*Washington's War on Nicaragua`*, South End Press, Boston, 1991.

The Lancet, Vol 341, March 27th, pg. 805 – 813, 1996

Thomas, H. *"The Cuba Revolution"*, Wiedenfeld & Nicolson, London, 1986.

UNESCO: *World Summit for Social Development - Cuba National Report.* Pg.103. Copenhagen. 1995

UNICEF : *State of the World's Children.* Paris, 1996.

UNICEF (with UNFPA, OPS-OMS, MINSAP*), "Cuba's Family Doctor Programme, Havana.*(English translation: Cynthia Selde), 1992

Urrutia, M *"Fidel Castro & Co. Inc - Communist Tyranny in Cuba"*. . pg.36-37. Frederick Praeger, New York, 1964.

Waller, J; Adams, L; Lyms, B; Redgrave, P and Schatzberger, P. *AIDS in Cuba – A Portrait of Prevention.* Cuba Solidarity Committee, London, 1993.

WHO, *Report 'Health Profile of the Dominican Republic for 1996'.* Geneva, 1997.

Williams, E., *From Columbus to Castro : The History of the Caribbean 1492-1969',* Andre Deutsch, London, 1970.

357

Work Plan for the Family Doctor Programme, Polyclinic and Hospital, Republic of
Cuba, MINSAP March 1988.

World Almanac (1990).

Wyden, P., *Bay of Pigs*, Jonathan Cape, London, 1979.

Zimbalist, Andrew (ed) *Cuba's socialist Economy: Entering the 1990s Boulder*,
Colorado, Lynne Rienner, 1989

Index

362

Los Cocos 169

Luanda 217-218, 223-225

Lung transplant 75, 202

Machismo 82, 129

Madrid 75

Malange 217-219, 223-224

Malaria 14-15, 17, 113, 128, 221, 323

Malformation 156, 159, 201, 285

Malnutrition 14, 44-45, 100, 212, 219, 262, 286

Mammograms 283

Manual labour 86-88

Mao Tse Tung 22, 135-136

Martí, José 21-22

Marxism 141, 226

Mater Misericordiam 68

Maternity 5, 107-108, 129-130, 156, 164, 213, 274, 290

Mathematics vii, viii, 88, 92, 103, 248, 251

Mazorra Hospital 105

Measles 54, 73, 102, 155, 223, 225, 270-271

Meat 41, 277

Medicaid & Medicare 247-247

Medical xviii, 7, 11, 48, 53, 56-57, 68, 73, 77-78, 83, 95, 111-112, 125, 144, 149, 186, 188, 196, 198-202, 208, 216, 230, 232, 243, 245-246, 257-258, 260, 269, 297, 334-335, 345

Medical Schools viii, 9, 17, 43-44, 56, 96, 110-111, 126, 140-141, 157, 179, 212, 230, 298

MEDICID system 201

Melagenina 235

Meningococcic Meningitis Type B 155, 263, 286, 324-325

Mental health 1, 105-106, 160, 171, 182

Methotrexate 265, 284

Mexico 4, 22, 28, 130, 292

Miami xii, 13, 47, 72, 102, 257, 300

Microsurgery 203

Milk xv, 41, 54, 87, 131-132, 221, 269, 271, 277

Mini-computer (CID-201) 201

Minister of Education 33, 80, 85-86, 95, 106, 124

Minister of Health 12, 48, 73, 102, 155, 223, 225, 270-271

MINSAP xvii, 5, 8, 14-15, 18, 62-34, 159, 164, 178-180, 182, 184-186, 188-189, 192-193, 195-196

Moncada 16, 26-27, 29-30, 35, 70

Quarantine   xviii, 2, 7, 170

Racism   51, 214

Radiation   208, 284, 287, 292

Radiology   290-291

Ration   146, 184-185, 278

RDA (vitamins)   87, 171

Reagan, President R.   xix, 204, 257

Renal transplant   203, 206

Republican (USA)   258

Research   2, 5-8, 43, 45, 93, 95, 99,
   107, 124-125, 153-155, 157,
   159, 161, 167, 175, 181, 186,
   197-198, 201-202, 204-207,
   210, 234-236, 246-247, 259,
   263, 267-268, 274-275, 279,
   281, 283, 291, 346-347

Respiratory Disorder Syndrome
   (RDS) 155

Reverse Cultural shock   226

Revolution   iv, vi, x, xi, xii, xiii, 2-4,
   10-13, 15-19, 21-25, 27-37,
   43-44, 46-47, 49-50, 53-54,
   56-57, 61-63, 67, 70, 72, 75,
   80, 82, 99, 101-102, 104,106-
   108, 112-117, 121, 126, 132,
   135-138, 140, 14, 150, 174,
   197, 199, 202, 205, 210, 212,
   215, 229-230

Ritalin   45

Rubella   75, 286, 325

Sanitation   55, 163

Sanatoria   163, 167, 169-172, 175,
   282

Santa Clara   108m 140

Santa Domingo (DR)   122

Santiago   6, 11, 26-27, 2, 37, 41, 47,
   53, 108, 119, 157, 164, 190-
   192, 203, 207, 221

Savimba, Jonas   216

Scabiosis   281

Schools   2, 11, 15, 35, 48, 69, 88,
   106, 110-111, 127, 130, 158,
   174, 181, 184, 186, 221, 224

Science   44, 88, 92, 103-104, 108,
   111, 125, 141, 151, 209, 236,
   298, 303

Sciences Citation Index   298

Scientific American   152

Secondary education   57, 94, 123

Selection Committee   50, 109

Sewer piping   153

Sex education   130, 163, 182, 193

Shipping   153, 261, 263, 269-270,
   273, 276-277, 291, 296, 299,
   301-302

Sierra Maestra   11, 30-31, 37

369

Tourism xvi, 3, 48, 100

Trading with the Enemy Act 4, 151-152, 205

Transplant 7, 153, 164, 203, 295-296

Trotsky, L 22, 58

Tuberculosis 54, 114, 286, 323-326, 346-347

Ultro-Micro Analytical Systems (UMAS) 6, 201

UNESCO 18, 39, 42-43, 58, 62, 64, 223

UNICEF 267

Upjohn 268-269, 282, 285, 289, 294, 297

Union of Soviet Socalist Republics (USSR) xiv, 106, 125, 140, 207, 229

UNITA 215-217

US Regulations 259, 265, 300

United Kingdom (UK) vi, x, xvii, 6, 8-9, 96-97, 110, 183, 239-240, 242-45, 247, 249, 251-256, 302

United States (US) iv, vi, ix, x, xi, xii, xiv, xv, xvi, xvii, xviii, xix, xx, 1-4, 6, 8, 13, 34, 36-37, 42, 44-47, 49, 51, 54-55, 61-62, 68, 75, 81, 96-97, 117,

125, 152, 155, 168-169, 174, 177, 183, 198, 211, 215-216, 229, 235, 239, 240-245, 247, 249-250, 252-254, 256-258, 261, 271, 273-277, 280-284, 287, 290-291, 293, 296-297, 300, 303-304

United Nations (UN) 234, 263, 302-304

Urrutia, Manuel 36

US Centres for Disease Control 279

US Commerce Department 260, 265-266, 274, 300

US Medical Board 45, 68

US Treasury 264-266, 273, 284, 299-301

Vaccination 10, 15, 54, 83, 123, 145, 149-150, 154-155, 160, 164-165, 268

Vietnamese xiii, 19

Vital statistics 51, 58, 61

Vitamins 171, 300

Voodoo 12, 37-38, 41

Washington, D.C. 62, 64, 260, 267

Whore-houses 40

World Health Organisation (WHO) 17-18, 58-59, 142, 155, 160,

STUDIES IN HEALTH AND HUMAN SERVICES

375